MRCGP
Practice Questions:
Applied Knowledge Test

Second Edition

Edited by
Rob Daniels MA (Cantab)
MB BChir MRCGP
General Practitioner

PasTest
Dedicated to your success

© 2011 PASTEST LTD
Egerton Court
Parkgate Estate
Knutsford
Cheshire
WA16 8DX

Telephone: 01565 752000

First Published 2008
Second Edition Published 2011

ISBN: 1905 635 664
978 1905 635 665

A catalogue record for this book is available from the British Library.

The information contained within this book was obtained by the author from reliable sources. However, while every effort has been made to ensure its accuracy, no responsibility for loss, damage or injury occasioned to any person acting or refraining from action as a result of information contained herein can be accepted by the publishers or author.

PasTest Revision Books and Intensive Courses

PasTest has been established in the field of undergraduate and postgraduate medical education since 1972, providing revision books and intensive study courses for doctors preparing for their professional examinations.

Books and courses are available for:
Medical undergraduates, MRCGP, MRCP Parts 1 and 2, MRCPCH Parts 1 and 2, MRCS, MRCOG, DRCOG, DCH, FRCA, Dentistry.

For further details contact:

PasTest, Freepost, Knutsford, Cheshire WA16 7BR

Tel: 01565 752000 Fax: 01565 650264

www.pastest.co.uk enquiries@pastest.co.uk

Text prepared by Carnegie Book Production, Lancaster

Printed and bound in the UK by Page Bros Ltd, Norwich

CONTENTS

ACKNOWLEDGEMENTS

We would like to acknowledge, with thanks, the following people who have contributed photographs:

Mr Peter Simcock, Consultant Ophthalmologist, Royal Devon & Exeter Hospital
Dr Chris Bower, Consultant Dermatologist, Royal Devon & Exeter Hospital
Mr Malcolm Hilton, Consultant Surgeon, Royal Devon & Exeter Hospital
Mr Ian Daniels, Consultant Surgeon, Royal Devon & Exeter Hospital
Townsend House Medical Partnership.

This book is dedicated to
all the editorial staff at PasTest,
who do all of the really hard work,
but get none of the credit

CONTRIBUTORS TO FIRST EDITION

Julius Bourke MBBS, MRCPsych
Specialist Registrar, General Adult Psychiatry and Neuropsychiatry
The Maudsley Hospital
London

Erika Damato MA (Cantab) MBBS MRCP
Medical Ophthalmology Registrar
Bristol Eye Hospital

Rob Daniels MA (Cantab) MB BChir MRCGP
General Practitioner
Devon

Alison Johnstone MBChB MRCGP DFFP
General Practitioner
Hampshire

Priya Joshi MB ChB DRCOG MRCGP
General Practitioner
Cambridge

Grant Neumegen MBChB (Otago) MRCGP
General Practitioner
Devon

Séamus Phillips MA BM MRCS DOHNS MSc
Otolaryngology SpR
South Thames Rotation

Suzanne Renshaw BM DRCOG MRCGP
General Practitioner
Hampshire

Andrew Rosewarne MBBS MRCS DFPP DCH MRCGP
General Practitioner
Exeter

Pinki Singh MBBS DGO DNB MRCOG
Specialist Registrar Obs & Gynae
Worcester (West Midlands Deanery)

Ramanathan Visvanathan BM BCh, FRCS (Irel, Eng, Ed), ILTM
Consultant Surgeon, Bronglais General Hospital, Wales
Honorary Senior Lecturer, Cardiff University

Amy Wilson MBChB MRCPCH
Paediatric Registrar
Manchester

Kurt Wilson BSc MBChB MRCGP
General Practitioner
Manchester

This edition provides exclusive access to all questions from this book online, see www.pastest.co.uk/onlineextras.

With 'Online Extras' you can practice questions online, helping you to acquire knowledge and build confidence for the computer-based AKT exam. You can analyse your strengths and weaknesses through detailed feedback and develop your revision strategy and exam technique. 'Online Extras' also compares your performance with that of your peers, helping you to see if you are performing at the right level.

PREFACE

This book was originally intended for candidates sitting the Applied Knowledge Test of the nMRCGP® exam, and was designed to complement the existing book of practice exams. We have found that the first edition has also proved popular with medical students and practicing GP's looking to explore areas of educational need. This edition has been revised and expanded and we hope you continue to find this book useful for whatever purpose you are using it. We are always keen to have feedback both good and bad and particularly welcome suggestions for changes in future editions, so please get in touch if you have any comments. Good luck with the exams.

Rob Daniels

At time of going to press every effort has been made to ensure content is accurate and up-to-date.

INTRODUCTION

This book was written as a companion title to *MRCGP® Practice Papers: Applied Knowledge Test* (9781905635597), and aims to provide a detailed, up-to-date revision resource that will allow both candidates for the MRCGP® and qualified GPs to test their skills in certain subject-based areas. This hopefully will help you to identify learning needs and focus your revision. The questions are all written by experienced clinicians who have a wealth of experience as generalists and also a special interest in their individual area, and are all written in the same format as the question types found in the Applied Knowledge Test (AKT) of the MRCGP® exam.

We have included questions on management, hot topics, algorithms, data interpretation and critical reading within the subject areas, which will provide practice for these areas of the exam. In writing subject-based chapters, there are of course some question types which do not fit in to a particular chapter, hence we have included a chapter on critical appraisal at the end. We have included a selection of questions on evidence based practice/hot topics, but would suggest the best way to prepare for this part of the exam is to attend a Hot Topics course or buy a Hot Topics book. Another effective way to prepare for this part of the exam is to form a journal club with other candidates and divide up the work of summarising key papers. We have also included a wide range of colour photographs and images to practice this question format, now used extensively in the AKT. The questions in this book are all based on commonly-occurring clinical situations, and we have taken every step to ensure they are concise, accurate and up-to-date, but if you disagree with anything, please let us know and we will endeavour to solve any controversy.

Good luck!

Rob Daniels

ABBREVIATIONS

ACE	angiotensin-converting enzyme
ACL	anterior cruciate ligament
ACTH	adrenocorticotrophic hormone
ADH	antidiuretic hormone
ADHD	attention deficit hyperactivity disorder
AF	atrial fibrillation
ALL	acute lymphoblastic leukaemia
ALP	alkaline phosphatase
ALT	alanine aminotransferase
AML	acute myeloid leukaemia
ARDS	acute respiratory distress syndrome
ARI	absolute risk increase
ARR	absolute risk reduction
AST	aspartate aminotransferase
BCC	basal-cell carcinoma
bd	*bis die* (twice daily)
BIPP	bismuth iodoform paraffin paste
BMI	body mass index
BP	blood pressure
BTS	British Thoracic Society
CBT	cognitive behavioural therapy
CC	case–control (study)
CER	control event rate
CHD	coronary heart disease
CI	confidence interval
CIN	cervical intraepithelial neoplasia
CK	creatine kinase
CKD	chronic kidney disease
CLL	chronic lymphoblastic leukaemia
CML	chronic myeloid leukaemia
CMV	cytomegalovirus
CNS	central nervous system
COC	combined oral contraceptive
COPD	chronic obstructive pulmonary disease

COX	cyclo-oxygenase
CREST	calcinosis, Raynaud's disease, (o)esophageal dysmotility, sclerodactyly and telangiectasia
CRP	C-reactive protein
CSF	cerebrospinal fluid
CT	computed tomography
CVD	cardiovascular disease
DEXA	dual-energy X-ray absorptiometry
DMARD	disease-modifying antirheumatic drug
DNA	deoxyribonucleic acid
DVT	deep vein thrombosis
EBV	Epstein–Barr virus
ECG	electrocardiogram
EER	experimental event rate
eGFR	estimated glomerular filtration rate
ENT	ear, nose and throat
EPA	Enduring Power of Attorney
ERCP	endoscopic retrograde cholangiopancreatography
ESR	erythrocyte sedimentation rate
FBC	full blood count
FEV_1	forced expiratory volume in 1 second
FRC	functional residual capacity
FSH	follicle-stimulating hormone
FVC	forced vital capacity
GFR	glomerular filtration rate
GGT	γ-glutamyltransferase
GMS	General Medical Services
GUM	genitourinary medicine
HELLP	haemolysis, elevated liver enzymes, low platelets
HIV	human immunodeficiency virus
HPV	human papillomavirus
HRT	hormone replacement therapy
HSP	Henoch–Schönlein purpura
ICU	intensive care unit
INR	international normalised ratio
IUCD	intrauterine contraceptive device
LDH	lactate dehydrogenase

LFTs	liver function tests
LH	luteinising hormone
LMWH	low-molecular-weight heparin
LPA	Lasting Power of Attorney
LVF	left ventricular failure
MA	meta-analysis
MAOI	monoamine oxidase inhibitor
MCH	mean corpuscular haemoglobin
MCV	mean corpuscular volume
MI	myocardial infarction
MMR	measles, mumps and rubella
MRI	magnetic resonance imaging
MRSA	methicillin-resistant *Staphylococcus aureus*
MSU	midstream urine
NICE	National Institute for Health and Clinical Excellence
NNT	number needed to treat
NSAID	non-steroidal anti-inflammatory drug
NSTEMI	non-ST-elevation myocardial infarction
OCD	obsessive–compulsive disorder
od	*omni die* (once daily)
PCL	posterior cruciate ligament
PCT	primary care trust
PCOS	polycystic ovary syndrome
PCR	polymerase chain reaction
PCT	primary care trust
PE	pulmonary embolus
PEFR	peak expiratory flow rate
PID	pelvic inflammatory disease
PMR	polymyalgia rheumatica
POP	progestogen-only pill
prn	*pro re nata* (when required)
PSA	prostate-specific antigen
PT	prothrombin time
PUVA	psoralens + UVA
QALY	quality-adjusted life-year
qds	*quarter die sumendum* (to be taken four times a day)
QOF	Quality and Outcomes Framework

RCT	randomised controlled trial
RICE	rest, ice, compression and elevation
RR	relative risk
RSV	respiratory syncytial virus
SCC	squamous-cell carcinoma
SLE	systemic lupus erythematosus
βhCG	beta-human chorionic gonadotrophin
SNRI	serotonin and norepinephrine reuptake inhibitor
SSRI	selective serotonin reuptake inhibitor
STEMI	ST-elevation myocardial infarction
STI	sexually transmitted infection
T3	triiodothyronine
T4	thyroxine
TB	tuberculosis
tds	*ter die sumendum* (to be taken three times a day)
TED	thromboembolic deterrent
TIA	transient ischaemic attack
TNF	tumour necrosis factor
TSH	thyroid-stimulating hormone
U&Es	urea and electrolytes
UTI	urinary tract infection
UTRI	upper respiratory tract infection
UVA	long-wavelength ultraviolet (light)
VEGF	vascular endothelial growth factor
WCC	white cell count
WOMAC	Western Ontario and McMaster Universities Index of Osteoarthritis

CHAPTER 1
CARDIOVASCULAR
SINGLE BEST ANSWER QUESTIONS

1.1 You see a newly diagnosed hypertensive patient for review after his baseline investigations. According to the Quality and Outcomes Framework (QOF), which one of the following statements is correct regarding assessment of new hypertensives?

☐ A Cardiovascular risk assessment must be carried out within 6 months of the date of diagnosis

☐ B Lifestyle advice must be given in the 3 months before or the 3 months after diagnosis of hypertension

☐ C Risk assessment must use the Framingham assessment tool

☐ D The QRISK assessment tool should be used for patients with pre-existing ischaemic heart disease

☐ E There must be a face-to-face assessment of cardiovascular risk

1.2 A national screening programme started in the UK in 2009 for abdominal aortic aneurysms. Which one of the following statements is correct regarding this process?

☐ A Aneurysms greater than 5 cm diameter will be referred for elective repair

☐ B Magnetic resonance imaging (MRI) is used in the screening process

☐ C Patients will be scanned every 5 years from age 50

☐ D Screening all men at 65 is estimated to reduce the rate of premature death from ruptured aortic aneurysm by 50%

☐ E The prevalence of abdominal aortic aneurysms greater than 5.5 cm diameter is 30% at age 65

1.3   One of your patients comes to see you after having primary coronary angioplasty for a non-ST-elevation myocardial infarction. He has been told that he has a drug-eluting stent and has been researching on the Internet about this. He is concerned about the possible adverse effects of this stent. Which one of the following statements is true regarding these stents?

☐   A   Drug-eluting stents are associated with a reduced rate of re-stenosis and a reduced rate of revascularisation procedures

☐   B   Drug-eluting stents are impregnated with clopidogrel, which reduces the rate of re-stenosis

☐   C   Patients with drug-eluting stents do not need to use clopidogrel and therefore have a lower risk of bleeding

☐   D   The drug used in the stent can cause systemic side-effects

☐   E   They reduce the rate of re-stenosis and are associated with lower risks of death and disability than bare metal stents

1.4   A 52-year-old man with controlled angina complains that he is getting nightmares, feels tired all the time and is impotent. You review his medication and note that he is on ramipril, isosorbide mononitrate, nebivolol and simvastatin. Which one of the following is the most appropriate management of this problem?

☐   A   Ask him to complete a PHQ-9 and return for review

☐   B   Counsel him about treatment for erectile dysfunction and start sildenafil

☐   C   Stop the nebivolol and arrange to review him in 2 weeks

☐   D   Stop the ramipril and replace it with an angiotensin II-receptor antagonist

☐   E   Stop the simvastatin for 4 weeks and review symptoms

1.5 Consider the following data from a review of statin trials:

Trial	Primary or secondary prevention?	Number of patients	Drug	Relative risk of cardiac event in treatment arm
4S	Secondary	4444	Simvastatin	0.66
GREACE	Secondary	1600	Atorvastatin	0.53
HPS	Secondary	20 356	Simvastatin	0.67
Jupiter	Primary	18 000	Rosuvastatin	0.56

Which one of the following statements is correct regarding the interpretation of this data?

A   Atorvastatin is the most cost effective option and should be used as first-line treatment for all patients

B   Rosuvastatin is the most effective statin in terms of reducing cardiovascular events

C   Rosuvastatin should be used as the first treatment in patients with established ischaemic heart disease

D   The data suggest a class effect

E   The GREACE trial is only small and the results are therefore not statistically significant

1.6 You see a 24-year-old woman with severe Raynaud syndrome. She has tried calcium-channel blockers in the past but was unable to tolerate these. She finds the winters very difficult to cope with and asks if there is any other drug that might help. Which one of the following would be appropriate?

A   B12

B   Bendroflumethiazide

C   Carbamazepine

D   Isosorbide mononitrate

E   Ramipril

1.7 A 52-year-old man with paroxysmal atrial fibrillation comes to see you requesting referral for ablation therapy which he has read about on the Internet. He is currently taking flecainide but finds that he is having to take increasing amounts of time off work and has been cardioverted three times. Which one of the following statements is correct about ablation for paroxysmal atrial fibrillation?

- [ ] A 76% of patients are successfully treated with this procedure
- [ ] B It is a first-line treatment for younger patients with paroxysmal atrial fibrillation
- [ ] C Serious side-effects are extremely rare
- [ ] D The procedure is usually carried out as an outpatient
- [ ] E Usually requires insertion of a pacemaker as part of the procedure

1.8 In which one of the following circumstances would it be appropriate to carry out 24-hour blood pressure recording?

- [ ] A In patients with palpitations
- [ ] B In patients with resistant hypertension despite medication
- [ ] C In patients with suspected orthostatic hypotension
- [ ] D In women with suspected pre-eclampsia
- [ ] E To confirm compliance with medication

1.9 With regard to the measurement of blood pressure (BP), which one of the following statements is correct?

- [ ] A Diastolic BP should be measured when flow sounds begin to muffle (Korotkoff 4)

- [ ] B Elevated blood pressure measurement due to 'white coat phenomenon' has a prevalance of 50%.

- [ ] C National Institute for Health and Clinical Excellence (NICE) recommend the use of ambulatory BP monitoring if previous readings have been very variable

- [ ] D On the first occasion the BP should be measured in both arms: the lower value should be used as the reference arm for future measurements

- [ ] E Specialist referral should be considered If there is a drop of more than 20 mmHg in systolic BP on standing, associated with symptoms of postural hypotension

1.10 The following results show the fasting lipid profile of a 35-year-old man who underwent routine testing as part of a general health check: total cholesterol 7.9 mmol/l, low-density lipoprotein (LDL) 4.9 mmol/l, high-density lipoprotein (HDL) 0.83 mmol/l, triglyceride 5.2 mmol/l. His father died of myocardial infarction (MI) at the age of 52. Which one of the following would be the most appropriate initial management?

- [ ] A Initiate dietary modification and monitor response by retest-ing in 3 months

- [ ] B Initiate treatment with a fibrate

- [ ] C Initiate treatment with simvastatin 10 mg od

- [ ] D Initiate treatment with simvastatin 80 mg od; further testing is not required

- [ ] E Refer for specialist opinion

1.11 A 65-year-old man has recently been discharged from hospital having suffered an ST-elevation MI. Coronary artery stenting was performed and he is now pain-free. He enquires whether he can drive his own car. Which one of the following is the most appropriate advice?

☐ A After an MI patients should not drive until they have undergone exercise or functional testing

☐ B Driving must cease for 6 months

☐ C Driving must cease for at least 4 weeks

☐ D The patient must notify the DVLA

☐ E The patient should be informed that the GP is obliged to inform the DVLA of this event

1.12 A 62-year-old woman has recently been discharged from hospital after an episode of non-ST-elevation acute coronary syndrome. She has no other significant medical conditions. Which one of the following would be the most appropriate antiplatelet therapy?

☐ A Aspirin 75 mg od

☐ B Aspirin 300 mg od for 1 month, then aspirin 75 mg alone

☐ C Clopidogrel 75 mg od for 12 months, then change to aspirin 75 mg od

☐ D Clopidogrel 75 mg od in combination with aspirin 75 mg od for 1 month, then aspirin 75 mg od alone

☐ E Clopidogrel 75 mg od in combination with aspirin 75 mg od for 12 months, then aspirin 75 mg od alone

1.13 A 47-year-old man has recently suffered an MI. He has no other significant conditions, and prior to this event was not taking medication or known to have cardiovascular disease. His BP is 135/80 mmHg and his fasting cholesterol is 4.8 mmol/l. Which of the following combinations of drugs would be most appropriate long-term treatment to reduce the risk of further events? Select one option only.

☐ A Atenolol and aspirin

☐ B Atenolol, candesartan, aspirin and atorvastatin

☐ C Atenolol, ramipril, clopidogrel and aspirin

☐ D Lercanidipine, atenolol, aspirin and simvastatin

☐ F Ramipril, atenolol, aspirin and simvastatin

1.14 A 67-year-old woman who underwent a hysterectomy 2 weeks ago presents with a 1-week history of pain in the left calf. There is no history of injury to the leg. On examination, her temperature is 37.7 °C, and the left calf is tender, with erythema but no swelling. The abdomen is soft, with tenderness and bruising around the suprapubic scar. Which one of the following would be the most appropriate initial management?

☐ A Request D-dimer

☐ B Request pelvic ultrasound

☐ C Request urgent Doppler ultrasound scan of the leg

☐ D Start oral flucloxacillin and penicillin V

☐ E Treat with a non-steroidal anti-inflammatory drug (NSAID)

1.15 A 64-year-old man who underwent mitral valve replacement 5 years ago has forgotten the advice he was given regarding the use of prophylactic antibiotics to prevent endocarditis when he undergoes dental treatment or other procedures. Which one of the following is the most appropriate advice?

☐ A Antibiotic prophylaxis is not recommended for routine procedures, but he should be advised about the importance of maintaining good oral health

☐ B He should receive antibiotic prophylaxis for any future dental or surgical procedures

☐ C He should receive antibiotic prophylaxis for any procedures on the gastrointestinal or genitourinary tracts

☐ D He should receive antibiotic prophylaxis for dental procedures only

☐ E He should use chlorhexidine mouthwash prior to dental treatment

1.16 A 42-year-old man of Asian origin attends for a general health check. He is a non-smoker, drinks 21 units of alcohol per week, is physically well, active, and enjoys regular moderate exercise and a healthy diet. His body mass index (BMI) is 27.2 kg/m². His BP, measured on three occasions, was 162/100 mmHg, 165/100 mmHg and 168/102 mmHg. Which one of the following would be the most appropriate initial management?

☐ A Advise about lifestyle modification and review in 6 months

☐ B Refer for investigation of a secondary cause of hypertension

☐ C Start a calcium-channel blocker

☐ D Start a thiazide diuretic

☐ E Start an ACE inhibitor

1.17 A 42-year-old woman has varicose veins which are normally asymptomatic. She presents with a 3-day history of moderately severe pain and erythema surrounding a superficial vein, below and medial to the right knee. On palpation, the varicose vein is hardened and tender; the rest of the calf is unremarkable. Which one of the following is the most appropriate management?

☐ A   Refer for surgical assessment

☐ B   Request a Doppler ultrasound scan of the leg

☐ C   Start oral flucloxacillin

☐ D   Treat with a NSAID and crêpe bandage

☐ E   Treat with topical corticosteroid

1.18 A 21-year-old female student with no significant medical history consults you 24 hours after collapsing in a shop. The event was witnessed by a friend, who reports that she suddenly became pale and clammy, lost consciousness and fell to the floor. There was a short episode of twitching of all four limbs. She regained consciousness after less than 1 minute, rapidly became orientated, and has felt well since the event. Neurological and cardiovascular examinations are normal, with a heart rate (HR) of 76/minute and BP of 120/65 mmHg. Which of the following is the single most likely diagnosis?

☐ A   Epilepsy

☐ B   Hyperglycaemia

☐ C   Neurocardiogenic syncope

☐ D   Paroxysmal arrhythmia

☐ E   Pseudoseizure

1.19 A 42-year-old man undergoes cardiovascular disease risk assessment. There is no significant family history. He smokes 20 cigarettes per day, has a BP of 155/90 mmHg, total cholesterol 7.2 mmol/l and HDL 1.4 mmol/l. His calculated risk of developing cardiovascular disease in the next 10 years is 14%. Which of the following is the recommended management? Select one option only.

- ☐ A Advise him to make changes to his lifestyle
- ☐ B Initiate treatment with a statin
- ☐ C Initiate treatment with an ACE inhibitor
- ☐ D No intervention
- ☐ E Refer for specialist opinion

1.20 A 72-year-old man who underwent coronary artery bypass surgery 5 years ago presents with intermittent cramp-like pain in the buttock, thigh and calf. The symptoms are worse on walking and relieved by rest. On examination, both legs are of normal colour, but the pedal pulses are difficult to palpate. Sensation is mildly reduced in the left foot. Which of the following is the single most appropriate action?

- ☐ A Advise him to reduce walking distance to prevent pain
- ☐ B Doppler ultrasound
- ☐ C Measure ankle:brachial systolic pressure index
- ☐ D Magnetic resonance imaging (MRI) of the lumbar spine
- ☐ E Referral for angiography

EXTENDED MATCHING QUESTIONS

THEME: CARDIOVASCULAR RISK ESTIMATION

Options

A ASSIGN

B Framingham

C JBS

D QRISK

For each of the statements below regarding estimation of cardiovascular risk, select the most appropriate option from the list above. Each option may be used once, more than once or not at all.

☐ **1.21** Based on population data for a predominantly white population and therefore can underestimate risk in patients from South Asia.

☐ **1.22** Estimates the impact of deprivation and body mass index on cardiovascular risk.

☐ **1.23** Cannot be used for patients with pre-existing ischaemic heart disease.

☐ **1.24** Designed to apply to Scottish populations.

THEME: VALVE DISEASE

Options

A	Aortic regurgitation	F	Mitral valve prolapse
B	Aortic sclerosis	G	Pulmonary regurgitation
C	Aortic stenosis	H	Pulmonary stenosis
D	Mitral regurgitation	I	Tricuspid regurgitation
E	Mitral stenosis	J	Tricuspid stenosis

For each of the scenarios below, select the most likely abnormality from the options above. Each option can be used once, more than once or not at all.

☐ **1.25** An 82-year-old man is noted incidentally to have an ejection systolic murmur. He is asymptomatic. Chest X-ray shows a calcified aortic valve.

☐ **1.26** A 78-year-old angina sufferer experiences episodes of syncope. On examination, there is an ejection systolic murmur which radiates to the carotids and apex.

☐ **1.27** A 72-year-old woman develops gradual-onset shortness of breath and fatigue. On examination, there is a displaced apex and a pansystolic murmur. She recalls having being treated for rheumatic fever in the past.

☐ **1.28** A 48-year-old man with a history of intravenous drug use complains of shortness of breath. On examination, there is oedema and a pansystolic murmur that is loudest at the left sternal edge.

☐ **1.29** A patient with Marfan syndrome develops shortness of breath and palpitations. On examination, there is a prominent pulse, a displaced apex and a high-pitched early diastolic murmur.

THEME: TREATMENT OF HYPERTENSION

Options

A	Amlodipine	**F**	Furosemide
B	Atenolol	**G**	Hydralazine
C	Bendroflumethiazide	**H**	No change indicated
D	Candesartan	**I**	Ramipril
E	Doxazosin	**J**	Specialist referral

Select from the options above the most appropriate treatment for each of the following scenarios. Each option can be used once, more than once or not at all.

☐ **1.30** A white 49-year-old man takes ramipril and amlodipine at their maximum doses for essential hypertension. His BP over the last 3 months has persistently been found to be between 148/92 mmHg and 154/96 mmHg.

☐ **1.31** A 56-year-old man of Afro-Caribbean origin takes bendroflumethiazide 2.5 mg od. His BP is persistently found to lie between 148/94 mmHg and 156/96 mmHg. He has a healthy diet and takes regular exercise.

☐ **1.32** A white 69-year-old man, who is otherwise well, takes atenolol and bendroflumethiazide for essential hypertension. His BP is 136/88 mmHg.

☐ **1.33** A 39-year-old businessman complains of daily headaches and stress at work. His BP is 186/116 mmHg and his urine is positive for protein on dipstick testing.

☐ **1.34** A previously well 42-year-old man has recently started taking an ACE inhibitor for essential hypertension. He complains of a dry cough, and has decided to stop his medication. On examination, his BP is 148/98 mmHg and auscultation of the chest is normal.

THEME: ANGINA

Options

A   Amlodipine 5 mg od

B   Anticoagulation with warfarin

C   Atenolol 100 mg od

D   Clopidogrel 75 mg od

E   Emergency hospital admission

F   Glyceryl trinitrate (GTN) 400 micrograms sublingually prn

G   Isosorbide mononitrate 20 mg bd

H   Lercanidipine 10 mg od

I   Nicorandil 5 mg od

For each of the scenarios below, select the most appropriate treatment from the list above. Each option can be used once, more than once or not at all.

☐ **1.35**   A 65-year-old man with a known diagnosis of angina experiences approximately one episode of chest pain on exertion per week, lasting less than 2 minutes. He is already prescribed aspirin, a β blocker and and an ACE inhibitor. He uses no other medication.

☐ **1.36**   A 48-year-old man is seen at the end of the morning surgery, having experienced four episodes of chest pain that morning. Each episode lasted for 15–20 minutes and radiated to the left arm. He smokes 20 cigarettes per day and has a family history of MI. He takes no regular medication. He is now pain-free, with a BP of 155/95 mmHg. Examination of the chest is normal.

☐ **1.37**   A 72-year-old woman with angina experiences chest pain three to four times per week. Episodes usually occur on exertion and are relieved by sublingual GTN. She takes no other medication.

☐ **1.38** A 79-year-old man with known left ventricular dysfunction requires further control of his angina despite the use of a long-acting nitrate. He takes no other medication.

☐ **1.39** A 59-year-old man with angina, for whom standard treatment with calcium antagonists, β blockers and long-acting nitrates has been unsuccessful.

THEME: COMMON INVESTIGATIONS IN CARDIOVASCULAR DISEASE

Options

A 24-hour electrocardiogram (ECG)

B Ambulatory BP monitoring

C Chest X-ray

D Coronary artery angiogram

E Echocardiogram

F Exercise ECG

G Fasting lipid profile

H Serum natriuretic peptides

I Serum troponin

J Thyroid function tests

K Tilt table test

For each of the following scenarios, select the most useful investigation from the list above.

☐ **1.40** A 29-year-old man with mild hypertension attends for a health check after his father died suddenly aged 48 years.

☐ **1.41** A 62-year-old man experiences very occasional central chest pain when he is out walking. This always resolves in less than 3 minutes after resting. He is otherwise well and takes no medication. Cardiovascular examination and ECG are normal.

☐ **1.42** A 42-year-old woman complains of a racing heart. These attacks are not associated with pain or shortness of breath. She feels that she has lost weight in recent months. An ECG shows sinus rhythm (100/minute) with a normal morphology.

☐ **1.43** A 53-year-old man with a history of hypertension complains of frequent episodes of dizziness and shortness of breath. These occur once or twice a day, and resolve spontaneously within 10–15 minutes. There is no history of chest pain, examination reveals sinus rhythm with a heart rate of 76/minute, sitting BP is 152/82 mmHg and standing BP is 149/79 mmHg. A 12-lead ECG is normal.

☐ **1.44** A 72-year-old man experienced an episode of central chest pain during the night. This woke him from his sleep and resolved after approximately 40 minutes. He comes to see you the following afternoon. A 12-lead ECG shows inverted T waves in leads V4, V5 and V6.

ALGORITHM QUESTIONS

THEME: RATE CONTROL FOR PERSISTENT AND PERMANENT ATRIAL FIBRILLATION (AF)

1.45–1.49

Options

A   Administer appropriate thromboprophylaxis

B   Attempt electrical cardioversion

C   Beta blocker and rate-limiting calcium antagonist

D   Beta blocker or rate-limiting calcium antagonist

E   Beta blocker or rate-limiting calcium antagonist with digoxin

F   Digoxin and class III antiarrhythmic

G   Flecainide

H   Rate control with digoxin alone

I   Rate-limiting calcium antagonist with digoxin

J   Specialist referral or consideration of other drugs

Complete the following algorithm, selecting options from the list above. Each option can be used once, more than once or not at all.

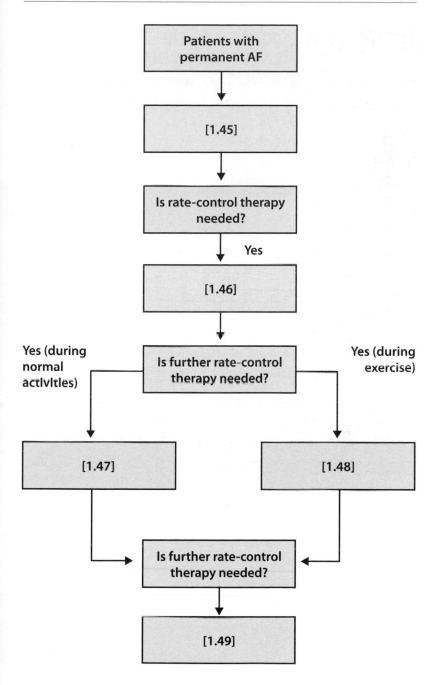

THEME: PHARMACOLOGICAL TREATMENT OF SYMPTOMATIC HEART FAILURE DUE TO LEFT VENTRICULAR SYSTOLIC DYSFUNCTION

1.50–1.55

Options

A ACE inhibitor

B Angiotensin II-receptor antagonist

C Beta blocker

D Digoxin

E Diuretic therapy

F Spironolactone

Complete the following algorithm, selecting options from the list above. Each option can be used once, more than once or not at all.

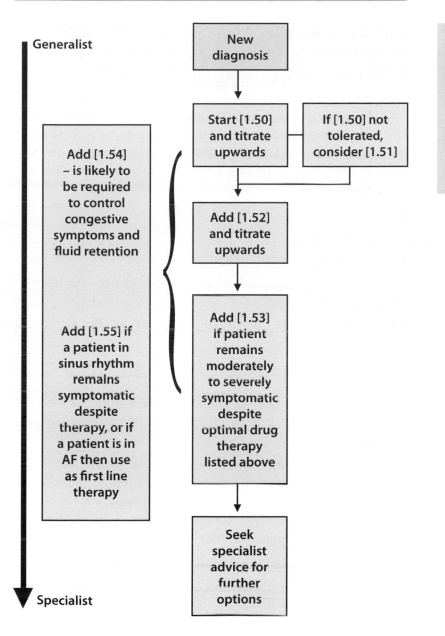

Generalist

New diagnosis

Start [1.50] and titrate upwards

If [1.50] not tolerated, consider [1.51]

Add [1.54] – is likely to be required to control congestive symptoms and fluid retention

Add [1.52] and titrate upwards

Add [1.55] if a patient in sinus rhythm remains symptomatic despite therapy, or if a patient is in AF then use as first line therapy

Add [1.53] if patient remains moderately to severely symptomatic despite optimal drug therapy listed above

Seek specialist advice for further options

Specialist

PICTURE QUESTION

1.56 A 78-year-old man with a history of atrial fibrillation treated with sotalol complains of recurrent syncopal episodes. Examination reveals atrial fibrillation with a rate of 84/minute and normal blood pressure. You ask your practice nurse to do an electrocardiogram (ECG) and while this is taking place he has another syncopal episode. A rhythm strip is obtained, which is shown below.

What would be the most appropriate action in this situation?

☐ A   Admit for pacemaker

☐ B   Check bloods to exclude myocardial infarction

☐ C   Give intravenous adrenaline and commence cardiopulmonary resuscitation (CPR)

☐ D   Start amiodarone

☐ E   Stop his beta blocker

1.57 A 78-year-old man is receiving treatment for a chronic ulcer, shown below.

Which one of the following is the most likely pathology?

☐ A Arterial ulcer
☐ B Marjolin's ulcer
☐ C Neuropathic ulcer
☐ D Rodent ulcer
☐ E Venous ulcer

DATA INTERPRETATION QUESTIONS

1.58 A 79-year-old man presents with a 1-month history of mild shortness of breath on exertion. On examination, his pulse is irregular with a rate of 90 beats per minute (bpm) at rest. A systolic murmur is heard on auscultation. His ECG is shown below.

Which one of the following would be most appropriate in his management?

☐ A   Amiodarone 200 mg od

☐ B   Aspirin 300 mg od

☐ C   Bendroflumethiazide 2.5 mg od

☐ D   Diltiazem hydrochloride 60 mg bd

☐ E   Furosemide 40 mg od

1.59 The following forest plot represents results from trials examining the effects of five different drugs (drugs F, G, H, I and J) on cardiovascular mortality.

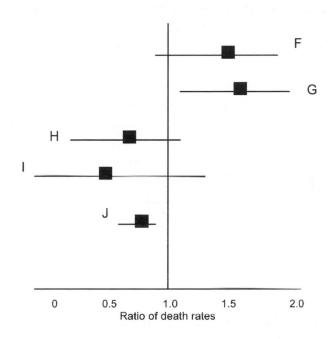

Which one of the following statements is correct?

- [ ] A   Drug F has a significant harmful effect
- [ ] B   Drug G is the most effective treatment in reducing mortality
- [ ] C   Drug I is shown to be the most effective treatment
- [ ] D   Drug J is shown to make the least overall difference to mortality
- [ ] E   Drug J is shown to significantly reduce mortality

HOT TOPICS/EVIDENCE BASED PRACTICE

1.60 Which one of the following was demonstrated by the Anglo-Scandinavian Cardiac Outcomes Trial (ASCOT) 2005?

☐ A Amlodipine plus perindopril has no effect on the onset of diabetes

☐ B Amlodipine plus perindopril reduced all-cause mortality and all coronary events

☐ C Amlodipine plus perindopril was equally as effective as atenolol plus bendroflumethiazide for reducing strokes

☐ D Atenolol has no significant effect on cardiovascular risk in hypertension

☐ E Thiazide diuretics are not well supported as a first-line therapy for hypertension

ANSWERS

1.1 E: There must be a face-to-face assessment of cardiovascular risk

The cardiovascular disease primary prevention indicators require that for patients with newly diagnosed hypertension there should be a face-to-face risk assessment using a validated tool (either QRISK, Framingham or JBS in England and Wales, or ASSIGN in Scotland) in the period from 3 months before diagnosis to 3 months after diagnosis, and lifestyle advice should be have been given in the past 15 months, although this does not need to be face to face. Patients with pre-existing cardiovascular disease are excluded from this indicator.

1.2 D: Screening all men at 65 is estimated to reduce the rate of premature death from ruptured aortic aneurysm by 50%

The National Screening Programme aims to screen all men in their 65th year by 2013. The prevalence of significant aneurysm in this age group is 4%. Those without significant aneurysms will be discharged, while those with aneurysms greater than 5.5 cm in diameter will be offered surgery. Those with small aneurysms will enter a follow-up programme. The mortality from elective surgery is 5–7%. Screening will be by ultrasound.

1.3 A: Drug-eluting stents are associated with a reduced rate of re-stenosis and a reduced rate of revascularisation procedures

Drug-eluting stents reduce re-stenosis and revascularisation rates but are associated with a slightly higher risk of death and all-cause mortality compared with bare metal stents (2.6% vs 1.3%). This can be reduced by the use of clopidogrel and aspirin, which are recommended in combination for the first 3–6 months after insertion. The stents release paclitaxel or sirolimus, which are antiproliferative but do not have systemic side-effects.

1.4   C: Stop the nebivolol and arrange to review him in 2 weeks

Beta blockers cause numerous side-effects, including erectile dysfunction, nightmares and reduced exercise capacity. They can also precipitate bronchospasm or heart failure. Depression is not uncommon in patients on beta blockers but usually resolves when these are stopped. Simvastatin can cause sleep dysfunction and erectile problems but in this patient the beta blocker is the most likely cause. Ramipril can cause a dry cough and in this situation it would be worth trying an angiotensin II-receptor antagonist but it would not help the symptoms this patient is suffering.

1.5   D: The data suggest a class effect

The table includes data from primary and secondary prevention trials and these cannot be directly compared. Of the three secondary prevention trials it looks as if atorvastatin could be more potent but without data on confidence intervals and P values this cannot be determined. Similarly, cost-effectiveness cannot be compared without data on cost of both drugs and outcome costs. Rosuvastatin seems to be the most potent but more data is needed on the other statins in primary prevention. The fact that all three drugs were associated with a reduction in risk suggests a class effect.

1.6   E: Ramipril

Calcium-channel blockers are the most commonly prescribed treatments for Raynaud's. Where these are ineffective or poorly tolerated, ACE inhibitors and angiotensin II-receptor antagonists can be helpful. There is also some evidence for vitamin E and vitamin C or fluoxetine. Where medical therapy is ineffective, surgical or medical sympathectomy should be considered. In secondary Raynaud's, treatment of the underlying condition might be useful. Where ischaemia is causing tissue loss prostacyclin therapy might be required.

1.7 A: 76% of patients are successfully treated with this procedure

Radiofrequency ablation via the femoral vein is carried out in patients who have refractory symptoms despite medical therapy or where medical therapy is contraindicated. It is combined with electrophysiological mapping of the heart to identify aberrant pathways and is usually carried out under sedation. Meta-analysis suggests success rates of 76% but the complication rate is 6%, with cardiac tamponade, transient ischaemic attack (TIA), oesophageal perforation and pulmonary vein stenosis all being reported.

1.8 B: In patients with resistant hypertension despite medication

Twenty-four-hour blood pressure recording should be considered in patients with resistant hypertension, suspected white-coat hypertension, variable blood pressure, suspected pregnancy-associated hypertension or where hypotension is suspected. It should not be used in suspected pre-eclampsia or palpitations. Suspected orthostatic hypotension should be investigated with tilt-table tests, while palpitations should be investigated with a 24 hour ECG.

1.9 E: Specialist referral should be considered if there is a drop of more than 20 mmHg in systolic BP on standing, associated with symptoms of postural hypotension

NICE advise specialist referral for patients with symptoms of postural hypotension when there is a drop of > 20 mmHg in systolic BP on standing. It is recommended that diastolic BP is measured when flow sounds disappear (Korotkoff 5). The prevalence of 'white coat hypertension' is 10% and, although useful in certain circumstances, NICE do not currently recommend ambulatory BP monitoring. After initial measurement in both arms, the side which measures highest should be used for future measurements.

1.10 A: Initiate dietary modification and monitor response by retesting in 3 months

The premature death (at 52 years) of this patient's father and his abnormal lipid profile suggest a diagnosis of familial hyperlipidaemia, of which there are several types. Combined elevation of cholesterol and triglycerides suggests familial combined hyperlipidaemia, which affects 0.5% to 1% of the population and approximately 15% of patients who have an MI under the age of 60. In the absence of other risk factors (smoking, diabetes, hypertension) he can safely be managed by diet and, if there is no response, with statins. Should other risk factors be present, these should also be addressed.

1.11 C: Driving must cease for at least 4 weeks

DVLA medical standards of fitness to drive state that driving of a private car (a group 1 vehicle) must cease for 4 weeks after an ST-elevation MI. All acute coronary syndromes, including MI, result in disqualification from driving group 2 vehicles (eg a heavy-goods vehicle or bus) for 6 months before relicensing.

1.12 E: Clopidogrel 75 mg od in combination with aspirin 75 mg od for 12 months, then aspirin 75 mg od alone

Current recommendations for antiplatelet therapy after a non-ST-elevation acute coronary syndrome are for dual therapy with clopidogrel and aspirin for 12 months, then aspirin alone (NICE, May 2007). The use of clopidogrel with aspirin increases the risk of bleeding, and there is no evidence of benefit beyond 12 months of the last event.

1.13 E: Ramipril, atenolol, aspirin and simvastatin

The recommended drug treatment for secondary prevention of MI is the combined use of a β blocker, an angiotensin-converting enzyme (ACE) inhibitor, a statin and aspirin. Statin treatment was previously only offered to patients with a cholesterol of > 5 mmol/l, but it has been shown that all patients with coronary heart disease (CHD) benefit from reduction in total cholesterol and LDL. Beta blockers are estimated to prevent deaths by 12/1000 treated/year. ACE inhibitors reduce deaths by 5/1000 treated in the first month post-MI, and trials show reduced long-term mortality for all patients.

1.14   C: Request urgent Doppler ultrasound scan of the leg

The most likely diagnosis is the postoperative complication, deep vein thrombosis (DVT). Typical features are unilateral leg pain, oedema, tenderness and warmth, and mild pyrexia, but clinical diagnosis is unreliable; D-dimer is unhelpful in the postoperative setting. All patients with suspected DVT should be referred for assessment. Treatment should be initiated immediately with low-molecular-weight heparin (LMWH), which is continued until oral anticoagulation with warfarin is in the therapeutic international normalised ratio (INR) range.

1.15   A: Antibiotic prophylaxis is not recommended for routine procedures, but he should be advised about the importance of maintaining good oral health

The use of prophylactic antibiotics to prevent endocarditis for patients with structural cardiac abnormalities and replacement valves has been long-standing, accepted medical practice, but there is little evidence of its effectiveness. Recommendations have recently been changed, based on the best available published evidence and multidisciplinary and expert consensus (NICE, March 2008).

1.16   E: Start an ACE inhibitor

This patient has a diagnosis of hypertension. With a BP of > 160/100 mmHg, he should be offered drug therapy. An ACE inhibitor is recommended as first-line treatment for patients younger than 55 years. Patients over the age of 55, and black patients of any age should initially be treated with a calcium-channel blocker or a thiazide diuretic.

1.17   D: Treat with a NSAID and crêpe bandage

These features are typical of superficial thrombophlebitis, which can usually be adequately treated with NSAIDs. A crêpe bandage will compress the vein and help prevent propagation of the thrombus. If phlebitis extends upwards in the medial thigh, towards the sapheno-femoral junction, refer for Doppler ultrasound as there is potential for extension into the femoral vein.

1.18   C: Neurocardiogenic syncope

These features are typical of neurocardiogenic (vasovagal) syncope. The condition is benign and can be triggered by the following factors: emotion, pain, fear and anxiety, micturition, defecation, dehydration, a warm environment and prolonged standing. Advice to patients should include avoidance of precipitating factors. Other methods of prevention include compression hosiery or voluntary forceful contraction of the limb muscles at the onset of symptoms.

1.19   A: Advise him to make changes to his lifestyle

Estimation of cardiovascular disease risk is recommended for patients aged over 40 years. The estimated risk can be used as an aid in making clinical decisions, but should not replace clinical judgement. It should not be used in patients with established cardiovascular disease (CVD), inherited dyslipidaemias, renal dysfunction or diabetes. It should not be used to decide whether to initiate antihypertensive therapy when the BP is persistently > 160/100 mmHg, or to decide whether to initiate lipid-lowering treatment when the total cholesterol to HDL ratio exceeds 6. In the absence of these conditions, treatment is recommended when the estimated CVD risk over 10 years is > 20%.

1.20   C: Measure ankle:brachial systolic pressure index

These symptoms are typical of intermittent claudication. The history and an ankle:brachial pressure index of < 0.9 support the diagnosis. Walking distance can be improved by exercise and patients should be encouraged to continue walking beyond the distance at which pain occurs. Referral to a vascular surgeon is indicated if symptoms are lifestyle-limiting. If there are bilateral symptoms, spinal stenosis should be considered.

THEME: CARDIOVASCULAR RISK ESTIMATION

1.21   B: Framingham

The Framingham risk assessment model is based on data from a predominantly white, middle-class population in North America, and is therefore less reliable at calculating risk in European or Asian populations.

1.22   D: QRISK

QRISK was developed from a database of UK patients and includes a large cohort from deprived areas. It is therefore more accurate in assessing risk in UK patients.

1.23   B: Framingham

Framingham is applicable only for primary prevention, not secondary, and should not be used in patients with pre-existing heart disease.

1.24   A: ASSIGN

ASSIGN was developed with the Scottish Intercollegiate Guidelines Network to address the fact that that Framingham model does not accurately assess risk in these patients.

THEME: VALVE DISEASE

1.25   B: Aortic sclerosis

Aortic sclerosis is age-related thickening of the aortic valve, often associated with calcification. It is not associated with outflow obstruction.

1.26   C: Aortic stenosis

Aortic stenosis presents with angina, shortness of breath, syncope or sudden death. Echocardiography is used to estimate the pressure gradient across the valve and severity of the condition. Surgery is considered for patients in whom the pressure gradient is > 50 mmHg. Treatment with ACE inhibitors should be avoided.

1.27   D: Mitral regurgitation

Complications of rheumatic fever include myocarditis and valvulitis, the mitral valve being the most commonly affected valve.

1.28   I: Tricuspid regurgitation

Intravenous drug users are susceptible to infective endocarditis. The right side of the heart can be involved by infection introduced into the venous circulation.

1.29   A: Aortic regurgitation

Marfan syndrome and Ehlers–Danlos syndrome are recognised causes of aortic regurgitation. The prominent pulse is referred to as a 'water-hammer' pulse. Other signs include visible neck pulsation and head-nodding in time with the pulse.

THEME: TREATMENT OF HYPERTENSION

1.30   **C:**   Bendroflumethiazide

1.31   **I:**   Ramipril

1.32   **H:**   No change indicated

1.33   **J:**   Specialist referral

1.34   **D:**   Candesartan

The guidance produced by NICE suggests a stepwise protocol for the treatment of hypertension, as follows:

	Patients aged < 55 years	Patients aged ≥ 55 years or black patients of any age
Step 1	A	C or D
Step 2	A + C or D	C or D + A
Step 3	A + C + D	A + C + D

A = ACE inhibitor (ALLRA if intolerant), C = Calcium channel blocker, D = Thiazide diuretic

Drug therapy should be offered to the following patients:

- Those with a persistent high blood pressure of 160/100 mmHg or more

- Those with a 10-year risk of CVD of > 20%, and persistent high blood pressure of ≥ 140/90 mmHg.

Patients should be referred immediately if there are signs of accelerated hypertension or if phaeochromocytoma is suspected.

THEME: ANGINA

1.35   **F:**   GTN 400 micrograms sublingually prn

1.36   **E:**   Emergency hospital admission

1.37   **C:**   Atenolol 100 mg od

1.38   **A:**   Amlodipine 5 mg od

1.39   **I:**   Nicorandil 5 mg od

For patients with mild angina with fewer than two attacks per week, 'as required' treatment with GTN is appropriate. Introduction of further treatments should be stepwise in the following order: 1) β blocker, 2) long-acting dihydropyridine calcium-channel blocker (eg amlodipine), and 3) long-acting nitrate.

In the presence of left ventricular dysfunction, long-acting nitrates are used first-line, with the addition of a long-acting dihydropyridine calcium-channel blocker if necessary. Nicorandil is recommended if standard treatment is unsuccessful but is contraindicated in left ventricular failure (LVF) and hypotension.

THEME: COMMON INVESTIGATIONS IN CARDIOVASCULAR DISEASE

1.40   **G:**   Fasting lipid profile

This family history (MI in a male aged < 55 or in a female aged < 65) suggests a possible diagnosis of familial hyperlipidaemia and relatives should be screened for this.

1.41   **F:**   Exercise ECG

The likely diagnosis is angina. Exercise testing is likely to reproduce symptoms, which can be associated with ischaemic changes on ECG.

1.42   J: Thyroid function tests

Hyperthyroidism is a common cause of tachycardia or palpitations, and should be screened for if patients experience these symptoms, particularly if there are other features of thyroid disease.

1.43   A: 24-hour ECG recording

These symptoms might be related to paroxysmal arrhythmia, which can be diagnosed by 24-hour ECG recording or using an event recorder.

1.44   I: Serum troponin

MI is a likely diagnosis. Troponin T and troponin I are released from cardiac muscle and reach a peak level within 6 9 hours after MI.

THEME: RATE CONTROL FOR PERSISTENT AND PERMANENT ATRIAL FIBRILLATION (AF)

1.45   A: Administer appropriate thromboprophylaxis

1.46   D: Beta blocker or rate-limiting calcium antagonist

1.47   E: Beta blocker or rate-limiting calcium antagonist with digoxin

1.48   I: Rate-limiting calcium antagonist with digoxin

1.49   J: Specialist referral or consideration of other drugs

[Based on NICE clinical guidance, *Atrial fibrillation*, June 2006.]

THEME: PHARMACOLOGICAL TREATMENT OF SYMPTOMATIC HEART FAILURE DUE TO LEFT VENTRICULAR SYSTOLIC DYSFUNCTION

1.50 **A:** ACE inhibitor

1.51 **B:** Angiotensin II-receptor antagonist

1.52 **C:** Beta blocker

1.53 **F:** Spironolactone

1.54 **E:** Diuretic therapy

1.55 **D:** Digoxin

[Based on NICE clinical guidance, *Management of adults in chronic heart failure in primary and secondary care,* July 2003.]

1.56 A: Admit for pacemaker

This ECG shows a 12-second episode of asystole. Atropine can be used if the episode is prolonged but a permanent pacemaker is needed. Amiodarone is used for atrial fibrillation, while adrenaline would be used in an arrest situation. If the patient collapses, basic life support should be instituted until he reaches hospital. Where pacing is not available, short-term treatment with isoprenaline might be helpful until definitive treatment is possible.

1.57 A: Arterial ulcer

Arterial ulceration typically occurs over the toes, heels and bony prominences of the foot and ankle. There is a 'punched out' appearance with well-demarcated edges. The surrounding skin is hairless and shows signs of atrophy. In contrast, venous ulcers tend to have smoothly sloping edges. A Marjolin's ulcer is a squamous-cell carcinoma arising within a pre-existing chronic ulcer. Neuropathic ulcers tend to occur on the sole of the foot and rodent ulcers (also known as 'basal-cell carcinoma' or BCC) occur in sun-exposed areas and have a characteristic rolled edge.

1.58 D: Diltiazem hydrochloride 60 mg bd

The ECG reveals AF with a rapid ventricular response. NICE clinical guidance on AF (2006) recommends that the most appropriate management strategy for this patient would be rate control with a rate-limiting calcium antagonist (or β blocker). Stroke risk stratification and anticoagulation is important, and it is likely that this patient would be a candidate for warfarin therapy (aged > 75 with clinical evidence of valve disease).

1.59 E: Drug J is shown to significantly reduce mortality

The forest plot represents results of studies shown as squares centred on the point estimate of the result of each study. The horizontal line represents the confidence interval (CI), usually a 95% CI. Statistical significance is only shown if the CI does not cross the line of no effect, which in this case is determined by ratio of death rate = 1.0. A ratio of < 1.0 shows a trend towards reduced mortality.

1.60 B: Amlodipine plus perindopril reduced all-cause mortality and all coronary events

In ASCOT, patients with hypertension were randomised into two groups. One group received atenolol with bendroflumethiazide if needed, and the other group received amlodipine with perindopril if needed. The trial was stopped early because the amlodipine-based arm of the trial was showing significantly lower rates of all-cause mortality and of all coronary events. In this group there was also a reduction in the onset of diabetes.

CHAPTER 2
DERMATOLOGY
SINGLE BEST ANSWER QUESTIONS

2.1 A 17-year-old boy comes to see you regarding his recurrent attacks of urticaria. Over the years he has tried excluding possible triggers but is now getting regular attacks. These involve itch and rash but he has no signs of angioedema. He has not tried any prescription medications yet. Which one of the following would be appropriate as the next step in his treatment?

- [ ] A Issue an EpiPen with advice on how to use it
- [ ] B Loratadine tablets
- [ ] C Montelukast tablets
- [ ] D Prednisolone to use orally when he develops attacks
- [ ] E Topical steroids to use for short periods

2.2 A 36-year-old businessman complains that he has suffered from sweaty palms for many years but is now finding this increasingly embarrassing in business meetings. He has a friend who has had successful treatment for this but is not sure what this was. He asks your advice. Which one of the following treatments is most effective for this condition?

- [ ] A Botox injections
- [ ] B Cervical sympathectomy
- [ ] C Excision of sweat glands
- [ ] D Topical aluminium hydroxide
- [ ] E Topical hydrocortisone

2.3 A 46-year-old man comes to see you regarding a rash he has developed on his elbows. He is otherwise well apart from a recent diagnosis of essential hypertension for which he has started atenolol. On examination he has well-defined, raised, scaly lesions. How would you treat this patient?

- [ ] A Prescribe Betnovate alone
- [ ] B Prescribe coal tar
- [ ] C Prescribe Dovobet (calcipotriol and betamethasone cream)
- [ ] D Refer for UV therapy
- [ ] E Stop his atenolol and prescribe emollients

2.4 A 24-year-old girl who has recently returned from a season as a holiday rep in Greece comes to see you regarding her florid genital warts. She is otherwise well and does not have any immunosuppressive illness. Which of the following is the most effective initial treatment option?

- [ ] A Cryotherapy
- [ ] B Diathermy
- [ ] C Imiquimod
- [ ] D Podophyllotoxin
- [ ] E Salicylic acid

2.5 Which one of the following is the most appropriate initial treatment for a patient presenting with palmar psoriasis?

- [ ] A Betamethasone valerate ointment
- [ ] B Hydrocortisone 1% ointment
- [ ] C Oral prednisolone
- [ ] D Regular emollients
- [ ] E Tacrolimus cream

2.6 Children with eczema are commonly seen in general practice. Which one of the following statements regarding NICE guidance is correct?

- [ ] A Moderately potent steroids can be used by children for facial eczema but not for more than 3 weeks continuously
- [ ] B Oral antihistamines are recommended routinely for childhood eczema
- [ ] C Potent topical steroids should never be used in children unless directed to do so by a specialist dermatologist
- [ ] D Topical tacrolimus can be used as an alternative to corticosteroids in children with mild eczema
- [ ] E When tachyphylaxis occurs, a different topical steroid of the same potency can be tried in children

2.7 You have been asked to teach foundation doctors at the practice. They wish to learn about acne vulgaris. Which one of the following statements is correct?

☐ A Minocycline is associated with a lower risk of systemic lupus erythematosus (SLE) than other tetracyclines

☐ B Systemic retinoids commonly cause suicidal behaviour if not administered with an antidepressant

☐ C Topical clindamycin should be avoided as it causes a high incidence of skin sensitisation

☐ D Topical retinoids are used to treat both inflammatory and non-inflammatory lesions in acne

☐ E Severe acne is diagnosed when both open and closed comedones are noted

2.8 A medical student has seen a 40-year-old man with prurigo nodularis. The medical student asks you to explain more about this condition. Which one of the following pieces of information is correct?

☐ A Hydrocortisone cream often worsens the condition

☐ B Patients with the condition often suffer with intense itch that lasts for about 1 day

☐ C The majority of patients have a personal or family history of atopy

☐ D The trunk is often the most affected area of the patient's body

☐ E Young children are more likely to be affected by prurigo nodularis than adults

EXTENDED MATCHING QUESTIONS

THEME: MANAGEMENT OF SKIN LESIONS

Options

A 5-Fluorouracil

B Cryotherapy

C Curettage

D Excision in primary care

E No treatment required

F Referral to secondary care

G Salicylic acid

H Topical steroids

For each of the dermatological lesions below, select the most appropriate management from the list above. Each option may be used once, more than once or not at all.

☐ **2.9** Pyogenic granuloma.

☐ **2.10** Squamous-cell carcinoma.

☐ **2.11** Actinic keratosis.

☐ **2.12** Seborrhoeic keratosis.

☐ **2.13** Keratin horn.

THEME: SKIN LESIONS

Options

A	Amelanotic melanoma	G	Nodular prurigo
B	Capillary haemangioma	H	Pyogenic granuloma
C	Dermatofibroma	I	Squamous-cell carcinoma
D	Melanoma	J	Superficial spreading basal-cell carcinoma
E	Molluscum contagiosum		
F	Nodular basal-cell carcinoma		

Choose the single most likely skin diagnosis from the list above for each of the following scenarios. Each option can be used once, more than once or not at all.

☐ **2.14** A 7-year-old girl sustained a trivial injury to her fingertip 3 weeks ago. Her mother noticed a small red lump on her fingertip the next day. She now has a 5-mm-wide, shiny, red, fleshy polypoid lesion on the dorsal aspect of her finger.

☐ **2.15** A 30-year-old lady presents with a 7-mm-diameter, firm, pink nodule on her thigh. It has been present for 6 months and has not changed in size recently. Squeezing the lesion causes dimpling of the overlying skin.

☐ **2.16** A 72-year-old renal transplant patient has an ulcerated lesion affecting the superior aspect of his left pinna. The ulcerated lesion is 15 mm in diameter and has rolled edges. The ulcer is partially covered in sloughy material.

☐ **2.17** An 8-year-old girl has a widespread papular rash on her arms and trunk. The papules are flesh-coloured and some are umbilicated. She has a past history of eczema.

☐ **2.18** A 55-year-old gardener presents with an ulcerated lesion above his left eye. It has slowly enlarged over the last 6 months and is now 1 cm in diameter. He complains that it bleeds from time to time. You note that the lesion has a pearly, rolled edge.

THEME: DIAGNOSIS OF SKIN CANCER

Options

A   Amelanotic melanoma

B   Bowen's disease

C   Invasive squamous-cell carcinoma

D   Keratoacanthoma

E   Lentigo maligna melanoma

F   Nodular basal-cell carcinoma

G   Superficial basal-cell carcinoma

H   Superficial spreading melanoma

For each of the scenarios below, select the single most likely diagnosis from the list of options above. Each option can be used once, more than once or not at all.

☐ **2.19** A 40-year-old white man has a skin lesion on his upper trunk that has a shiny, dark-pink appearance and some moderate scaling. The lesion is now 2 cm in diameter. It has been slowly enlarging in size over the past 14 months. The lesion bleeds easily.

☐ **2.20** A 62-year-old woman has been attending the local dermatology department regarding her left leg. She has a well-demarcated skin lesion, 3 cm in diameter, on the shin. The lesion is red and scaly. She has a skin biopsy taken and you are told that the cancer is 'in situ'.

☐ **2.21** A 68-year-old woman has had a brown lesion affecting her right cheek for the past 7 years. The lesion has poorly defined margins and is about 25 mm in diameter. The brown discoloration is variable in shade and a dark-brown nodule has developed within the lesion recently.

PICTURE QUESTIONS

2.22 A 23-year-old man complains of an intensely itchy rash on the palms of his hands. This came on without any obvious cause about 2 weeks ago and was initially painful. It is now very itchy and keeping him awake at night. His hand is shown below.

What is the most likely diagnosis?

☐   A   Contact dermatitis
☐   B   Eczema
☐   C   Hand, foot and mouth disease
☐   D   Pompholyx
☐   E   Scabies

2.23 An 87-year-old man complains of a rash on his chest, back and stomach. He has tried emollients and antihistamines without any luck. The rash is shown below.

What is the most likely diagnosis?

☐ A Contact dermatitis
☐ B Erythema annulare
☐ C Erythema chronicum migrans
☐ D Erythema nodosum
☐ E Urticaria

2.24 This 73-year-old patient has had a rash on the palms of both hands for the past few months. It is not itchy. Recently, he has been treated with an antifungal cream for a rash on the soles of his feet but it made no difference. He does not have skin lesions elsewhere and is otherwise well. He has recently started taking atenolol for angina.

The single most likely diagnosis is:

- [ ] A   Contact dermatitis
- [ ] B   Eczema
- [ ] C   Fixed drug eruption
- [ ] D   Psoriasis
- [ ] E   Tylosis

2.25 A 14-year-old girl presented with erythematous patches affecting the dorsal aspect of both feet (shown below). The rest of her skin was clear. The rash was itchy. She had recently bought some new shoes and the rash appeared shortly after she had worn them.

Select the single most likely diagnosis from the following list:

- A   Allergic contact dermatitis
- B   Eczema
- C   Irritant contact dermatitis
- D   Perniosis (chilblains)
- E   Tinea pedis

2.26 A pensioner asks you whether you can arrange to have this lesion on his back treated (shown below). He is not sure how long it has been there but he complains that it is now catching on his clothes.

What is the single most appropriate course of action?

☐   A   Refer to a local minor surgery service for complete excision with 2-mm borders

☐   B   Refer to a local minor surgery service for shave excision

☐   C   Refer to dermatology for a routine opinion

☐   D   Refer to dermatology for an urgent outpatient opinion

☐   E   Treat with 5-fluorouracil cream

2.27 This 60-year-old lady has recently started to take treatment for a severe unilateral headache associated with scalp tenderness. She returns a few weeks later because she is unhappy with lesions she has developed on both forearms (see below). Her headache has gone.

Which of the following medications is most likely to have been prescribed for her headache and caused her skin problem? Select one option only.

- ☐ A   Ibuprofen
- ☐ B   Paracetamol
- ☐ C   Pizotifen
- ☐ D   Prednisolone
- ☐ E   Sumatriptan

2.28 A 54-year-old gentleman took paracetamol after a minor injury 3 months ago. He developed a pruritic, oval skin lesion on his right shoulder. The lesion gradually resolved after he stopped the paracetamol. He recently restarted paracetamol for a headache. He quickly developed a recurrent skin lesion affecting his right shoulder (shown below).

Which one of the following options is the most likely skin diagnosis? Select one option only.

- [ ] A Drug hypersensitivity syndrome
- [ ] B Drug-induced photosensitivity
- [ ] C Fixed drug eruption
- [ ] D Gout
- [ ] E Mycetoma

2.29 An 81-year-old man has a skin lesion on dorsal aspect of his right forearm, shown below. It is not painful or itchy. He first noticed it when it was a few millimetres in diameter and it has slowly increased in size over at least a year. The skin lesion is hard to see and feels rough on palpation.

Which one of the following options is the most likely diagnosis:

- A Actinic keratosis
- B Discoid lupus
- C Keratoacanthoma
- D Seborrhoeic keratosis
- E Squamous cell carcinoma

ANSWERS

2.1   B: Loratadine tablets

Urticaria has multiple causes and avoidance can be difficult if an obvious precipitant cannot be identified. Symptomatic treatment with oral antihistamines is usually sufficient to control symptoms of simple urticaria but where there is associated angioedema parenteral epinephrine might be needed. Montelukast in association with antihistamines can be useful in refractory cases but is ineffective as monotherapy. In severe cases not responding to oral antihistamines short courses of steroids orally might be needed but topical steroids are not effective.

2.2   A: Botox injections

Botulinum toxin injections are effective treatment for this condition but require repeated treatment every 4–6 months. They are effective for axillary, palmar and facial sweating. With prolonged use they can cause the production of antibodies, which reduce their efficacy. An alternative treatment is iontophoresis. Aluminium hydrochloride is useful for axillary hyperhidrosis but is less so for sweating of the hands and often leaves a residue.

2.3   E: Stop his atenolol and prescribe emollients

Beta blockers are common precipitants of psoriasis and in this case it is appropriate to stop the beta blocker and try emollients. If the rash fails to resolve a course of calcipotriol could be useful, but Dovobet is usually only necessary in severe or recurrent psoriasis. UV therapy and coal-tar treatment are seldom used but can be needed in refractory cases.

2.4   C: Imiquimod

Imiquimod can be applied by patients themselves and has been demonstrated to be effective in outpatient settings. Sixteen weeks of treatment achieves clearance in 75% of patients. Patients should take steps to avoid pregnancy during treatment and partners should be screened. When they have a very large number of warts they should be referred to a local genitourinary medicine (GUM) clinic. Genital warts often coexist with other sexually transmitted diseases (STDs) and consideration should be given to testing for these. Diathermy and cryotherapy are better suited to keratinised warts.

2.5   A: Betamethasone valerate ointment

The British Association of Dermatology recommends using potent topical steroids as part of the initial treatment of palmar psoriasis. Keratolytic agents, such as salicylic acid in Lassar's paste, might be required to remove scale from hyperkeratotic skin. Tars and vitamin D analogues can also help. Palms and soles can be difficult areas to treat, and the patient should be referred to a dermatologist if initial treatments fail after 2–3 months or if there is diagnostic uncertainty. Specialists may recommend treatments including clobetasol propionate under occlusion or PUVA.

2.6   E: When tachyphylaxis occurs, a different topical steroid of the same potency can be tried in children

NICE produced guidance covering the management of children with eczema in December 2007. Emollients are used on a regular basis in mild, moderate and severe eczema. Guidance suggests that emollient treatment should continue even when the eczema is clear. Topical steroids of higher potency might be required during exacerbations of eczema. When tachyphylaxis is suspected, a different drug of equal steroidal potency can be tried rather than stepping up steroidal treatment. Topical steroids of mild, moderate and potent strengths are discussed further in the guidelines. All are recommended for use by primary care in specific situations. It is recommended that very potent steroids are only commenced by specialist dermatology teams.

2.7   D: Topical retinoids are used to treat both inflammatory and non-inflammatory lesions in acne

Acne vulgaris is commonly seen and the majority of patients can be managed in primary care. Closed and open comedones occur in mild acne, and represent non-inflammatory lesions. Inflammatory lesions occur where the wall of closed comedones has ruptured and secondary inflammation has occurred. Infection with *Propionibacterium acnes* has been implicated. Topical treatments are useful for mild to moderate acne. Topical retinoids are used to treat both inflammatory and non-inflammatory lesions but are contraindicated in pregnancy. Oral antibiotics are often prescribed for moderate acne and combat inflammatory lesions. Nodular and cystic lesions are seen in severe acne; the patient should be referred to a dermatologist.

2.8   C: The majority of patients have a personal or family history of atopy

Prurigo nodularis is an intensely itchy skin condition of unknown aetiology. Adults are affected more frequently than children and the condition is equally distributed between males and females. Affected individuals are likely to have a personal or family history of atopy; up to 80% have a positive history compared with 25% of the normal population. Nodular, itchy lesions, 1–2 cm in diameter, are symmetrically distributed, particularly on the extensor limb surfaces. Itching is often difficult to treat and is commonly a long-standing problem. High-potency corticosteroids can be tried to treat itchy lesions, under occlusive dressings to increase absorption. Many topical and systemic treatments have been tried in the past with limited success.

THEME: MANAGEMENT OF SKIN LESIONS

2.9   D: Excision in primary care

Pyogenic granulomas are inflammatory reactions to minor trauma such as thorns. They develop over about 7 days and should be excised for histological confirmation of diagnosis and the base curetted. They do not usually resolve spontaneously.

2.10   F: Referral to secondary care

Squamous-cell carcinomas should be excised, but this should not be done in primary care as these tumours are more likely to metastasise than basal-cell carcinomas.

2.11   A: 5-Fluorouracil

Actinic keratosis can be treated with topical 5-FU, diclofenac gel or cryotherapy. Resistant cases are sometimes treated with excision. These lesions are thought to be precursors of squamous-cell carcinoma so treatment should be active.

2.12   E: No treatment required

No treatment is required for simple seborrhoeic keratoses. If they irritate or catch on clothes or where there is uncertainty over diagnosis, curettage with histological confirmation would be appropriate.

2.13   C: Curettage

Curettage and histological confirmation of the diagnosis is appropriate to exclude underlying squamous-cell carcinoma, although these lesions usually have a typical appearance.

THEME: SKIN LESIONS

2.14   H: Pyogenic granuloma

These benign lesions are common in children and young adults. They grow rapidly over a period of a few weeks. Predisposing factors include minor trauma, infection and pregnancy. The lesions are removed by shave excision or curettage, but can recur.

2.15   C: Dermatofibroma

Dermatofibromas are benign skin lesions. They are more common in women than men and tend to occur on the lower limbs. It was thought that these lesions were precipitated by minor trauma or insect bites but this is now disputed. Dimpling on squeezing is a helpful pointer to the diagnosis. No treatment is required unless the diagnosis is in doubt or the lesion is cosmetically unacceptable.

2.16   I: Squamous-cell carcinoma

Squamous-cell carcinoma develops in areas of sun-exposed skin. Transplant recipients taking who are immunosuppressants are at particularly high risk of these lesions. Squamous-cell carcinomas are more common than basal-cell carcinomas in this group of patients. Squamous-cell carcinomas can metastasise and are more aggressive if the patient is immunosuppressed.

2.17   E: Molluscum contagiosum

Molluscum contagiosum is caused by a pox virus and is common in young children. The rash is usually asymptomatic but can be itchy and can persist for several monthis. It is often more widespread in patients with eczema. Patients with human immunodeficiency (HIV) infection can present with extensive molluscum.

2.18   F: Nodular basal-cell carcinoma

Chronic sun exposure is a well-recognised risk factor for basal-cell carcinoma (BCC). BCC is the most common skin cancer in white people. Metastases are exceedingly rare but local invasion and damage can be extensive. Nodular BCC commonly affects the face and lesions have a pearly, rolled edge. Superficial spreading BCCs are more commonly found on the trunk and shoulders.

THEME: DIAGNOSIS OF SKIN CANCER

2.19   G: Superficial basal-cell carcinoma

BCC is the commonest type of skin cancer in white people. Lesions develop after long-term sun exposure in susceptible individuals (fair hair, poor skin tanning and blue eye colour are all risk factors). Facial lesions are the most common and are usually nodular in nature. Lesions on the trunk are usually superficial BCCs. Superficial BCCs are erythematous, flat, shiny and pink in appearance, with moderate scaling. They are slow-growing lesions and metastases are exceedingly rare. Lesions tend to occur in younger patients than those affected by nodular BCC. Treatment is by surgical excision or topical treatment with 5-fluorouracil cream.

2.20   B: Bowen's disease

Bowen's disease is squamous-cell carcinoma in situ, involving the epidermis. It usually presents as a slowly enlarging, well-demarcated, erythematous lesion. It most commonly affects elderly women. Most lesions present on the lower leg. The diagnosis is usually made clinically but it can be biopsied. Treatment options include surgical excision, topical 5-fluorouracil or radiotherapy. Overall, the prognosis is very good.

2.21   E: Lentigo maligna melanoma

Lentigo maligna presents as a slow-growing area of pigmented skin affecting sun-exposed areas. Usually, the lesion has poorly defined borders and is brown in colour. The brown pigmentation is usually variable in tone throughout the lesion. The lesion is premalignant and often grows slowly over many years. New nodular lesions, which are often dark-brown or black in nature, can develop within lentigo maligna lesions. These lesions represent invasive melanoma and are known as 'lentigo maligna melanoma'.

2.22   D: Pompholyx

This is a typical appearance for pompholyx, with painful, itchy vesicles on the palms (and sometimes soles). It is difficult to treat without potent topical steroids but usually subsides over 2–3 weeks. Potassium permanganate can be used for treatment if vesicles break down and, in refractory cases, topical calcineurin inhibitors, Botox or PUVA (psoralen plus UVA) can be effective.

2.23   B: Erythema annulare

This annular and erythematous rash is erythema annulare. It affects all ages and usually starts as a small papule which slowly enlarges to form a ring while the central area clears. The rash is not usually very itchy but does persist. It is often idiopathic but can be associated with underlying malignancy (particularly where there are multiple concentric, whirling rings), tuberculosis, liver disease and Graves' disease. Patients should have blood tests, ultrasound of the liver and a chest X-ray if there is suspicion of underlying disease. The rash usually settles spontaneously, but this can take up to 12 months. Topical steroids might be helpful in speeding resolution.

2.24   D: Psoriasis

The patient has well-demarcated, hyperkeratotic areas on the palms of his hands. The soles of his feet have also been affected. Inspection of his palms reveals silvery scaling.

Psoriasis can be precipitated by medications and worsened by medication and alcohol. Drugs implicated include β blockers, chloroquine and lithium. Stress and withdrawal of oral corticosteroids are other precipitants. The lack of itch makes eczema and contact dermatitis unlikely.

2.25   C: Irritant contact dermatitis

Allergy and irritants can both trigger contact dermatitis. Irritant contact dermatitis is usually well demarcated and itchy and often has a glazed appearance; there can be some surface scaling. Causes include exposure to detergents and damage due to repeated friction and sweating. On further questioning the patient admitted that her new shoes felt too tight and had been rubbing.

2.26   B: Refer to a local minor surgery service for shave excision

This is seborrhoeic keratosis, a benign epidermal tumour common in the elderly. Note the characteristic stuck-on appearance and rough, warty surface. Treatment is not necessary unless the lesion is bothering the patient. Troublesome lesions can be removed by shave excision or curettage; smaller lesions can by treated with cryotherapy.

2.27   D: Prednisolone

This is steroid-induced purpura. She has been receiving prednisolone in high doses for giant-cell arteritis. Systemic steroids alter connective tissue surrounding skin capillaries, causing fragility. This leads to the extravasation of blood under the skin.

2.28   C: Fixed drug eruption

Fixed drug eruptions manifest as painful oval or round lesions. They characteristically occur at the same site 30 minutes to 8 hours after taking the medication responsible. The lesions sometimes blister and occur most commonly on the hands, feet, glans penis and lips. Many drugs have been implicated.

2.29   A: Actinic keratosis

Actinic keratosis is a premalignant skin lesion. The rough, keratotic lesions are often only a few millimetres in diameter. They are often easier to feel than to see. They enlarge to a few centimetres in diameter in some cases and can progress to squamous-cell carcinoma (usually over a period of several years); regression of the lesion is also possible. The lesions are most common in fair-skinned adults over the age of 40; ultraviolet light exposure is recognised as a strong risk factor. Lesions most commonly affect the face, ears or bald scalp skin.

CHAPTER 3
ENDOCRINOLOGY
SINGLE BEST ANSWER QUESTIONS

3.1 You arrange a routine pelvic X-ray for a patient with painful hips. The report comments on likely Paget's disease. You arrange some blood tests, which show a raised calcium level. Which of the following is the most appropriate management in this patient?

- [ ] A Calcitonin
- [ ] B Intravenous bisphosphonate
- [ ] C No treatment required
- [ ] D Oral bisphosphonate
- [ ] E Simple analgesia

3.2 You see a 57-year-old postmenopausal lady who has just had a DEXA scan carried out at a local private hospital as part of a well woman check. The results show that she has a T score of –1.8. She has a normal diet, normal BMI, exercises most days and does not smoke. You review her medical records and these show that she has no major previous medical history. Routine blood tests are carried out, which are normal. She would like to be treated. Which one of the following is the most appropriate management?

- [ ] A Calcium and vitamin D supplements
- [ ] B No treatment required
- [ ] C Oral bisphosphonate
- [ ] D Teriparatide
- [ ] E Three-monthly intravenous bisphosphonate

3.3 A 78-year-old man with advanced prostate cancer has become increasingly confused over the last 2 weeks. He reports constipation and passing urine more frequently, and has felt nauseous. He has no signs of infection and urine testing is negative. He is taking ibuprofen and paracetamol for backache and is on luteinising hormone-releasing hormone (LHRH) injections for his cancer but takes no other medications. Clinical examination is unremarkable. What is the single most likely cause of his symptoms?

- [ ] A Cerebral metastases
- [ ] B Diabetes mellitus
- [ ] C Hypercalcaemia
- [ ] D Hyperkalaemia
- [ ] E Infection

3.4 A 46-year-old man complains of problems with erections. He has been through a divorce after a long and unhappy marriage and has now started a new relationship. His new partner is frustrated by his erectile problems and would like him to try Viagra. His previous medical history is unremarkable, he takes no regular medications and he has no children. He is a new patient so you undertake a physical examination and you note that he has small testes and less body hair than you might expect in a man of his age. Which of the following would be the most appropriate next step in his management?

- [ ] A Check FSH and testosterone levels
- [ ] B Prescribe sildenafil at 25 mg initially and review in 2 weeks
- [ ] C Prescribe testosterone supplements
- [ ] D Refer for psychosexual counselling
- [ ] E Start treatment with LHRH analogues

3.5 A 39-year-old woman joins your practice after relocating to the area. She comes to see you for a new patient check and to pick up her medication. She has diabetes mellitus, for which she takes metformin, and severe asthma, which has caused her to be admitted to hospital on several occasions. Her previous doctor was in the habit of giving her a supply of oral steroids to keep at home, allowing her to manage her asthma symptoms with minimal input from the practice. You note that she has acne and is obese, and that she has hirsutism, dark skin and abdominal striae. Which one of the following is the most likely cause of these symptoms?

- A   Addison's disease
- B   Cushing's disease
- C   Cushing syndrome
- D   Hypopituitarism
- E   Polycystic ovary syndrome

3.6 A 27-year-old woman of South Asian origin is brought to see you complaining of chronic pain in her legs. This seems to have started insidiously and there is no history of trauma. She lives according to strict cultural rules and wears full Muslim dress. You arrange for an X-ray and blood tests. These both show evidence of osteomalacia. What would be the most appropriate next step in her management?

- A   Arrange for DEXA scan
- B   Investigate for causes of vitamin D deficiency
- C   Prescribe bisphosphonates
- D   Prescribe calcium and vitamin D supplements
- E   Refer to social services

3.7 In diabetic patients with microalbuminuria, which one of the following interventions is most appropriate to reduce the risk of progression to chronic renal failure?

☐ A   Angiotensin-converting enzyme (ACE) inhibitor

☐ B   Beta blocker

☐ C   Calcium-channel blocker

☐ D   Direct renin inhibitor

☐ E   Thiazide diuretic

3.8 A healthy 16-year-old girl became concerned about a prominence in her neck, which was found to be a smooth, diffuse, non-tender enlargement of the thyroid gland. Which one of the following is the most likely diagnosis?

☐ A   Colloid goitre

☐ B   Endemic goitre

☐ C   Physiological goitre

☐ D   Thyroglossal cyst

☐ E   Thyroid nodule

3.9 A 62-year-old man with a long-standing goitre complains of recent onset of pain in the neck and hoarseness. Examination reveals a firm swelling in the left lobe of the thyroid and Horner syndrome on that side. Select the single most likely diagnosis from the list below.

☐ A   Carcinoma of the thyroid

☐ B   Colloid goitre

☐ C   Endemic goitre

☐ D   Postviral thyroiditis

☐ E   Thyroid nodule

3.10 A 70-year-old-woman was found to have an asymptomatic swelling of the thyroid gland on a routine visit to her doctor. She recalled that in her youth several members of her community had similar neck swellings which were said to be caused by the water. Select the single most likely diagnosis from the list below.

- [ ] A   Endemic goitre
- [ ] B   Graves' disease
- [ ] C   Physiological goitre
- [ ] D   Thyroglossal cyst
- [ ] E   Thyroid nodule

3.11 A 33-year-old woman presents with a 6-month history of breast tenderness, localised to the upper outer quadrant of her right breast. She has been on oral contraception intermittently for nearly 15 years. Clinically, the breast has a nodular feeling but no lumps or lymph nodes are palpable. Select the single most likely diagnosis from the list below.

- [ ] A   Benign breast change
- [ ] B   Breast carcinoma
- [ ] C   Fibroadenoma
- [ ] D   Haematoma
- [ ] E   Paget's disease

3.12 A 55-year-old man presents with a painful swelling of the left breast disc. There is no past history of breast disease. He is currently on hormone therapy for prostatic cancer. From the list below select the single most likely cause of his symptoms.

- [ ] A   Benign breast change
- [ ] B   Breast carcinoma
- [ ] C   Fibroadenoma
- [ ] D   Gynaecomastia
- [ ] E   Mondor's disease

3.13 A 21-year-old woman presents with a non-tender, firm, mobile 2-cm lump in the upper inner quadrant of the right breast. She has been on oral contraception for 5 years. Select the single most likely cause of her symptoms from the following options.

☐ A Benign breast change

☐ B Breast carcinoma

☐ C Fibroadenoma

☐ D Galactocoele

☐ E Gynaecomastia

3.14 A 79-year-old woman in a residential home was found by her carers to have a painless lump in the lower inner quadrant of the left breast. Clinically, there is a 4-cm lump adherent to the overlying skin, with nipple retraction on extending the arm. Select the single most likely diagnosis from the list below.

☐ A Breast carcinoma

☐ B Breast cyst

☐ C Fat necrosis

☐ D Fibroadenoma

☐ E Mondor's disease

EXTENDED MATCHING QUESTIONS

THEME: BLOOD TESTS IN ENDOCRINOLOGY

Options

A   Addison's disease

B   Clinical hypothyroidism

C   Cushing's disease

D   Hypercalcaemla

E   Hyperparathyroidism

F   Hyperthyroidism

G   Hypocalcaemia

H   Hypopituitarism

I   Menopausal

J   Subclinical hypothyroidism

For each of the blood result profiles below, select the most likely diagnosis from the list above. Each option may be used once, more than once or not at all.

☐   **3.15**   Raised TSH, normal T4.

☐   **3.16**   Low sodium, raised potassium, raised ACTH with low cortisol.

☐   **3.17**   Raised follicle-stimulating hormone (FSH), low oestrogen.

☐   **3.18**   Low levels of T4, T3, TSH, prolactin, sodium and potassium.

☐   **3.19**   Low TSH, raised T4.

THEME: BREAST PAIN

Options

A	Benign breast change	**F**	Breast hypertrophy
B	Blunt injury	**G**	Gynaecomastia
C	Breast abscess	**H**	Haematoma
D	Breast carcinoma	**I**	Mondor's disease
E	Breast engorgement	**J**	Shingles (herpes zoster)

For each of the scenarios described below, select the most appropriate diagnosis from the list above. Each option can be used once, more than once or not at all.

☐ **3.20** A 19-year-old man complains of a diffuse swelling and discomfort of the right breast over a 9-month period. Clinically and on ultrasound scanning there is no discrete lesion.

☐ **3.21** A 22-year-old woman presents in the immediate postpartum period with moderately severe bilateral breast pain and swelling; she is unable to initiate lactation.

☐ **3.22** A 53-year-old woman presents with a 4-day history of severe left-sided breast pain and the appearance of a red rash and blisters over the breast.

☐ **3.23** A 16-year-old girl complains of progressive dragging pain in both breasts, which have increased in size over the past 15 months.

☐ **3.24** A 38-year-old woman who underwent excision of a large fibroadenoma of the left breast 10 days ago complains of pain, swelling and bruising at the operation site.

THEME: NIPPLE DISCHARGE

Options

A	Duct ectasia	F	Paget's disease of the nipple
B	Duct papilloma	G	Papillary carcinoma
C	Galactocoele	H	Prolactinoma
D	Juvenile mammary hyperplasia	I	Tuberculosis (TB) of the breast
E	Mammilary fistula	J	Virginal hypertrophy

For each of the scenarios described below, select the most appropriate diagnosis from the list above. Each option can be used once, more than once or not at all.

☐ **3.25** A 27-year-old woman developed a breast abscess during lactation, which was incised and drained. Some days later she was draining milk through the partially healed wound.

☐ **3.26** A 34-year-old woman with oligomenorrhoea complains of bilateral creamy nipple discharge over a 5-month period. There is no previous history of breast lesions or hormonal treatment.

☐ **3.27** A 38-year-old woman complains of unilateral bloodstained nipple discharge and is found to have an underlying lump; there are palpably enlarged axillary nodes on that side.

☐ **3.28** An 18-month-old male infant presents with an enlarged breast from which a milky fluid is being expressed.

☐ **3.29** A 56-year-old woman complains of itchiness and excoriation of the right nipple, with a serosanguinous discharge, over an 8-week period.

THEME: BREAST INFLAMMATION

Options

A   Acute mastitis

B   Benign breast change (aberration of normal development and involution or ANDI)

C   Breast abscess

D   Breast carcinoma

E   Breast engorgement

F   Breast hypertrophy

G   Eczema

H   Mondor's disease

I   Paget's disease of the nipple

J   TB of the breast

For each of the scenarios described below, select the most appropriate diagnosis from the list above. Each option may be used once, more than once or not at all.

☐ **3.30**   A 43-year-old female asylum seeker from Sudan complains of a chronic cough and progressive swelling and pain in the right breast. Further questioning reveals febrile episodes, malaise, weakness and loss of weight.

☐ **3.31**   A 19-year-old woman, breastfeeding 3 months postpartum, presents with a painful, reddened and indurated area of the right breast.

☐ **3.32**   A 63-year-old woman presents with a 4-month history of itching, redness and scaling over the left nipple that has not responded to topical steroid applications.

☐ **3.33** A 36-year-old woman presents with a 3-month history of painful nodularity in the upper half of the left breast, with cyclical changes in her symptoms. An ultrasound scan reveals multiple benign cysts.

☐ **3.34** A 34-year-old woman who is breastfeeding presents with a very painful, red, fluctuant swelling in the inferior aspect of the right breast. She has a mild pyrexia.

ALGORITHM QUESTIONS

THEME: THE MANAGEMENT OF PATIENTS WITH LOW THYROID-STIMULATING HORMONE (TSH) LEVELS

3.35–3.39

Options

A   Goitre

B   Signs of Graves' disease

C   Endemic goitre

D   Repeat in 3 months or if there are symptoms

E   Subacute thyroiditis

F   Consider referral for radioiodine uptake scan

G   Graves' disease

H   Thyroidectomy

I   Carbimazole therapy

J   Levothyroxine therapy

The following flowchart describes the management of patients with low thyroid-stimulating hormone (TSH) levels. Complete the flow chart from the list of options above. Each option can be used once, more than once or not at all.

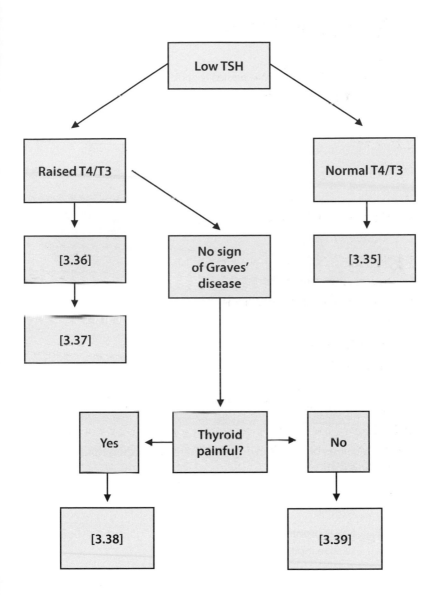

PICTURE QUESTION

3.40 A 34-year-old woman who has recently arrived from India comes for a new patient check. Her appearance is shown below.

Which one of the following statements regarding this situation is correct?

- [ ] A If the she is asymptomatic, no treatment or investigation is needed
- [ ] B She is probably suffering from endemic goitre and should receive iodine supplementation
- [ ] C She should be referred for surgical assessment
- [ ] D She should be started on carbimazole
- [ ] E She should have thyroid function tests carried out and if these are normal she can be reassured

DATA INTERPRETATION QUESTION

3.41 A 46-year-old woman presents with a 3-month history of weight gain, tiredness and irritability with night sweats. She reports that her periods have been rather irregular for the last 6 months but that she had not had any missed periods. She says that she is not depressed. Blood tests are taken which give the following results:

Haemoglobin	13.2 g/dl
White cell count	$5.2 \times 10^9/l$
Platelet count	$232 \times 10^9/l$
Glucose	4.8 mmol/l
TSH	6.4 mU/l (normal range 0.5–4.5 mU/l)
FT4	11 pmol/l (normal range 10–24 pmol/l)
FSH	2.5 U/l
βhCG	< 1 U/l

FT4, free thyroxine; FSH, follicle-stimulating hormone; βhCG, beta human chorionic gonadotrophin.
Normal range for FSH: follicular phase = 3.5–12.5 U/l; ovulatory phase = 4.7–21.5 U/l; luteal phase = 1.7–7.7 U/l; postmenopausal range = 25.8–134.8 U/l.

What is the single most likely diagnosis?

- [ ] A Clinical hypothyroidism
- [ ] B Depression
- [ ] C Hyperthyroidism
- [ ] D Perimenopause
- [ ] E Pregnancy

HOT TOPICS/EVIDENCE BASED PRACTICE

3.42 **Which one of the following statements is true regarding recent developments in the management of diabetes in pregnancy?**

☐ A Mild gestational diabetes should be monitored initially rather than treated aggressively

☐ B Pregnancy outcomes are similar in diabetic and non-diabetic women

☐ C Screening for gestational diabetes based on clinical risk factors is more effective than universal screening

☐ D The rates of caesarean section in diabetic women are approximately double that in non-diabetic women

☐ E Two-thirds of pregnant diabetics have an $HbA_{1c} > 7\%$ in the first trimester

ANSWERS

3.1   D: Oral bisphosphonate

Asymptomatic Paget's does not need treatment unless it is likely to lead to complications (eg Paget's disease affecting the skull or long bones). Where fractures occur, there is significant pain or hypercalcaemia, the treatment of choice is an oral bisphosphonate. There are no significant advantages in most patients for parenteral rather than oral preparations.

3.2   A: Calcium and vitamin D supplements

This patient has osteopenia rather than osteoporosis. Treatment should be aimed at lifestyle measures, calcium supplementation and reassurance. Where there are underlying risk factors such as coeliac disease these should be treated. Bisphosphonates are only indicated in otherwise healthy patients where osteoporosis is confirmed, or for prophylaxis in patients on steroids. Teriparatide is only useful in patients who do not respond to bisphosphonates.

3.   C: Hypercalcaemia

Hypercalcaemia causes constipation, nausea, polyuria, confusion, depression, lethargy, weakness and bone pain. When chronic it can cause renal stones. Calcium levels greater than 3.5 mmol/l can cause renal failure and arrythmias. Treatment is aimed at removing causes where appropriate, rehydration and, if necessary, bisphosphonates. In cases due to primary hyperparathyroidism referral for surgical treatment is necessary and in cases where the hypercalcaemia is due to haematological malignancy steroids can be helpful.

3.4   A: Check FSH and testosterone levels

This patient has symptoms of hypogonadism. This can be primary (eg due to orchitis or testicular torsion) or secondary, due to pituitary failure. Checking FSH levels will differentiate between these two causes. Testosterone supplements will probably be needed but these should only be prescribed after specialist assessment. Sildenafil is unlikely to be effective. A drug history should be taken to exclude reversible causes such as steroids, spironolactone or drugs of abuse such as marijuana. Counselling might be needed if the hypogonadism is irreversible as sterility is likely. LHRH analogues cause a reversible hypogonadism.

3.5   C: Cushing syndrome

This patient has symptoms of glucocorticoid excess, with metabolic and soft-tissue changes. The majority of cases of this are secondary to prescribed medication, usually for arthritis or asthma. The diagnosis can be confirmed with a dexamethasone suppression test. Primary Cushing's disease is rare and is caused by pituitary-dependent adrenal hyperplasia. Treatment of Cushing syndrome should be by gradual reduction of steroids and replacement where possible with steroid-sparing agents. Addison's disease is caused by a deficiency of steroids and causes low blood pressure, lassitude and depression.

3.6   B: Investigate for causes of vitamin D deficiency

Osteomalacia is characterised by abnormal mineralisation of bone and is usually caused by vitamin D deficiency in adults. It can be difficult to differentiate from osteopenia and osteoporosis but there are typically Looser's zones evident on X-ray and blood tests reveal reduced calcium, phosphate and vitamin D levels with raised alkaline phosphatase. It is often caused by low sunlight or poor diet, but investigation should aim to exclude secondary causes such as coeliac disease or inherited disorders of vitamin D metabolism. Treatment is usually with dietary supplements once other causes have been excluded.

3.7 A: Angiotensin-converting enzyme (ACE) inhibitor

Patients with evidence of diabetic nephropathy should be treated with an ACE inhibitor or an angiotensin II-receptor antagonist at the highest tolerated dose, with a target blood pressure of 130/80 mmHg. Several different drug classes are often needed to reach the target blood pressure.

3.8 C: Physiological goitre

Asymptomatic enlargement of the thyroid gland can occur at puberty or during pregnancy, when there is an increased physiological stimulation of the thyroid gland.

3.9 A: Carcinoma of the thyroid

Thyroid carcinoma, particularly anaplastic and medullary lesions, invade the larynx and the cervical sympathetic chain, leading to pain, hoarseness and Horner syndrome.

3.10 A: Endemic goitre

Iodine-deficiency (endemic) goitres contain acini distended with colloid. They are also referred to as 'colloid goitres' and are caused by mineral deficiencies in the natural water. Iodised table and cooking salt provides the required iodine.

3.11 A: Benign breast change

Painful nodularity of the breast (unilateral or bilateral) is characteristic of benign breast change (sometimes referred to as 'abnormalities of normal development and involution' or ANDI, 'fibroadenosis' or 'fibrocystic change'). It affects a third of all women and often causes anxiety in premenopausal women. The symptoms can be cyclical and evening primrose oil provides symptomatic relief.

CHAPTER 3 ANSWERS

3.12   D: Gynaecomastia

A breast lump in a male can be a discrete lesion in the breast disc or a diffuse enlargement. The latter is associated with oestrogenic activity in adolescence, in liver disease or during hormonal treatment of prostatic cancer.

3.13   C: Fibroadenoma

Fibroadenomas are not uncommon in premenopausal women and are usually transient. They are small mobile lumps with a smooth surface. However, once they exceed 3 cm in size they rarely regress; rarely, they may grow into a giant fibroadenoma or a phyllodes tumour.

3.14   A: Breast carcinoma

A solid lump with overlying skin tethering or nipple retraction is clinically diagnostic of an infiltrating ductal carcinoma. In the elderly these tumours are usually slow-growing and slow to metastasise. They are usually hormone receptor-sensitive and respond well to tamoxifen, letrazole or anastrazole therapy.

THEME: BLOOD TESTS IN ENDOCRINOLOGY

3.15   J: Subclinical hypothyroidism

Subclinical hypothyroidism is associated with raised TSH with normal T4 and T3 levels. These patients should be monitored over time as a significant number will become overtly hypothyroid in time.

3.16   A: Addison's disease

Addison's disease is due to adrenal failure, so ACTH is elevated with a normal or low serum cortisol. A short Synacthen test will often confirm hypoadrenalism.

3.17   I: Menopausal

Luteinising hormone (LH) and follicle-stimulating hormone (FSH) levels are raised in testicular and ovarian failure, in association with low levels of oestrogen or testosterone.

3.18   H: Hypopituitarism

Hypopituitarism should be suspected in patients with signs of hypothyroidism, hypogonadism or growth hormone deficiency; these patients also often have diabetes insipidus. The diagnosis can be confirmed by a combined pituitary test.

3.19   F: Hyperthyroidism

Raised T4 with suppressed TSH is diagnostic of primary hyperthyroidism. Low TSH with normal T4 and T3 is usually caused by excess thyroxine replacement or high-dose steroids.

THEME: BREAST PAIN

3.20   G: Gynaecomastia

Gynaecomastia in adolescence is due to unopposed oestrogenic activity; it is usually self-limiting and resolves following puberty. Occasionally the swelling persists and when it is cosmetically unacceptable it is treated by subcutaneous mastectomy.

3.21   E: Breast engorgement

Breast engorgement in the early postpartum period is not uncommon in primips; it is also associated with a poor suckling reflex or inverted nipples.

3.22 J: Shingles (herpes zoster)

Herpes zoster infection presents as a linear subcutaneous rash with overlying blisters along intercostal dermatomes; the breast is not affected. However, the diagnosis can be difficult prior to the appearance of the rash and if there is no history of the infection.

3.23 F: Breast hypertrophy

'Virginal hypertrophy' is a rare condition in the postpubertal female and can involve one or both breasts. It is treated by reduction mammoplasty.

3.24 H: Haematoma

Postoperative haematoma or a seroma following surgery on the breast usually resolves, provided the collection is small and uninfected; large collections can require repeated aspiration.

THEME: NIPPLE DISCHARGE

3.25 E: Mammilary fistula

Communication of a milk duct with an abscess cavity that is drained during lactation results in milk discharging through the wound. A mammilary fistula will heal once breastfeeding is stopped and when there is no residual infection.

3.26 H: Prolactinoma

A prolactin-secreting tumour of the pituitary presents with a history of headaches, nipple discharge, oligomenorrhoea and infertility. Bromocriptine lowers prolactin levels and shrinks large tumours, which can subsequently be treated by trans-sphenoidal surgery or radiotherapy.

3.27   G: Papillary carcinoma

Ductal papilloma or papillary carcinoma can ulcerate and cause bleeding. Papillomas are treated by duct excision (microdochotomy). The finding of a papillary carcinoma or invasive ductal carcinoma requires a wide excision or mastectomy with axillary staging.

3.28   C: Galactocoele

Galactocoele (milk cyst) in infants is a feature of mammary hyperplasia due to maternal hormones. Galactocoeles usually resolve following cessation of breast stimulation and rarely require surgical excision. Mammary hyperplasia in childhood is managed symptomatically. Any form of surgery may result in breast maldevelopment in puberty.

3.29   F: Paget's disease of the nipple

Nipple excoriation is either eczema or Paget's disease. The former responds to topical steroids in 4–6 weeks. Failure to respond to steroids or destruction of the nipple skin requires biopsy for confirmation of Paget's disease, which is treated by simple mastectomy.

THEME: BREAST INFLAMMATION

3.30   J: TB of the breast

TB of the breast is usually an extension of primary lung disease. The breast becomes enlarged, indurated and painful. Later, cold abscesses form and discharge to the skin surface as persistent sinuses. In the early stages, anti-TB chemotherapy resolves the lung disease and the breast inflammation. Patients who develop breast distortion with sinus formation might require mastectomy.

3.31   A: Acute mastitis

Acute mastitis occurring during lactation is a pyogenic Gram-positive infection acquired from the infant's mouth through a cracked nipple. Stopping feeding from the inflamed breast and broad-spectrum antibiotic therapy lead to rapid resolution.

3.32   I: Paget's disease of the nipple

Paget's disease of the nipple is a subepidermoid carcinoma arising in the nipple–areola complex that invades the underlying breast tissue. It is not under hormonal influence and is treated by simple mastectomy.

3.33   B: Benign breast change (ANDI)

Benign breast change (fibroadenosis) is caused by an abnormal sensitivity of breast tissue to cyclical changes in ovarian oestrogen and progesterone production. It is associated with oral contraceptive and hormone replacement therapy.

3.34   C: Breast abscess

Breast abscess is a sequel of acute pyogenic mastitis and occurs rarely in the non-lactating breast. Inflammatory carcinoma can present as an acute mastitis or rarely as an abscess.

THEME: THE MANAGEMENT OF PATIENTS WITH LOW THYROID-STIMULATING HORMONE (TSH) LEVELS

3.35   **D**   Repeat in 3 months or if there are symptoms

3.36   **B**   Signs of Graves' disease

3.37   **G**   Graves' disease

3.38   **E**   Subacute thyroiditis

3.39   **F**   Consider referral for radioiodine uptake scan

3.40   **C:**   She should be referred for surgical assessment

All patients with goitre should have their thyroid function tested. Where there is asymmetry, referral is indicated to exclude cancer. Hyperthyroidism is treated with carbimazole initially, although levothyroxine supplementation is often required later under a 'block and replace' regime. Diffuse enlargement with normal thyroid function is usually due to endemic goitre.

3.41   **D:**   Perimenopause

Blood tests are unreliable in diagnosing the perimenopause and clinicians should rely on a menstrual history and exclusion of other possible causes. Overt hypothyroidism is unlikely with a T4 in the normal range. Hyperthyroidism would generally cause a raised T4 and suppressed TSH, while pregnancy would cause a raised βhCG. Oestradiol levels are unhelpful for diagnosing and monitoring the menopause.

3.42   E: Two-thirds of pregnant diabetics have an HbA$_{1C}$ > 7% in the first trimester

Pregnancy care for diabetic women should start before conception, with joined-up care involving primary care, obstetricians and endocrinologists. Close control of diabetes is associated with lowered perinatal mortality and lowered risk of congenital malformation. The ACHOIS trial (the Australian Carbohydrate Intolerance Study) demonstrated the benefits of treating mild gestational diabetes, and therefore supports the argument for universal screening, particularly because relying on clinical risk factors alone has been shown to miss up to 50% of cases of gestational diabetes in some groups. The caesarean section rate is 60–70% in diabetic women and current NICE guidelines suggest women should be offered delivery at 38 weeks to reduce the risk of shoulder dystocia and subsequent emergency section.

CHAPTER 4
EAR, NOSE AND THROAT
SINGLE BEST ANSWER QUESTIONS

4.1 A 53-year-old woman returns from ENT Outpatients, where she was told she has no evidence of sinus disease. She complains of daily pain in the side of her face and has seen her dentist and had a full panel of blood tests, which have all failed to show a cause for her facial pain. She is thoroughly fed up and demands you do something. Which one of the following would be appropriate?

- [ ] A   Prescribe amitriptyline
- [ ] B   Prescribe capsaicin
- [ ] C   Refer her for counselling
- [ ] D   Refer her for MRI scanning
- [ ] E   Refer her for physiotherapy

4.2 A 49-year-old man complains of sore gums. These have been bleeding and sore intermittently for years. In spite of this, he has not seen a dentist for 20 years. Examination reveals receding gums with evidence of recent bleeding. Which of the following would be appropriate in this situation?

- [ ] A   Advise the patient to use chlorhexidine mouthwash twice a day
- [ ] B   Prescribe amoxicillin 250 mg tds for 1 week
- [ ] C   Prescribe erythromycin 250 mg qds for 1 week
- [ ] D   Prescribe metronidazole 400 mg tds for 1 week
- [ ] E   Refer the patient to oral surgery

4.3 A 67-year-old woman complains of 3 weeks of reduced hearing in one ear following an upper respiratory tract infection. She says her head feels as if it is in a bucket. On examination she has no evidence of acute infection in her middle or outer ear but does have clinical evidence of a middle ear effusion. She is otherwise well, and 2 months prior to this she had a full ENT assessment for reduced smell, which was normal. Which one of the following management strategies is effective in this situation?

☐   A   Nasal steroids

☐   B   Oral decongestant

☐   C   Otovent device

☐   D   Reassurance that her symptoms should resolve within 1–2 weeks

☐   E   Refer for grommets

4.4 A 28-year-old man complains of reduced hearing in his right ear. On examination you cannot see any signs of acute infection, but both drums look dull. You carry out tuning fork tests. Rinne's test shows that bone conduction is heard better than air conduction on that side while Weber's test localises to the right ear. Rinne's test on the left shows air conduction better than bone conduction. What sort of hearing loss is present?

☐   A   Left-sided conductive hearing loss

☐   B   Left-sided sensorineural hearing loss

☐   C   Non-organic hearing loss

☐   D   Right-sided conductive hearing loss

☐   E   Right-sided sensorineural hearing loss

4.5 A 19-year-old student is diagnosed with tonsillitis and starts antibiotic therapy. Twenty-four hours later she presents to the out-of-hours service with fever, ear pain, dysphagia and trismus. On examination her uvula is displaced away from the midline and her tonsils appear asymmetrically enlarged. What is the most likely diagnosis?

- [ ] A   Epiglottitis
- [ ] B   Glandular fever
- [ ] C   Lemierre syndrome
- [ ] D   Quinsy
- [ ] E   Tonsillar lymphoma

4.6 A 16-year-old schoolboy complains of flu-like symptoms, sore throat and enlarged glands in his neck. On examination he has a temperature of 38.5°C, significantly enlarged lymph nodes in his neck, enlarged tonsils with white exudate, and a yellowish tinge to his skin. Abdominal examination reveals some tenderness in the right upper quadrant. What is the most likely diagnosis?

- [ ] A   Epstein–Barr virus infection
- [ ] B   Hepatitis A
- [ ] C   Quinsy
- [ ] D   Streptococcal tonsillitis
- [ ] E   Viral sore throat

4.7 Acute otitis media in a non-allergic child is initially treated with which one of the following antibiotics?

- [ ] A   Ciprofloxacin
- [ ] B   Amoxicillin
- [ ] C   Erythromycin
- [ ] D   Metronidazole
- [ ] E   Phenoxymethylpenicillin (penicillin V)

4.8 Asymmetrical tonsil enlargement in a 40-year-old man is best treated with which of the following options?

☐ A Antifungals

☐ B Antibiotics

☐ C Referral for biopsy

☐ D Steroids

☐ E Watch and wait

4.9 A patient presents with a watery noise on inspiration, and is also noted to have large inflamed tonsils. How is this noise best described? Select only one option.

☐ A Hypernasal speech

☐ B Rhonchi

☐ C Stertor

☐ D Stridor

☐ E Wheeze

4.10 A patient presents with an inability to swallow, a 'hot potato' voice, and an asymmetrical tonsillitis. What is the single most effective treatment?

☐ A Analgesia

☐ B Antibiotics

☐ C Drainage of abscess

☐ D Oral steroids

☐ E Watch and wait

4.11 A red swelling is seen in the lower lateral wall of a patient's nose on anterior rhinoscopy. It is sensitive to the touch and seems to be obstructing the airway. What is it most likely to be?

- [ ] A Foreign body
- [ ] B Inferior turbinate
- [ ] C Inflammatory nasal polyp
- [ ] D Middle turbinate
- [ ] E Superior turbinate

4.12 A child presents with a 3-cm swelling to the left of the midline in the lower part of the anterior triangle of the neck. It moves with swallowing and tongue protrusion. What is it most likely to be?

- [ ] A Branchial cyst
- [ ] B Lymph node
- [ ] C Thyroglossal cyst
- [ ] D Thyroid cyst
- [ ] E Sebaceous cyst

4.13 A 54-year-old man with a BMI of 22 kg/m² complains of snoring and waking up at night. He is tired during the daytime, and his partner says that he seems to stop breathing for up to a minute every night. What is the most appropriate first-line treatment?

- [ ] A Advice on lifestyle changes and weight loss
- [ ] B Advise the use of ear plugs
- [ ] C Refer for a sleep study
- [ ] D Refer for surgery
- [ ] E Refer to a dentist for a mandibular advancement splint device

CHAPTER 4 QUESTIONS

4.14 A 6-year-old girl has a 1-year history of 30-dB conductive hearing loss, flat tympanograms and poor school performance. What is the single most appropriate next-stage treatment?

☐   A   Adenoidectomy

☐   B   Bilateral grommet insertion

☐   C   Conservative treatment

☐   D   Nasal decongestants

☐   E   Tonsillectomy

EXTENDED MATCHING QUESTIONS

THEME: DRUG MANAGEMENT OF ENT DISEASE

Options

A   Amoxicillin

B   Betnesol

C   Ciprofloxacin drops

D   Doxycycline

E   Erythromycin

F   Mometasone nasal spray

G   Montelukast

H   Penicillin V

I   Sofradex

J   Sterimar

For each of the scenarios described below, select the most appropriate treatment option from the list above. Each option may be used once, more than once or not at all.

☐ **4.15**   A 4-year-old boy complains of earache on one side. Examination shows a red, dull, bulging eardrum on that side. He has a temperature of 39.2°C and looks unwell.

☐ **4.16**   A 24-year-old woman with long-standing perennial rhinitis not helped by antihistamines.

☐ **4.17**   A 19-year-old man with a history of a chronically discharging ear. A swab is sent which shows *Pseudomonas* species.

☐ **4.18**   A 51-year-old woman who is on a long-term nasal steroid spray complains of a blocked nose, reduced smell and taste. Examination reveals bilateral nasal polyps.

THEME: LUMPS IN THE NECK

Options

A Branchial cyst

B Carotid body tumour/ chemodectoma

C Inflammatory cervical lymphadenopathy

D Metastasis of neoplastic disease

E Pleomorphic adenoma of the parotid

F Sebaceous cyst

G Submandibular gland stone

H Thyroglossal cyst

I Thyroid nodule

J Tuberculosis

K Virchow's node

Select the single most likely diagnosis in each of the cases described below from the list of options above.

☐ **4.19** A 25-year-old man presents with a 3-cm, slowly enlarging mass anterior to the sternocleidomastoid. It does not move with swallowing and has no overlying punctum. Fine needle aspiration (FNA) reveals straw-coloured fluid.

☐ **4.20** A 45-year-old lady has a lump 3 cm to the left of the midline, low in the anterior triangle of the neck. The lump moves with swallowing but not on tongue protrusion.

☐ **4.21** A 54-year-old, non-smoking man presents with a rubbery lump just below and in front of his right ear.

☐ **4.22** A 35-year-old man presents with an intermittent anterior triangle lump just below the mandible, which increases in size after eating, but then reduces again, accompanied by a strange taste in the mouth.

☐ **4.23** A 60-year-old Nepalese man presents with a pulsatile mass in the anterior triangle.

THEME: TINNITUS

Options

A	Acute otitis media	**G**	Otosclerosis
B	Chronic secretory otitis media	**H**	Physiological tinnitus
C	Dural arteriovenous fistula	**I**	Presbyacusis-related tinnitus
D	Hypertension	**J**	Schizophrenia
E	Ménière's disease	**K**	Vestibular schwannoma
F	Myoclonus of stapedius muscle		

Select the single most likely diagnosis in each case described below from the list above.

☐ **4.24** A 75-year-old man has a 2-year history of progressive unilateral sensorineural hearing loss, balance disturbance and constant high-frequency tinnitus.

☐ **4.25** A 45-year-old man has a progressive conductive hearing loss with normal eardrums, and a constant tinnitus over a period of 3 years. He mentions that his hearing is better in noisy surroundings.

☐ **4.26** A 30-year-old woman suffers a severe otitis externa, and gradually develops a pulsatile whooshing noise in one ear over the following 6 months.

☐ **4.27** A 65-year-old woman describes a progressive drop in her hearing and a constant high-pitched noise in both ears. Pure-tone audiogram reveals a 40-dB sensorineural loss, which is symmetrical and worse at high frequencies.

☐ **4.28** The parents of a 7-year-old boy complain of his reduced performance in class and his need to turn the TV up loud. He complains of a 'popping noise' in one ear. He has bilateral flat tympanograms.

ALGORITHM QUESTION

4.29 The following algorithm applies to patients presenting with a complaint of dizziness:

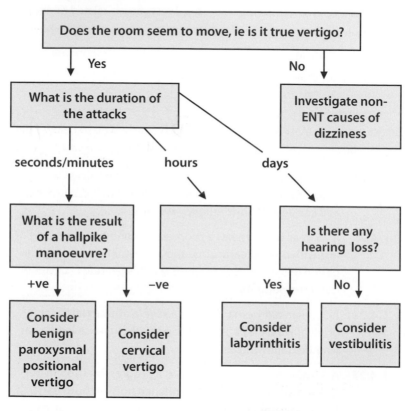

What is the missing diagnosis to be considered?

- ☐ A Cardiac failure
- ☐ B Epilepsy
- ☐ C Head injury
- ☐ D Hypotension
- ☐ E Ménière's disease

PICTURE QUESTIONS

4.30 An 86-year-old gentleman is seen for a new patient check. While talking to him you notice a swelling in front of and inferior to the right ear. He tells you that this has been slowly growing for 10 years. On examination the swelling is firm but non-tender and mobile. He has no other findings of note. The swelling is shown below.

What is the most likely diagnosis?

☐ A Acute bacterial parotitis
☐ B Adenocarcinoma
☐ C Lymphoma
☐ D Mumps
☐ E Parotid adenoma

4.31 A 35-year-old surfer complains of blocked ears after surfing. On examination you note the appearance below.

Which one of the following is the most likely diagnosis?

☐ A   Chronic otitis externa

☐ B   Chronic suppurative otitis media

☐ C   Exostoses

☐ D   Keratosis obturans

☐ E   Osteomas

4.32 A 10-year-old girl complains of earache and a discharge from her ear and she has a fever. On examination you note the appearance below.

What is the single most likely diagnosis?

- [ ] A   Acute otitis externa
- [ ] B   Acute tympanic membrane perforation
- [ ] C   Chronic otitis externa
- [ ] D   Chronic tympanic membrane perforation
- [ ] E   Glue ear

4.33 A 27-year-old man with itchy ears has had several courses of ear drops over the last 3 months. He now complains of recurrent itchiness. On examination you note the appearance below.

What is the most appropriate treatment?

☐ A Betnesol drops

☐ B Ciprofloxacin drops

☐ C Clotrimazole drops

☐ D Locorten-Vioform drops

☐ E Sofradex ear drops

4.34 A 21-year-old girl has just returned from a holiday in Greece, where she developed a very painful ear. She has been taking regular ibuprofen, paracetamol and codeine from a local pharmacy, but to no effect. On examination her ear has the appearance shown below.

What is the diagnosis?

- A   Acute otitis externa
- B   Chronic suppurative otitis media
- C   Fungal otitis externa
- D   Otitis media with effusion
- E   Otitis media with perforation

4.35 A 23-year-old woman attends for a diving medical she has been told she will need before she can start a divemaster course. During the course of the medical you notice the appearance below in her left ear.

What is the underlying diagnosis?

- ☐ A   Acute otitis media
- ☐ B   Aural polyp
- ☐ C   Cholesteatoma
- ☐ D   Tympanic membrane perforation
- ☐ E   Tympanic membrane retraction

4.36 This picture shows the right tympanic membrane in a patient who presented with an acute loss of hearing after having a painful ear for some days.

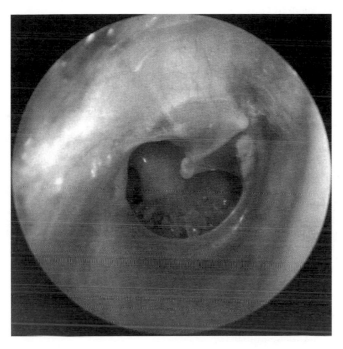

What is the most likely diagnosis?

☐ A   Cholesteatoma
☐ B   Otitis externa
☐ C   Otitis media
☐ D   Otosclerosis
☐ E   Tympanosclerosis

DATA INTERPRETATION QUESTION

4.37 A 45-year-old man presents with left ear discharge after swimming. The swab from this discharge shows the following results:

Organism: *Pseudomonas aeruginosa*

Sensitivity:

- Penicillin – resistant

- Neomycin – resistant

- Framycetin – resistant

- Metronidazole – resistant

- Ciprofloxacin – sensitive

What is the single best treatment?

- [ ] A   Intravenous co-amoxiclav
- [ ] B   Oral ciprofloxacin
- [ ] C   Oral co-amoxiclav
- [ ] D   Topical aluminium acetate eardrops
- [ ] E   Topical ciprofloxacin eyedrops used as eardrops

HOT TOPICS/EVIDENCE BASED PRACTICE

4.38 The National Prospective Tonsil Audit (Royal College of Surgeons, 2005) looked at the incidence of post-tonsillectomy haemorrhage. Which one of the following statements about the results is true?

☐ A 'Hot' dissection techniques (eg diathermy) led to a lower rate of postoperative haemorrhage than 'cold' techniques (eg scissors and ties)

☐ B Postoperative antibiotics were shown to influence the incidence of haemorrhage

☐ C The higher the grade of surgeon, the less likely a postoperative haemorrhage

☐ D The total rate of postoperative haemorrhage was 3.5%

☐ F The total rate of return to theatre for arrest of haemorrhage was 3.5%

CHAPTER 4 QUESTIONS

ANSWERS

4.1   A: Prescribe amitriptyline

Atypical facial pain often improves with a low-dose antidepressant or anticonvulsant. Patients often need to have this therapy explained and in particular they should be reassured that this is not being prescribed as an antidepressant but for chronic pain. Where there is difficulty coming to terms with the pain, counselling might be appropriate once all therapeutic options have been explored. Capsaicin is efficacious in some patients with post-herpetic neuralgia.

4.2   A: Advise the patient to use chlorhexidine mouthwash twice a day

Chronic gingivitis is best treated by referral to a general dental practitioner for regular oral hygiene, together with flossing and chlorhexidine mouthwash. Where there is acute infection, amoxicillin, erythromycin or metronidazole might be indicated. Referral to oral surgery would only be necessary in a severe infection (eg Vincent's angina).

4.3   C: Otovent device

Middle ear effusions are often seen on a background of acute upper respiratory tract infection and are typically unilateral. They can take several months to clear, but this can be improved with an Otovent device. Grommets might be necessary for refractory cases. Nasal decongestants and steroids are ineffective. Patients presenting with acute middle ear effusions in adulthood should have nasendoscopy performed to exclude postnasal space lesions.

4.4   D: Right-sided conductive hearing loss

In the presence of a conductive hearing loss bone conduction is better than air, while a sensorineural hearing loss causes air and bone conduction both to be reduced. In a unilateral conductive hearing loss Weber's test localises to the affected side, and in a unilateral sensorineural loss it localises to the good side.

4.5   D: Quinsy

This presentation is typical of quinsy, or peritonsillar abscess. Treatment usually involves intravenous antibiotics and fluids and incision of the abscess if it does not settle. Interval tonsillectomy is offered in most centres. Epiglottitis affects the epiglottis rather than the uvula and a lymphoma would not normally present over such a short period. Glandular fever does not usually cause significant asymmetry, while Lemierre syndrome causes more widespread disease throughout the mediastinum and patients are usually much more unwell.

4.6   A: Epstein–Barr virus infection

Epstein–Barr virus causes glandular fever. Most patients develop a sore throat, fever, malaise and cervical lymphadenopathy. Hepatosplenomegaly is not uncommon and most patients develop transient abnormalities of liver function. Treatment is supportive and most patients make a full recovery. Complications include cranial nerve palsies, encephalitis and splenic rupture, but these are rare. The symptoms usually last 2–4 weeks but up to 50% of patients report ongoing fatigue, which can take months to resolve.

4.7   B: Amoxicillin

For uncomplicated acute otitis media where bacterial infection is suspected amoxicillin is the first choice, unless there is a history of penicillin allergy, in which case erythromycin should be used.

4.8   C: Referral for biopsy

Asymmetrical tonsil enlargement in adults is suspicious of neoplasia, and biopsy is needed, as well as imaging of the head and neck.

4.9   C: Stertor

Proximal airway obstruction due to enlarged tonsils creates a noise that is very different from stridor, which tends to originate from the larynx or below. Wheeze and rhonchi come from the parenchyma of the lung, and hypernasal speech suggests incompetence of closure of the palate against the back of the pharynx.

4.10   C: Drainage of abscess

This is probably a quinsy (peritonsillar abscess) and represents a collection around the tonsil capsule secondary to a tonsillitis. The uvula is displaced and one side of the oropharynx is enlarged and might be pointing. Drainage via needle and scalpel incision can provide speedy relief. Steroids, antibiotics and analgesia will also help in the longer term, but are unlikely to be effective unless drainage has been performed first.

4.11   B: Inferior turbinate

Inferior turbinates are commonly mistaken for other pathologies on examination. Superior turbinates are rarely visible on anterior rhinoscopy, and middle turbinates are higher up and further back. Polyps are insensate and light in colour. If the inferior turbinates are large enough to obstruct the airway, treatment with nasal steroids may help.

4.12   C: Thyroglossal cyst

The thyroglossal cyst is a remnant of the thyroglossal duct, which descends from the tongue via the hyoid and neck to the thyroid during development. There can be a connection to the hyoid bone which explains its pattern of movement. Treatment is with surgical excision via Sistrunk's procedure.

4.13   C: Refer for a sleep study

Surgery for snoring is controversial, and evidence on its effectiveness is conflicting – some surgery might provide short-term help with snoring, but problems tend to recur. Any surgery should be carefully targeted at the source of the snoring. Lifestyle changes and earplugs will be ineffective with this patient. A mandibular advancement device might help, depending on the site of snoring, but with a clear history of daytime somnolence and apnoea, a sleep study should be performed first – night-time continuous positive airway pressure (CPAP) might be all that is necessary to improve the patient's quality of life.

4.14   B: Bilateral grommet insertion

Typically, glue ear produces a 20-40-dB conductive loss with flat tympanograms – it is most common in children aged between about 3 years and 8 years, and tends to improve with time, although if it starts to affect development intervention is indicated. Some think that supplementing grommet insertion with adenoidectomy, especially in younger children, prevents recurrence.

THEME: DRUG MANAGEMENT OF ENT DISEASE

4.15   A: Amoxicillin

Acute otitis media in a child who is unwell should be treated with antibiotics. If the child is not unwell a symptomatic approach might be appropriate, with the option of returning for antibiotics should the patient worsen.

4.16   F: Mometasone nasal spray

Second-line treatment in patients with rhinitis who have tried oral antihistamines is a nasal steroid. This can also help with ocular symptoms.

4.17   C: Ciprofloxacin drops

Pseudomonas is often seen in patients with discharging ears and topical ciprofloxacin will often cure this. An alternative is Sofradex but there are theoretical arguments against using this in patients without an intact tympanic membrane.

4.18   B: Betnesol

A short course of nasal steroid drops will often shrink nasal polyps, affording symptomatic relief in patients who are not fit for or who do not wish to have surgery. Mometasone nasal spray is licensed for the treatment of nasal polyps and is often effective in patients with smaller polyps and useful for preventing recurrence.

THEME: LUMPS IN THE NECK

4.19   A: Branchial cyst

Branchial cysts originate from the 2nd, 3rd and 4th branchial grooves, and generally present in the 3rd decade when the embryological space fills with straw-coloured fluid. Treatment is surgical removal, as there is a small possibility that the cyst coexists with carcinoma.

4.20   I: Thyroid nodule

Thyroid lumps typically present in middle-aged women, and are investigated by ultrasound scanning and FNA. Excision might be required if neoplasia cannot be excluded.

4.21   E: Pleomorphic adenoma of the parotid

Pleomorphic adenomas can be found in any of the salivary glands, but are most common in the parotid. They are benign tumours but will continue to grow if not fully excised, and will eventually cause cosmetic and nerve damage. Complete excision, usually via a superficial parotidectomy, is therefore advised.

4.22   G: Submandibular gland stone

The submandibular gland is intermittently being blocked by a stone in the submandibular duct, which might be visualised on sialogram or ultrasound. Treatment can be conservative, with sialagogues and hydration. If problems persist, removal of the stone via the mouth or of the whole gland is indicated.

4.23   B: Carotid body tumour/chemodectoma

The carotid bifurcation lies in the anterior triangle, and contains the carotid body, which may produce the rare chemodectoma. It is more common in those who have been living at high altitude.

THEME: TINNITUS

4.24   K: Vestibular schwannoma

Vestibular schwannomas (acoustic neuromas) are rare. They are visible on MRI scans of the internal auditory meati and are benign tumours of the cerebellopontine angle which cause their effects by exerting pressure on the surrounding structures. Treatment can be conservative, surgical or with radiotherapy.

4.25   G: Otosclerosis

Otosclerosis is more frequently diagnosed in women than men and the risk is increased in patients with a positive family history. It involves the replacement of mature otic capsule bone with woven bone, and leads to sclerosis of the ossicles and so a largely conductive loss, with no tympanic membrane fluid visible. Treatment can be conservative, with a hearing aid, but a stapedectomy is often performed. Women of child bearing age should wait until they have completed their family as the disease can progress in pregnancy.

4.26   C: Dural arteriovenous fistula

Rarely, severe ear disease can affect the vessels around the ear lying close to the dura, leading to the formation of arteriovenous connections and consequent unilateral transmitted tinnitus. Appropriate imaging is required and any treatment must be conducted in a specialist centre

4.27   I: Presbyacusis-related tinnitus

Symmetrical sensorineural loss in older people is most likely to be due to presbyacusis, and can be accompanied by bilateral tinnnitus at a frequency similar to that lost. If findings are symmetrical, further investigation is not required.

4.28   B: Chronic secretory otitis media

The popping noise represents the movement of fluid behind the eardrum, and may be present in CSOM. There is usually a 20-40-dB conductive hearing loss. Treatment can be conservative initially, but if there is no improvement after a few months, grommets might provide a solution.

4.29   E: Ménière's disease

Ménière's disease characteristically comes in attacks lasting for hours at a time. There is often a warning of aural fullness before an attack. At the time of an attack there can be nausea, tinnitus and hearing loss, classically low-frequency – the symptoms initially resolve after the attacks but over time can become permanent. Ménière's disease is treated with caffeine and salt restriction, rehabilitation, and betahistine. It is relatively uncommon, and other causes of dizziness should be carefully considered. In particular, a careful history should be taken to find out whether the patient suffers with true vertigo (a hallucination of movement).

4.30   E: Parotid adenoma

The most likely diagnosis in this case is a parotid adenoma. These account for 90% of benign parotid tumours and are typically in the lower pole of the parotid. They are benign but can cause local damage to the facial nerve. They grow slowly and elderly patients might not require treatment. The diagnosis should be confirmed by fine-needle aspiration. Malignant tumours of the parotid tend to present more acutely due to rapid growth. Lymphomas tend to be more aggressive and often have a rubbery feel.

4.31   C: Exostoses

Exostoses of the external auditory meatus are common in people who are frequently exposed to cold water (eg surfers and swimmers). They are smooth, bony swellings arising from the canal wall, and can grow until they meet in the middle. They frequently trap water and wax once they reach a certain size and removal might be indicated for this reason. Osteomas are benign tumours of bone and are not usually multiple. Chronic otitis externa tends to produce an atrophic appearance, with scaling and tenderness or itching. Keratosis obturans is a condition where hard plugs of wax are found in the canal lumen.

4.32   B: Acute tympanic membrane perforation

The history of fever and otalgia followed by otorrhoea suggests an acute otitis media followed by perforation. The discharge is thin and mucoid, which suggests middle-ear involvement rather than otitis externa, which causes a much thicker discharge that seldom runs from the ear. Chronic perforations can behave in this way but usually follow water exposure or coryza rather than an acute febrile illness. The tympanic membrane usually heals in 4–6 weeks.

4.33   C: Clotrimazole drops

This is a fungal otitis externa. Treatment is with 2 weeks of antifungal therapy and management of underlying risk factors such as diabetes and excessive use of antibiotic or steroid preparations. Microsuction might be necessary where there is a lot of exudate.

4.34   A: Acute otitis externa

The presence of pain, particularly when moving the tragus, with creamy, thick exudate and meatal oedema is typical of otitis externa. The discharge in a tympanic membrane perforation tends to be more mucoid while in otitis media with effusion there is no exudate in the canal. Fungal otitis externa shows typical spores and hyphae.

4.35   D: Tympanic membrane perforation

This shows a large central perforation without evidence of cholesteatoma. Small retraction pockets can look like perforations but in this example the middle ear mucosa is clearly visible. Aural polyps tend to be peripheral and are often granulomatous with an angry red appearance. Cholesteatoma usually appears as crusting and exudate in the attic.

4.36   C: Otitis media

This patient has most probably suffered from an acute middle ear infection, resulting in a perforation and discharge and later resolution of symptoms. Cholesteatoma usually causes a painless perforation which tends to be peripheral. Otitis externa rarely causes a perforation. Otosclerosis is a disease of the ossicles and causes a slowly progressive conductive hearing loss, and tympanosclerosis causes a conductive loss which is usually stable.

4.37   E: Topical ciprofloxacin eye drops used as ear drops

The presence of discharge after swimming suggests otitis externa. This is best treated with topical drops. Ciprofloxacin eye drops used as ear drops is the usual way to treat this infection. The patient should also be asked to keep his ears dry, and oral ciprofloxacin can be considered as a second-line treatment.

4.38   D: The total rate of postoperative haemorrhage was 3.5%

Around 40 000 UK cases were followed after tonsillectomy. Findings were that 3.5% suffered a post-tonsillectomy haemorrhage – for cold techniques the figure was 1.7%, whereas for hot techniques it was 4.6%. The total rate of return to theatre was around 1%. The effect of antibiotics was not assessed. There was no significant differences in outcomes between different grades of surgeon.

CHAPTER 5
GASTROENTEROLOGY
SINGLE BEST ANSWER QUESTIONS

5.1   A 67-year-old man has been discharged from hospital after
      being treated for pneumonia. He has now developed a profuse
      watery diarrhoea, but has had no vomiting. There is no blood in
      the stool but he is febrile, tachycardic and hypotensive. What is
      the most likely cause?

☐   A   *Campylobacter*
☐   B   *Clostridium difficile*
☐   C   *Escherichia coli*
☐   D   Norovirus
☐   E   Rotavirus

5.2   A 27-year-old woman requests testing for coeliac disease. She
      does not have any diarrhoea but says that wheat makes her feel
      uncomfortable. Which one of the following would be the most
      appropriate initial test according to NICE guidance?

☐   A   Blood test for antigliadin antibodies
☐   B   Blood test for IgA tissue transglutaminase (tTGA)
☐   C   Blood test for IgG endomysial antibodies (EMA)
☐   D   Referral for oesophagogastroduodenoscopy
☐   E   Test stool for faecal fats

5.3 You are updating the practice protocol for the investigation of change in bowel habit and want to base this on the NICE guidance. Which one of the following scenarios should prompt a referral under the 2-week rule?

- [ ] A A 28-year-old man with 6 weeks of loose stools; examination and blood tests are normal

- [ ] B A 34-year-old woman with 3 months of discomfort in her right iliac fossa; examination is normal, as are blood tests

- [ ] C A 36-year-old woman noted on routine blood testing to have a haemoglobin of 10.6 g/dl

- [ ] D A 45-year-old man who has routine blood tests showing a haemoglobin of 10.5 g/dl; he is otherwise well and examination is unremarkable

- [ ] E A 66-year-old man with 3 weeks of loose stools, but no bleeding or anal symptoms; blood tests and examination are normal

5.4 A 52-year-old alcoholic has just been discharged from hospital after an admission with an upper gastrointestinal bleed secondary to oesophageal varices. He tells you that he has definitely stopped drinking now and asks what his chances are of having a further episode of bleeding. Which one of the following statements is correct regarding the risk of re-bleeding?

- [ ] A Alcoholism is associated with a better prognosis than other causes of portal hypertension

- [ ] B Bleeding in association with signs of liver failure has a good prognosis once the cause of the liver failure is addressed

- [ ] C If he can abstain from alcohol the risk of re-bleeding is minimal

- [ ] D Mortality for subsequent bleeds is 90%

- [ ] E The risk of re-bleeding is > 90% at 2 years

5.5 An 85-year-old lady with a previous history of peripheral vascular disease and hypertension presents with acute severe abdominal pain and loose bowels. The pain is colicky but examination findings are unremarkable apart from some tenderness In her abdomen, and an irregular pulse that has not been noted before. A rectal examination reveals bloodstained mucus. Which one of the following statements is correct regarding this presentation?

- [ ] A Bloodstained mucus is likely to be due to haemorrhoids
- [ ] B Mesenteric ischaemia should be considered
- [ ] C The absence of any significant examination findings suggests that serious disease is unlikely
- [ ] D The most likely diagnosis is diverticulitis
- [ ] E The most likely diagnosis is irritable bowel syndrome (IBS) and the patient should be given mebeverine

5.6 A 3-year-old boy is brought in by his mother after swallowing a battery from a watch. On examination he is well, with no drooling, respiratory symptoms or abdominal tenderness. What would the most appropriate management be?

- [ ] A Admit under the general surgeons for endoscopy
- [ ] B Ask the parents to check stools to confirm passage
- [ ] C Prescribe laxatives
- [ ] D Reassure the mother that it should pass and that no further action is needed
- [ ] E Refer for abdominal X-ray

5.7   One of your patients has been diagnosed with coeliac disease. Which one of the following can she eat normally?

- ☐   A   Barley
- ☐   B   Porridge oats
- ☐   C   Rice
- ☐   D   Rye
- ☐   E   Wheat

5.8   Which of the following statements about Crohn's disease is true? Select one option only.

- ☐   A   Active disease should be treated initially with mesalazine
- ☐   B   Anti-mycobacterial therapies are an effective treatment if used early
- ☐   C   Anti-TNFα therapy is associated with remission rates of 80%
- ☐   D   Crohn's disease only affects the colon
- ☐   E   Patients should be referred early for surgery

5.9   Which one of the following statements about ulcerative colitis is true? Select one option only.

- ☐   A   Is always associated with perianal fistulas
- ☐   B   Mesalazine should always be prescribed generically
- ☐   C   Oral steroids are the mainstay of maintenance therapy
- ☐   D   Patients with ulcerative colitis should have regular colono-scopic follow-up to identify malignant change
- ☐   E   Ulcerative colitis can affect any part of the gastrointestinal tract

5.10 A 4-month-old, full-term male infant presents with a 6-week history of regurgitation of feeds. He is otherwise well, with a normal growth chart. Select the single most appropriate diagnosis from the options below.

- [ ] A   Annular pancreas
- [ ] B   Duodenal atresia
- [ ] C   Gastro-oesophageal reflux
- [ ] D   Gastroschisis
- [ ] E   Hypertrophic pyloric stenosis

5.11 A 4-year-old boy presents with a 3-day history of colicky central abdominal pain and bile-stained vomiting. The abdomen feels full and tender. Digital rectal examination reveals an empty rectum with red-jelly-like mucus on the glove. Select the single most likely diagnosis.

- [ ] A   Annular pancreas
- [ ] B   Intestinal duplication
- [ ] C   Intussusception
- [ ] D   Malrotation syndrome
- [ ] E   Midgut volvulus

5.12 A 5-year-old boy is seen with an 8-hour history of colicky central abdominal pain and vomiting. He presents with a tender, irreducible lump in the left groin that extends into the scrotum. Select the single most likely diagnosis.

- [ ] A   Appendicitis
- [ ] B   Incarcerated hernia
- [ ] C   Intussusception
- [ ] D   Malrotation
- [ ] E   Mesenteric thrombosis

5.13 A 9-year-old child gives a 2-day history of intermittent abdominal pain that shifts to the right lower quadrant, preceded by nausea. She is mildly pyrexial with a tachycardia. Select the single most likely diagnosis from the list below.

- ☐ A Appendicitis
- ☐ B Incarcerated hernia
- ☐ C Intussusception
- ☐ D Malrotation
- ☐ E Mesenteric thrombosis

5.14 A 67-year-old Welsh sheep farmer presents with a 9-month history of malaise, tiredness and abdominal discomfort. On examination, his liver is enlarged and tender. An ultrasound scan of the liver reveals a 7-cm cystic lesion in the right lobe that contains numerous 'daughter cysts'. Select the single most likely diagnosis from the list below.

- ☐ A Bladder worm infection
- ☐ B Cystic echinococcosis
- ☐ C Tapeworm infection
- ☐ D Guinea worm
- ☐ E Filariasis

5.15 A 39-year-old woman who works in a dairy presents with a 9-month history of poor appetite, malaise and weight loss. Abdominal radiography reveals mesenteric nodal calcifications. There is a history of unpasteurised cheese consumption. Select the single most likely diagnosis from the list below.

- ☐ A Abdominal tuberculosis
- ☐ B Actinomycosis
- ☐ C Enteric *Staphylococcus aureus* infection
- ☐ D Hydatid disease
- ☐ E Trypanasomiasis

5.16 A 36-year-old restaurateur was diagnosed with typhoid infection. Despite long-term antibiotic therapy, he was found to have persistent positive typhoid stool cultures. Which one of the following is the most appropriate management option in this situation?

- ☐ A Change antibiotic therapy
- ☐ B Elective cholecystectomy
- ☐ C Reassure and discharge
- ☐ D Resect infected bowel
- ☐ E Stop all treatment and reassess in 6 months

5.17 A 29-year-old woman who has returned to the UK after a brief working holiday in the Far East presents with a 4-week history of intermittent abdominal cramps and bowel hurry. A barium enema reveals superficial scattered mucosal ulcers and segmental narrowing of the colon. Select the single most likely diagnosis from the list below.

- ☐ A Abdominal tuberculosis
- ☐ B Amoebic ulceration
- ☐ C Cholera
- ☐ D Enteric *Staphylococcus aureus* infection
- ☐ E *Strongyloides stercoralis*

5.18 A 35-year-old woman presents with a 3-day history of upper abdominal pain that radiates to the right side, associated with nausea and bloating. She is febrile and has upper abdominal tenderness and guarding. Select the single most likely diagnosis from the list below.

- [ ] A   Appendicitis
- [ ] B   Cholecystitis
- [ ] C   Ectopic pregnancy
- [ ] D   Mesenteric thrombosis
- [ ] E   Visceral perforation

5.19 A 74-year-old woman on long-term diclofenac for rheumatoid arthritis presents with abdominal pain. She is hypotensive with a rapid pulse and epigastric tenderness. Select the single most likely diagnosis from the list below.

- [ ] A   Acute pancreatitis
- [ ] B   Appendicitis
- [ ] C   Cholecystitis
- [ ] D   Intussusception
- [ ] E   Visceral perforation

EXTENDED MATCHING QUESTIONS

THEME: ABNORMAL LIVER FUNCTION

Options

A	Acute pancreatitis	**E**	Gilbert syndrome
B	Anticonvulsant use	**F**	Hepatitis A
C	Fatty liver	**G**	Hepatitis B
D	Gallstones	**H**	Nephrotic syndrome

For each of the scenarios below, select the most likely diagnosis from the list of options above. Each option may be used once, more than once or not at all.

☐ **5.20** A 19 year-old man has blood tests carried out after a viral illness. These show a normal full blood count (FBC), negative Monospot and a raised bilirubin. All other tests are normal.

☐ **5.21** A 7-year-old boy comes to you with weight gain and oedema after an upper respiratory tract infection. Blood tests show a low albumin.

☐ **5.22** A 44-year-old, poorly controlled type 2 diabetic has routine blood tests that show a raised alanine aminotransferase (ALT). Her other liver function tests are normal. Clinical examination is unremarkable. Reviewing previous results, you find that her ALT has been raised for approximately 18 months.

☐ **5.23** A 26-year-old epileptic has routine bloods carried out which show a raised gamma-glutamyltransferase (GGT). He denies drinking and the FBC and ALT, alkaline phosphatase (ALP) and bilirubin are all normal.

THEME: DIARRHOEA

Options

A *Campylobacter*

B *Clostridium difficile*

C *Cryptosporidium*

D Norovirus

E Rotavirus

F *Salmonella*

G *Shigella*

For each of the descriptions below, select the most appropriate causative agent from the list above. Each option may be used once, more than once or not at all.

☐ **5.24** Causes diarrhoea by contamination of drinking water with agricultural waste, usually cow slurry.

☐ **5.25** Usually spread by poultry and milk, it is the commonest notified cause of diarrhoea in the UK.

☐ **5.26** Causes epidemics of gastroenteritis in children.

☐ **5.27** Causes watery diarrhoea and abdominal cramps, progressing to bloody diarrhoea.

☐ **5.28** Highly infectious, with aerosol transmission; causes projectile vomiting.

THEME: ACUTE ABDOMEN

Options

A	Appendicitis	**G**	Mesenteric thrombosis
B	Cholecystitis	**H**	Ruptured ectopic pregnancy
C	Incarcerated hernia	**I**	Septic abortion
D	Intussusception	**J**	Urinary tract infection
E	Malrotation	**K**	Visceral perforation
F	Meconium ileus		

For each of the descriptions below, select the most appropriate diagnosis from the list of options above. Each option may be used once, more than once or not at all.

☐ **5.29** A 6-year-old girl complains of 24 hours of generalised abdominal pain. On examination she is diffusely tender with some guarding. Urine dipstick testing is positive for nitrites.

☐ **5.30** A 28-year-old woman is admitted with a 14-hour history of sudden onset of severe lower abdominal pain with nausea and retching. Her last normal period was 10 weeks ago. Her pulse is 120 bpm and her BP is 90/70 mmHg.

☐ **5.31** A 4-year-old boy is seen with an 8-hour history of colicky central abdominal pain and vomiting. He presents with an irreducible lump in the left groin, extending into the scrotum.

☐ **5.32** An 18-month-old toddler who has been on a weaning diet becomes fretful, clutches his abdomen and cries out. He refuses feeds and passes loose motions containing bloodstained mucus.

☐ **5.33** A 7-day-old male neonate has not opened his bowels since birth. Symptoms of bowel obstruction develop, with bile-stained vomiting. Respiratory investigations suggest cystic fibrosis.

THEME: OESOPHAGEAL LESIONS

Options

A   Achalasia

B   Barrett's oesophagus

C   Boerhaave syndrome

D   Cirrhosis of the liver

E   Globus hystericus

F   Oesophageal ring

G   Sliding hiatus hernia

For each of the statements below, select the most appropriate diagnosis from the list above. Each option can be used once, more than once or not at all.

☐ **5.34**   **Predisposes to adenocarcinoma.**

☐ **5.35**   **Causes progressive dysphagia to solids.**

☐ **5.36**   **Causes severe retrosternal pain, leading to hypotension and shock.**

☐ **5.37**   **Causes waterbrash.**

☐ **5.38**   **Associated with oesophageal varices.**

THEME: STOMACH

Options

A Erosive gastritis

B Gastric carcinoma

C Gastrocolic fistula

D *Helicobacter pylori*

E Hourglass stomach

F Hypertrophic pyloric stenosis

G Peptic ulcer disease

H Post-cibal syndrome

I Teapot stomach

For each of the scenarios described below, select the most appropriate diagnosis from the list above. Each option may be used once, more than once or not at all.

5.39 A 3-month-old baby presents with vomiting after feeds, insatiable appetite and poor weight gain. The mother has noticed a palpable lump in the upper abdomen after feeds.

5.40 A 38-year-old stockmarket trader with a history of 'hunger pains' is admitted following an episode of haematemesis.

5.41 A 19-year-old male student presented with a 7-month history of dyspepsia; gastroduodenoscopy revealed no obvious mucosal lesion. Antral biopsies were diagnostic, however, and he was commenced on medication.

5.42 A 78-year-old man with a 9-month history of poor appetite and weight loss has developed faeculent vomiting. Barium meal investigation reveals barium in the transverse colon.

THEME: LIVER DISEASE

Options

A Acute calculous cholecystitis

B Acute cholangitis

C Acute liver failure

D Biliary atresia

E Biliary stricture

F Cirrhosis

G Gallstone ileus

H Wilson's disease

I Hepatocellular carcinoma

J Liver abscess

For each of the scenarios described below, select the most appropriate diagnosis from the list above. Each option can be used once, more than once or not at all.

☐ **5.43** A 39-year-old man with a history of alcoholism complains of malaise, anorexia and weight loss. Clinically, he has a firm, enlarged liver, a palpable spleen and moderate ascites.

☐ **5.44** A 44-year-old Northern European with a dusky complexion presents with painful arthritic swelling of both knees and a 3-month history of polyuria and polydypsia. He has a 15-cm, firm hepatomegaly with cutaneous signs of chronic liver disease.

☐ **5.45** A 42-year-old woman is admitted with severe right sided abdominal pain that is radiating to the back, with nausea and retching some hours following a meal. She is tender in the right upper quadrant and inflammatory markers in her peripheral blood are raised.

☐ **5.46** A 46-year-old woman with known gallstones is admitted acutely ill with progressive jaundice, upper abdominal pain and rigors. She has been confined to bed for the past 4 days.

☐ **5.47** A 67-year-old woman from a psychiatric unit gives a vague history of intermittent upper and central abdominal pain with episodes of nausea and vomiting. Plain abdominal X-ray (AXR) shows moderately dilated small-bowel loops, a 4-cm opacity in the right lower quadrant and possibly air in the biliary tree.

ALGORITHM QUESTIONS

THEME: MANAGEMENT OF HAEMORRHOIDS

5.48–5.52

Options

A 1st/2nd degree

B 4th degree

C Antimuscarinics

D Fibre

E Haemorrhoidectomy

F Increased fluids

G Ligation/injection

H Loperamide

I Non-prolapsing piles

J Prolapsing piles

K Reassurance

L Sphincterotomy

M Topical diltiazem

N Topical GTN

Complete the following algorithm for the management of haemorrhoids, from the list of options above. Each option may be used once, more than once or not at all.

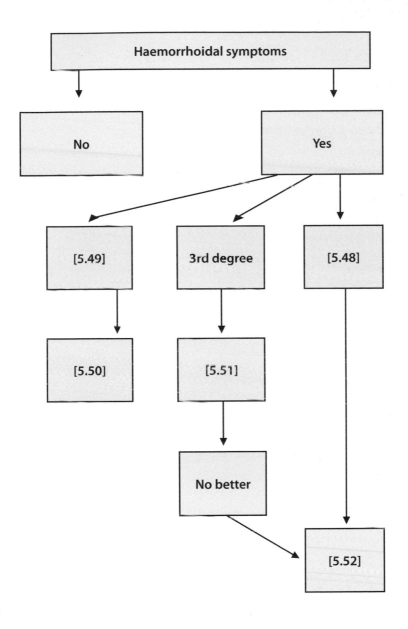

THEME: INVESTIGATION OF ABNORMAL LIVER FUNCTION TESTS (LFTS)

5.53–5.57

Options

A   Cytomegalovirus (CMV)

B   Epstein–Barr virus (EBV)

C   Hep A Ag

D   Hep A IgM

E   Hep Bs Ag

F   Hep C Ab

G   Hep D serology

H   Hep E serology

Consider the following flow chart for the investigation of abnormal liver function tests. For each missing step in the flow chart, select the single most appropriate option from the list above. Each option can be used once, more than once or not at all.

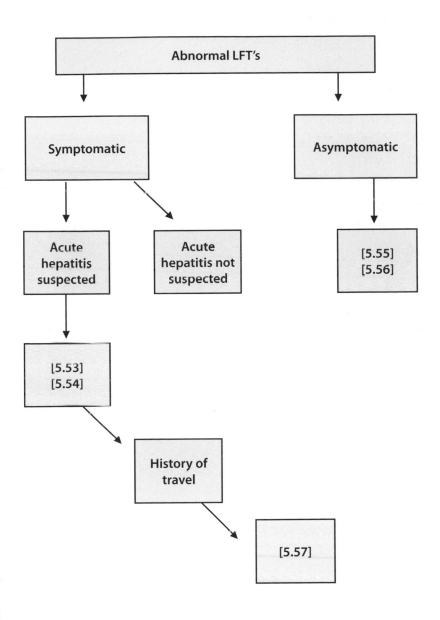

PICTURE QUESTIONS

5.58 A 33-year-old woman has a violent coughing fit and shortly afterwards notices an unusual rash over her lower abdomen. Her abdomen is shown below:

Which one of the following is the single most likely underlying diagnosis?

☐ A   Disseminated intravascular coagulation (DIC)
☐ B   Haemophilia
☐ C   Psoas abscess
☐ D   Rectus sheath haematoma
☐ E   von Willebrand's disease

5.59 A 42-year-old man complains of fresh bleeding after defecation, discomfort, itching and intermittent soiling of his underwear with mucus. On examination of his anus you note the appearance below:

Which one of the following is the most likely diagnosis?

- [ ] A   Anal fissure
- [ ] B   Condyloma acuminata
- [ ] C   Crohn's disease
- [ ] D   Haemorrhoids
- [ ] E   Squamous-cell carcinoma of the anus

DATA INTERPRETATION QUESTION

5.60 A new test has been developed to pick up asymptomatic bowel cancer. This involves patients sending specimens of stool for analysis for dyskaryotic epithelial cells. It is reported by its inventors to be non-invasive and therefore safe and accurate. Initial trial data are shown below:

Total number of samples submitted	1000
Number suitable for analysis	500
Number of samples which tested positive	50
Number of true positives (confirmed by colonoscopy)	25
Total number of diagnoses in patients who submitted suitable sample	30
Number of false negatives	5
Number of diagnoses in all patients participating in trial	60

Which one of the following statements is true regarding this data?

- [ ] A For patients submitting a suitable sample, the sensitivity of the test is 25/30, ie 83%

- [ ] B For patients submitting a suitable sample, the sensitivity of the test is 25/50, ie 50%

- [ ] C For patients submitting a suitable sample, the sensitivity of the test is 50/500, ie 10%

- [ ] D For patients submitting a suitable sample, the specificity of the test is 25/30, ie 83%

- [ ] E The data suggest that this test will make a significant impact on early diagnosis of bowel cancer

HOT TOPICS/EVIDENCE BASED PRACTICE

5.61 Which one of the following statements about the initial management of dyspepsia in primary care is correct?

☐ A 20% of the UK population take long-term prescription drugs for dyspepsia

☐ B Costs are greater at 1 year for test and treat compared with empirical treatment due to the relatively high cost of antibiotics compared with generic proton-pump inhibitors

☐ C Endoscopy is more cost-effective than empirical treatment in the long term

☐ D Eradication of *Helicobacter pylori* might reduce the long-term incidence of cancer

☐ E Test and treat at initial consultation is more effective at 1 year than acid suppression alone

ANSWERS

5.1   B: *Clostridium difficile*

Watery diarrhoea starting after recent antibiotic therapy is usually caused by *Clostridium difficile*. The commonest implicated antibiotics are amoxicillin, ampicillin, clindamycin and cephalosporins. Treatment consists of stopping the offending antibiotics, metronidazole or oral vancomycin, fluid replacement and barrier nursing. Toxic megacolon can occur and this should be managed surgically. *Campylobacter* causes a diarrhoeal illness that is usually associated with eating chicken, while norovirus causes a transient diarrhoeal and vomiting illness. Rotavirus usually affects children.

5.2   B: Blood test for IgA tissue transglutaminase (tTGA)

NICE guidance suggests first-line testing should be for tTGA. If IgA deficiency is suspected, EMA testing can be used. Positive testing on these should prompt referral for biopsy. False-negative results can be seen in patients who have abstained from gluten for some time. Antigliadin antibodies have low specificity and sensitivity and are now not used routinely. Faecal fat is non-specific sign of malabsorption and can be positive in chronic pancreatitis or following gastrectomy.

5.3   D: A 45-year-old man who has routine blood tests showing a haemoglobin of 10.5 g/dl; he is otherwise well and examination is unremarkable

NICE guidance suggests referral in the following situations:

- People aged 40 years and older, reporting rectal bleeding with a change of bowel habit for 6 weeks

- People aged 60 years and older, with rectal bleeding persisting for 6 weeks without anal symptoms

- People aged 60 ears and older, with a change in bowel habit to looser stools for 6 weeks or more without rectal bleeding

- People of any age with a right lower abdominal or rectal mass

- Men with iron-deficiency anaemia and a haemoglobin of 11 g/dl or below

- Non-menstruating women with a haemoglobin of 10 g/dl or below.

5.4   E: The risk of re-bleeding is > 90% at 2 years

Poor prognostic factors in variceal bleeding are encephalopathy, hypoalbuminaemia, jaundice and ascites. The mortality rate in first bleeds is 40–70% and from subsequent bleeds is 30%. Almost all patients will have re-bleeding within 2 years. Abstaining from alcohol helps slow the progression of underlying liver disease but will not reverse portal hypertension.

5.5   B: Mesenteric ischaemia should be considered

The presentation of acute severe abdominal pain in an arteriopath, out of keeping with clinical findings, should suggest the possibility of ischaemic bowel. Initially there are few signs but, later on, bloodstained mucus, signs of bowel obstruction and shock are common. The prognosis is poor due to late diagnosis. Diverticulitis generally causes milder pain with more of a change in bowel habit while IBS would not normally cause severe pain.

5.6 A: Admit under the general surgeons for endoscopy

Batteries are prone to leakage in the gut and should be removed as soon as possible to avoid potentially fatal complications. Smooth objects such as coins will usually pass normally, as will objects such as safety pins once they reach the stomach safely. X-rays are not usually needed if there are no signs of obstruction.

5.7 C: Rice

Patients with coeliac disease should avoid wheats, rye and barley but can eat rice and maize. Some coeliac patients are sensitive to pure oats but many patients can take these without any problem, although commercially available oats such as porridge oats are usually contaminated with wheat during the milling process, so patients should try and obtain pure oats.

5.8 C: Anti-TNFα therapy is associated with remission rates of 80%

Mesalazine is no better than placebo in the management of active disease. Its main use is in prevention of relapse after surgery. Infliximab is an effective anti-TNFα therapy in up to 80% of cases, but only 24% are steroid-free. Surgery should be reserved for patients who do not respond to steroids, methotrexate or infliximab. Antibiotics should only be used for septic complications and perianal disease. Crohn's disease can affect any part of the gastrointestinal tract from the mouth to the anus.

5.9 D: Patients with ulcerative colitis should have regular colonoscopic follow-up to identify malignant change

Ulcerative colitis only affects the large bowel, while Crohn's disease can affect any part of the gastrointestinal tract. Mesalazine should be prescribed by brand. Ulcerative colitis is associated with bowel cancer and so patients should be regularly screened with colonscopy. In most patients the disease can be controlled with mesalazine and where steroids are needed topical steroids such as Predfoam enemas should be used to reduce systemic effects. Perianal fistulas are associated with Crohn's disease.

5.10   C: Gastro-oesophageal reflux

Gastro-oesophageal reflux is normal in the newborn, due to a 'physiological' hiatus hernia. The gastro-oesophageal sphincter is underdeveloped at birth; mothers learn to 'burp' their babies after feeds by holding them up and patting them on the back to bring up wind and prevent regurgitation. Where violent vomiting after each meal occurs, together with weight, loss pyloric stenosis should be suspected.

5.11   C: Intussusception

Intussusception in children usually occurs during weaning and is thought to be due to lymphoid hyperplasia in the small intestine. This acts as a nidus for the intussusception. A tender mobile mass might be palpable in the upper abdomen.

5.12   B: Incarcerated hernia

Inguinal hernias in early childhood are caused by the virtual apposition of the external and internal rings during development of the inguinal canal. The processus vaginalis is also patent, providing access of abdominal contents to the scrotum.

5.13   A: Appendicitis

Acute appendicitis in children must be distinguished from acute mesenteric adenitis caused by systemic viral infections and urinary tract infections. In adolescent girls, mid-cycle pain, twisted ovarian cysts or ruptured ovarian follicles can mimic acute appendicitis.

5.14   B: Cystic echinococcosis

Hydatid disease is of insidious onset, with an incubation period of many years. It can involve any organ, with cyst formation. Appropriate imaging and immunological tests confirm the diagnosis. Solitary cysts are surgically removed and widespread disease might respond to oral mebendazole or albendazole therapy. Bladder worm, guinea worm and filariasis are all tropical infections; tapeworm usually affects the bowel only.

5.15   A: Abdominal tuberculosis

Abdominal TB is acquired through the consumption of infected milk or milk products and leads to caseation in mesenteric, portal or splenic lymphatic tissue; these lesions can eventually heal with calcification.

5.16   B: Elective cholecystectomy

The reservoir of infection in typhoid is in the gallbladder. Cholecystectomy eliminates the faeco–oral infectivity of the carrier. T-tube drainage of the common bile duct might be required to confirm eradication of infection.

5.17   B: Amoebic ulceration

Entamoeba histolytica is acquired through the faeco–oral route in endemic regions and causes colonic mucosal ulceration and granuloma formation.

5.18   B: Cholecystitis

Tenderness in the gallbladder area, a tender, palpable gallbladder or a positive Murphy's sign are all suggestive of acute calculous cholecystitis. An ultrasound scan would exclude empyema of the gallbladder, confirm stones in the gallbladder and exclude duct stones and pancreatitis.

5.19   E: Visceral perforation

Peptic perforation is a complication of peptic ulcer disease and is associated with anti-ulcer therapy non-compliance, alcohol abuse, long-term steroids and NSAIDs. A rare cause is gastrinoma (an islet-cell tumour), which stimulates gastric hypersecretion, causing multiple ulcers.

THEME: ABNORMAL LIVER FUNCTION

5.20   E: Gilbert syndrome

Gilbert syndrome causes isolated hyperbilirubinaemia, often after a mild illness. It is of no clinical significance and can be confirmed by taking blood before and after a 24-hour period of starvation.

5.21   H: Nephrotic syndrome

Nephrotic syndrome causes a low albumin level due to renal loss. Other causes of low albumin include starvation and burns. High albumin levels might be seen in dehydration.

5.22   C: Fatty liver

Fatty liver can be seen in alcohol abuse, diabetes and obesity; less commonly, it is seen in chronic disease, pregnancy and malnutrition. ALT is typically raised and GGT and bilirubin levels are usually normal, although the ALP can be elevated. Treatment usually consists of weight reduction and improved glycaemic control. Abstinence should be encouraged in cases of alcoholic fatty liver.

5.23   B: Anticonvulsant use

GGT can be raised with phenytoin or barbiturate use or, more commonly, with alcohol abuse. The absence of other markers of alcohol abuse, such as a raised mean corpuscular volume (MCV), suggests the cause is anticonvulsants. GGT can also be elevated in hepatobiliary disease and is particularly useful in children, in whom a raised ALP could be due to growth. A raised GGT with raised ALP suggest a hepatic cause, while a raised ALP in isolation suggests a non-hepatic cause (eg growth spurt).

CHAPTER 5 ANSWERS

THEME: DIARRHOEA

5.24   C: *Cryptosporidium*

Cryptosporidium causes a self-limiting diarrhoeal illness in children and the immunocompromised. Treatment with spiramycin might be needed in patients with reduced immunity.

5.25   A: *Campylobacter*

Campylobacter can cause malaise, diarrhoea and abdominal pain. It is self-limiting but in some cases prolonged carriage occurs. Patients with this disease who work in certain environments (eg care homes) should stay off work until free from infection. Where necessary, treatment is with erythromycin.

5.26   E: Rotavirus

Rotavirus is the commonest cause of gastroenteritis in children in the UK. Epidemics tend to occur in winter and spring, with fewer cases in the summer. Treatment is supportive.

5.27   G: *Shigella*

Shigella causes dysentery and in the UK outbreaks have been seen in nurseries, psychiatric facilities and care homes. It causes a bloody diarrhoea after an incubation period of 48 hours. Treatment is supportive; ciprofloxacin is useful in those who are immunocompromised or severely affected.

5.28   D: Norovirus

Norovirus causes epidemics of gastroenteritis and often causes epidemics on cruise ships, in schools and in hospitals. Symptoms usually settle with conservative treatment in 48 hours.

THEME: ACUTE ABDOMEN

5.29   A: Appendicitis

Appendicitis typically starts with vague abdominal pain that tends to localise to the right iliac fossa over 12–24 hours. Nitrites have low specificity for urinary tract infection. A pelvic appendix can mimic a urinary tract infection.

5.30   H: Ruptured ectopic pregnancy

Sudden onset of severe, persistent abdominal pain with hypotension and peritonism in a woman of childbearing age strongly suggests a ruptured ectopic pregnancy. A pelvic ultrasound scan will confirm the diagnosis.

5.31   C: Incarcerated hernia

Inguinal hernia in early childhood is caused by the virtual apposition of the internal and external rings during the development of the inguinal canal. The processus vaginalis is also patent, providing access of abdominal contents to the scrotum.

5.32   D: Intussusception

Intussusception in childhood is usually caused by hyperplasia of submucosal lymphoid tissue due to changes in bowel flora during weaning. The intussusception is initially intermittent but bowel obstruction rapidly supervenes which leads to ischaemia of the intussuscepted loop.

5.33   F: Meconium ileus

Meconium ileus is caused by inspissated meconium impacting in the terminal ileum and results from changes in bowel mucus associated with cystic fibrosis. If colonic washouts fail to restore patency, surgical evacuation is required.

THEME: OESOPHAGEAL LESIONS

5.34   B: Barrett's oesophagus

Columnar epithelial dysplasia in the distal oesophagus is associated with chronic reflux and peptic oesophagitis and predisposes to adenocarcinoma.

5.35   A: Achalasia

A developmental or acquired motility disorder characterised by narrowing of the distal oesophagus, with hypertrophy of the circular muscle layer.

5.36   C: Boerhaave syndrome

Oesophageal tear following forceful retching or vomiting results in mediastinitis and shock. Diagnosis is by the finding of gas in the mediastinum on chest X-ray (CXR) and computed tomography (CT). Endoscopic visualisation is unreliable and is contraindicated.

5.37   G: Sliding hiatus hernia

The symptom of acid reflux. Incompetence of the cardio-oesophageal sphincter leads to reflux oesophagitis and hiatus hernia; fibrotic narrowing can result in oesophageal stenosis.

5.38   D: Cirrhosis of the liver

Bleeding from gastro-oesophageal varices is a feature of portal hypertension from cirrhosis; clinical signs of liver failure might also be present.

THEME: STOMACH

5.39   F: Hypertrophic pyloric stenosis

Hypertrophy of the circular muscle fibres of the pylorus produces intermittent gastric outlet obstruction in neonates and infants; it is treated by pyloromyotomy (Ramstedt's operation).

5.40   G: Peptic ulcer disease

Benign peptic ulcer disease is characterised by dyspeptic periodicity and weight gain. Gastroduodenoscopy and mucosal biopsy confirms the diagnosis before anti-ulcer treatment is commenced. A coexisting *Helicobactor pylori* infection must be treated.

5.41   D: *Helicobacter pylori*

Non-ulcer dyspepsia is usually associated with *H. pylori* (type 2) gastritis. Diagnosis is made on mucosal biopsy or urease breath test.

5.42   C: Gastrocolic fistula

Gastrocolic fistula is caused by advanced gastric or colonic tumour in the elderly; Crohn's disease is a rare cause in the younger age group. Resection of the diseased bowel and fistula relieves symptoms in both instances.

THEME: LIVER DISEASE

5.43   F: Cirrhosis

In cirrhosis, cutaneous signs are spider naevi, caput medusae, skin bruising, pigmentation and purpuric rash. The uncongugated plasma bilirubin can be raised, with raised liver enzymes and a low albumin.

5.44   H: Wilson's disease

Wilson's disease (hepatolenticular degeneration) is an autosomal recessive disorder of defective copper metabolism in the liver, resulting in copper deposition in tissues. Chelating agents (eg penicillamine) control disease progression and liver transplantation is indicated for advanced disease.

5.45   A: Acute calculous cholecystitis

Ultrasound of the gallbladder would confirm the presence of gallstones in an inflamed, thick-walled gallbladder. Liver function is usually unaffected if the biliary tree is free of stones or inflammation.

5.46   B: Acute cholangitis

Cholangiohepatitis is an ascending infection of the biliary tree caused by calculus obstruction and would lead to inflammation of the liver parenchyma and microabscess formation. Urgent decompression of the biliary tree by percutaneous catheterisation, endoscopic drainage or surgical drainage is required.

5.47   G: Gallstone ileus

Gallstone ileus is a rare complication of cholelithiasis, where the gallstone erodes into the adjacent duodenum. The clinical picture is that of small-bowel obstruction, which requires surgical relief. Removal of the diseased gallbladder or closure of the choledochoduodenal fistula is not usually indicated.

THEME: MANAGEMENT OF HAEMORRHOIDS

5.48 **B:** 4th degree

5.49 **A:** 1st/2nd degree

5.50 **G:** Ligation/injection

5.51 **G:** Ligation/injection

5.52 **E:** Haemorrhoidectomy

THEME: INVESTIGATION OF ABNORMAL LIVER FUNCTION TESTS

5.53 **D:** Hep A IgM

5.54 **E:** Hep Bs Ag

5.55 **E:** Hep Bs Ag

5.56 **F:** Hep C Ab

5.57 **H:** Hep E serology

5.58 **D:** Rectus sheath haematoma

This is the typical appearance of a rectus sheath haematoma, which usually occurs spontaneously after coughing or vomiting. It is usually caused by blood leaking from the inferior epigastric artery, and usually settles spontaneously.

5.59   D: Haemorrhoids

This is a typical appearance of third-degree piles. Typical symptoms are itching and irritation, dull ache, bleeding, sensation of a lump, and soiling. They are classified as 'first degree' if they are within the anal canal, 'second degree' if they come down with bowel motions but return afterwards, and 'third degree' if they are down all the time.

5.60   A   For patients submitting a suitable sample, the sensitivity of the test is 25/30, ie 83%

Sensitivity = 100 × true positive/(true positive + false negative)

Specificity = 100 × true negative/(true negative + false positive)

The fact that half of all samples were unsuitable suggest that this test is unlikely to be useful on a population basis, because this resulted in 30 diagnoses being missed.

5.61   D: Eradication of *Helicobacter pylori* might reduce the long-term incidence of cancer

Three per cent of the population take long-term drugs for dyspepsia at an estimated annual cost of £500 million. Endoscopy is the least cost-effective option when compared with test and treat or empirical treatment. Eradication of *H. pylori* in high-risk patients has reduced the incidence of gastric cancer. The MRC-CUBE trial (Multicentre Randomised Controlled Trial of ^{13}C Urea Breath Testing and *H. pylori* Eradication for Dyspepsia in Primary Care) demonstrated equivalent cost-effectiveness for test and treat and empirical treatment and therefore supported initial empirical treatment. The researchers concluded that the decision to test for *H. pylori* should be made with the patient.

CHAPTER 6
GENETICS
SINGLE BEST ANSWER QUESTIONS

6.1 You see the parents of a 30-month-old boy who are concerned about his development. He was born at term after a normal delivery and initially seemed to be developing normally but they have now become concerned that he is not walking as well as he should. He falls frequently and when he stands he has to push himself up with his hands. Examination shows some wasting of his quadriceps and hypertrophy of his calves. What is the single most likely diagnosis?

- [ ] A   Cerebral palsy
- [ ] B   Down syndrome
- [ ] C   Duchenne muscular dystrophy
- [ ] D   Motor neurone disease
- [ ] E   Myotonic muscular dystrophy

6.2 A 49-year-old smoker has just been diagnosed with emphysema, and has been found to have alpha-1-antitrypsin deficiency. Which one of the following is a correct description of the aetiology of the emphysema?

- [ ] A   Environmental
- [ ] B   Multifactorial
- [ ] C   New mutation
- [ ] D   Single gene effect
- [ ] E   Sporadic

6.3 A 27-year-old woman comes to see you after a second spontaneous miscarriage. She is concerned that there could be an underlying reason for this and asks you what is likely to have caused her miscarriage. Which one of the following statements is true regarding spontaneous miscarriage?

☐ A 90% of early spontaneous miscarriages are chromosomally abnormal

☐ B If the parents are healthy, there is unlikely to be a hereditary component

☐ C Maternal age is not associated with risk of miscarriage

☐ D There are no effective treatments for recurrent miscarriage

☐ E Spontaneous miscarriage occurs in 50% of pregnancies

6.4 Which one of the following statements about cystic fibrosis is true?

☐ A 98% of male patients are infertile

☐ B It is transmitted as an X-linked recessive trait

☐ C The disease is common in Asians and Afro-Caribbeans

☐ D The incidence of cystic fibrosis in the UK is 1 in 10 000 live births

☐ E The prevalence of carriers is 1 in 200 in the UK

6.5 A 39-year-old lady with two children by her first marriage comes to see you to discuss pre-conception counselling now that she is to remarry. She is particularly concerned about the risk of Down syndrome. Which one of the following statements is true regarding this situation?

- [ ] A   All women with a risk greater than 1 in 400 should be offered chorionic villus sampling (CVS)
- [ ] B   Nuchal translucency testing has 98% sensitivity and specificity for Down syndrome
- [ ] C   The risk at age 40 is 1 in 30
- [ ] D   The risk of Down syndrome is negligible below the age of 30
- [ ] E   The risk of having a baby with Down syndrome is significantly greater In parents who have already had a Down syndrome pregnancy

6.6 A 46-year-old man comes to see you to discuss his recent diagnosis of Huntington's chorea. He was adopted and has no knowledge of his genetic family. He has two teenage sons and lost his wife 3 years ago to breast cancer. Which of the following statements is true regarding this situation? Select one option only.

- [ ] A   If his teenage sons show no signs of chorea, they can be reassured
- [ ] B   Testing the children to see if they will develop the condition is not possible
- [ ] C   The average life expectancy from diagnosis is 25 years
- [ ] D   The condition is inherited as an autosomal dominant trait and the risk of his sons developing the condition is 1 in 2
- [ ] E   This condition usually presents in the late teens

6.7 **Which of the following statements is true about Turner syndrome? Select one option only.**

☐ A Affected individuals tend to be tall with hyperextensible joints

☐ B Affected patients have the karyotype 47XXX

☐ C The external genitalia are characteristically abnormal

☐ D The incidence is 1 in 5000 live births

☐ E Turner syndrome is invariably associated with mental retardation

6.8 **Which one of the following statements about genetic counselling in primary care is true? Select one option only.**

☐ A Family trees are not helpful in counselling families affected by Down syndrome

☐ B Families with conditions with variable penetrance, eg tuberous sclerosis, can be successfully counselled in primary care

☐ C Genetic counselling is a complex field and there is no place for genetic counselling in primary care

☐ D Risk is best expressed as percentages (eg 0.1%), rather than as proportions (eg 1 in 1000)

☐ E Two generations of a family tree are sufficient to identify a genetic predisposition

6.9   A family who have recently joined your list come to see you to discuss phenylketonuria. The parents are unaffected but have had a son who has been diagnosed on the basis of a neonatal heel-prick test. They wish to discuss the risks relating to further pregnancies. Which one of the following statements about this situation is true?

☐   A   Because the parents are unaffected the affected son is the result of a new mutation and the recurrence risks are very rare

☐   B   Phenylketonuria is an autosomal dominant trait so the lack of the disease in either parent suggests that the stated father is not the biological father

☐   C   Phenylketonuria is an autosomal recessive trait, so both parents must be carriers

☐   D   The risk of a future child being a carrier is 1 in 4

☐   E   The risk of another child having phenylketonuria is 1 In 2

6.10   Premature baldness is inherited as an X-linked recessive condition. Which one of the following statements about risk to future generations is true?

☐   A   Where the father is affected and the mother is not a carrier, there is a 100% risk of an affected son

☐   B   Where the father is affected and the mother is not a carrier, there is no risk of an affected son

☐   C   Where the mother is a carrier and the father is unaffected, there is a 50% risk of any offspring being a carrier

☐   D   Where the mother is a carrier and the father is unaffected, there is a 100% risk of an affected son

☐   E   X-linked dominant conditions do not cause disease in females

EXTENDED MATCHING QUESTIONS

THEME: MODES OF INHERITANCE

Options

A   Autosomal dominant

B   Autosomal recessive

C   Chromosomal translocation

D   Non-dysjunction

E   X-linked dominant

F   X-linked recessive

For each of the conditions below, select the most appropriate inheritance pattern from the list above. Each option may be used once, more than once or not at all.

☐   **6.11**   **Cystic fibrosis.**

☐   **6.12**   **Duchenne muscular dystrophy.**

☐   **6.13**   **Klinefelter syndrome.**

☐   **6.14**   **Huntington's disease.**

THEME: DISORDERS OF X AND Y CHROMOSOMES

Options

A   Fragile X syndrome

B   Klinefelter syndrome

C   Noonan syndrome

D   Testicular feminisation syndrome

E   Triple X syndrome

F   Turner syndrome

G   Turner syndrome mosaic

For each of the descriptions below, select the most appropriate diagnosis from the list above. Each option may be used once, more than once or not at all.

☐ **6.15**   A 16-year-old girl is being investigated for primary amenorrhoea. She is of normal height and, apart from lack of secondary sexual characteristics, is normal in appearance and has normal IQ. An ultrasound shows no sign of ovaries.

☐ **6.16**   A 17-year-old boy is brought to see you because of gynaecomastia. He is tall, but has minimal male secondary sexual characteristics and has small firm testes on examination. His mother reports that he has had developmental delay in the past and behavioural problems.

☐ **6.17**   A 14-year-old girl is seen with her mother. She has always struggled to keep up at school but is now getting teased on account of her short stature, webbed neck and delayed puberty. Her previous medical history includes repair of coarctation of the aorta in childhood.

☐ **6.18**   A 17-year-old girl comes to see you regarding primary amenorrhoea. She is otherwise healthy and has normal secondary sexual characteristics. A blood test shows raised LH and FSH and an ultrasound test shows an absent uterus and ovaries.

THEME: DIAGNOSTIC TESTS IN GENETICS

Options

A Amniocentesis

B Carrier testing

C Chorionic villus sampling (CVS)

D Fetoscopy

E Fluorescent in-situ hybridisation

F Guthrie test

G Heel-prick test

H Karyotyping

I Triple test

J Ultrasound

For each of the conditions affecting babies described below, select the most appropriate diagnostic or screening test from the list above. Each option can be used once, more than once or not at all.

- [ ] **6.19** Hypothyroidism.
- [ ] **6.20** Tay–Sachs disease.
- [ ] **6.21** Phenylketonuria.
- [ ] **6.22** Congenital cardiac disease.
- [ ] **6.23** Thalassaemia major.

THEME: CANCER GENETICS

Options

A   Acoustic neuroma

B   Acute lymphoblastic leukaemia

C   Colonic cancer

D   Gastrointestinal Maltoma

E   Glioma

F   Kaposi's sarcoma

G   Meningioma

H   Non-Hodgkin's lymphoma

I   Oesophageal cancer

J   Retinoblastoma

K   Small-cell lung cancer

L   Thyroid cancer

For each of the genetic conditions described below, select the tumour that is most commonly associated with that condition from the list above. Each option can be used once, more than once or not at all.

☐ **6.24**   **Neurofibromatosis.**

☐ **6.25**   **Tuberous sclerosis.**

☐ **6.26**   **Down syndrome.**

☐ **6.27**   **Familial adenomatous polypsosis.**

☐ **6.28**   **Multiple endocrine neoplasia.**

TABLE QUESTIONS

THEME: ANTENATAL TESTING

6.29–6.33

Options

A   0%

B   0.01%

C   0.25%–0.5%

D   0.5–1%

E   5%

F   10–12 weeks

G   10–13 weeks

H   15–18 weeks

I   15–20 weeks

J   18–20 weeks

K   Diagnostic

L   Screening

The local midwives have constructed an information pack about antenatal testing to include in their booking information packs. Complete the table below from the list of options given. Each option may be used once, more than once or not at all.

Investigation	Screening or diagnostic test?	Gestation	Risk of adverse effects
Nuchal translucency	[6.29]		
Chorionic villus sampling		[6.30]	[6.31]
Amniocentesis			[6.32]
Triple test	[6.33]		
Anomaly scan			

PICTURE QUESTION

6.34 A patient has had the lesions shown in the photograph below all over his body since childhood. He does not know anything about his family history because he was adopted at the age of 3 months. His wife is not affected. He is planning a family and consults you for advice as to whether their children are likely to be affected.

Which one of the following statements is true regarding the risk of passing the condition to any children?

- [ ] A The condition is a spontaneous condition rather than genetic, so there is no risk of transmission to offspring
- [ ] B The risk of affected offspring is 50%
- [ ] C The risk of affected offspring is 100%
- [ ] D The risk of children being carriers is 25%
- [ ] E The risk of male children being carriers is 100%

DATA INTERPRETATION QUESTION

6.35 A couple attend for pre-conception counselling after having two children affected by a genetic disease. They would like to have a third child but are concerned about the risk of recurrence. Their families pedigree is shown below:

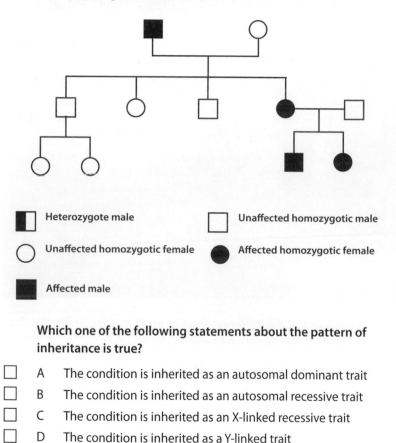

■ Heterozygote male   □ Unaffected homozygotic male

○ Unaffected homozygotic female   ● Affected homozygotic female

■ Affected male

Which one of the following statements about the pattern of inheritance is true?

- [ ] A The condition is inherited as an autosomal dominant trait
- [ ] B The condition is inherited as an autosomal recessive trait
- [ ] C The condition is inherited as an X-linked recessive trait
- [ ] D The condition is inherited as a Y-linked trait
- [ ] E The condition is sporadic rather than an inherited trait

HOT TOPICS/EVIDENCE BASED PRACTICE

6.36 Which one of the following statements about stem cell research in the UK is true?

☐ A It is currently legal to select embryos for implantation so that their cells can be used for treating siblings with genetic diseases

☐ B Fetal stem cells have been used successfully for the treatment of Parkinson's disease for several years

☐ C Stem cells can only be found in embryos or umbilical cord blood

☐ D Stem cells for research are extracted from in-vitro fertilisation (IVF) embryos before they are implanted into the womb

☐ E Stem cells have been shown to reverse the progress of Alzheimer's disease

ANSWERS

6.1   C: Duchenne muscular dystrophy

Duchenne muscular dystrophy is an X-lined trait that usually manifests from 18 months of age but is typically not diagnosed until the age of 4–5 years. It causes progressive weakness, starting in the legs, and most patients are wheelchair-bound by the age of 20. Myotonic dystrophy has an onset from late teens onwards and is characterised by hypogonadism, cataracts, weakening and wasting of sternocleidomastoid in particular. Motor neurone disease affects adults while cerebral palsy is non progressive and usually present from birth.

6.2   B: Multifactorial

Patients with alpha-1 antitrypsin deficiency are at increased risk of heart and lung problems. The condition is inherited as a co-dominant trait, ie heterozygotes have 50% of normal enzyme activity, while homozygotes have only 10% normal activity. The development of emphysema depends on the enzyme activity and environmental insult, so development of pulmonary complications frequently occurs in the third and fourth decade in smokers, later in non-smokers. Homozygotes are also prone to cirrhosis and hepatocellular carcinoma. Treatment is aimed at avoiding smoking and in some centres recombinant alpha-1-antitrypsin is used.

6.3 E: Spontaneous miscarriage occurs in 50% of pregnancies

While spontaneous miscarriage occurs in 50% of all pregnancies, most occur in the first 14 days after conception and only 15% of these have been noticed by the mother, the rest occurring so close to an expected period as to seem like a late period. Around 60% of early miscarriages are associated with a chromosomal abnormality while 20% of miscarried fetuses are structurally abnormal (eg anencephalic). Higher maternal age is associated with increased risk. In cases of recurrent miscarriage, 5–10% of couples will carry a balanced translocation that does not affect them but does affect their gametes. A number of maternal conditions are associated with recurrent miscarriage, including systemic lupus erythematosus, uncontrolled hypertension, antiphospholipid syndrome, and treatment of these can improve the prospects of a successful pregnancy.

6.4 A: 98% of male patients are infertile

Cystic fibrosis is the commonest inherited condition in the UK and is transmitted as an autosomal recessive trait. The gene is carried by 1 in 25 people in the UK, but is rare in non-whites. The incidence is 1 in 2000 live births. Ninety-eight per cent of male patients are infertile and now that the life expectancy is well into the thirties, fertility counselling plays an increasingly important role in the management of patients.

CHAPTER 6 ANSWERS

6.5   E: The risk of having a baby with Down syndrome is significantly greater in parents who have already had a Down syndrome pregnancy

Most cases of Down syndrome are due to non-dysjunction during meiosis, although some parents carry a balanced translocation, which puts them at high risk. Karyotyping of parents should be considered after a Down syndrome pregnancy to exclude this risk. Nuchal translucency is a useful screening tool but is not specific for Down syndrome and can be a sign of Edwards syndrome amongst others. It is therefore used as a screening test rather than a diagnostic test. In combination with serum screening as part of the 'integrated test', it is more sensitive and specific. Women with a risk of 1 in 200 or worse will usually be offered diagnostic tests such as CVS or amniocentesis. The risk of carrying a Down syndrome baby is 1 in 1400 at 25, 1 in 900 at 30, 1 in 400 at 35, 1 in 100 at 40 and 1 in 30 at 45. More babies are born with Down syndrome to women under 30 than to women over 40 due to the higher number of births in this age group.

6.6   D: The condition is inherited as an autosomal dominant trait and the risk of his sons developing the condition is 1 in 2

Huntington's chorea usually manifests between 30 and 50 years of age and usually starts with chorea, with typical hemiballismus. Dementia develops later on, although there is often good insight, which leads to significant depression and suicide. The inheritance is autosomal dominant, giving offspring a 50% chance of developing the disease and their children a 25% chance of inheriting the disease, rising to 50% if their father develops the condition. The gene has been identified, so diagnosis is possible and although there is no cure this can be helpful in family planning.

6.7   D: The incidence is 1 in 5000 live births

Turner syndrome (45X) is seen in 1 in 5000 live births. Affected patients are often short, with wide-spaced nipples and a webbed neck. Coarctation of the aorta can occur and internal genitalia are abnormal, although the external genitalia and vagina are usually normal. This can present late as primary amenorrhoea. Oestrogen supplementation from puberty will encourage the development of normal secondary sexual characteristics. Mental retardation is more commonly seen with Klinefelter syndrome in men. Many women with Turner syndrome live a normal life, albeit an infertile one.

6.8   A: Family trees are not helpful in counselling families affected by Down syndrome

Three generations of a family tree are needed, together with racial background, to identify genetic predisposition. Down syndrome arises in the parent as a balanced translocation (rare, < 1% of cases) or spontaneously during meiosis, so family history is irrelevant. A basic working knowledge of genetics should be sufficient for GPs to advise on inheritance risks of different disorders, particularly with regard to pre-conception counselling. Conditions with variable penetrance or complex inheritance should be dealt with by the genetic counselling service because prediction of risk is complicated. Most people understand risk better as a proportion (eg 1 in 20 children would be affected and 19 in 20 would not be affected), rather than as a percentage (eg 5% are affected).

6.9   C: Phenylketonuria is an autosomal recessive trait, so both parents must be carriers

Phenylketonuria is an autosomal recessive disorder which affects 1 in 10 000 live births. The risk of recurrence of the condition is 1 in 4 and risk of future children being carriers is 1 in 2, while the risk of having a child free from the gene is 1 in 4. Screening at birth is important because early phenylalanine exclusion will lead to normal mental development. Where unusual patterns of inheritance are seen, the possibility of biological versus stated parenthood should be considered but there are many other causes, such as incomplete penetrance and new mutation, so this area is best broached by an expert rather than risk causing offence.

6.10   B: Where the father is affected and the mother is not a carrier, there is no risk of an affected son

X-linked recessive conditions usually result in affected males or female carriers. All female offspring of an affected male will have an affected X chromosome and if his partner is a carrier, 50% of her offspring will have a second copy of the gene, ie 50% of female offspring will have the disease.

The scenarios are best considered by drawing a 2 × 2 box where 'X' is an X chromosome carrying the gene, while 'x' is one that does not, while 'y' is a normal Y chromosome. A carrier female would be xX, an affected male Xy, an affected female XX and an unaffected female xx, while an unaffected male is xy:

Situation 1 – carrier female and affected male:

	X	**y**
X	XX	Xy
x	xX	xy

Therefore, of the offspring, 1 in 4 is XX, ie an affected female, 1 of 4 is Xy, ie an affected male, 1 in 4 is xX, ie a carrier female and 1 in 4 is xy, ie an unaffected male.

Situation 2 – normal female and affected male:

	X	y
x	xX	xy
x	xX	xy

Of these offspring, 2 in 4 offspring and all female children are carrier females (Xx), while 2 in 4 offspring are unaffected males (all male children).

Situation 3 – carrier female and unaffected male:

	x	y
X	Xx	Xy
x	xx	xy

These offspring therefore have a 1 in 4 risk of being a carrier female, a 1 in 4 risk of being an affected male, a 1 in 4 risk of being an unaffected male, and a 1 in 4 risk of being a female non-carrier.

THEME: MODES OF INHERITANCE

6.11   B: Autosomal recessive

Cystic fibrosis is inherited as an autosomal recessive with a 1 in 4 risk of two carriers having an affected child, a 2 in 4 risk of having a carrier child and a 1 in 4 risk of an unaffected child.

6.12   F: X-linked recessive

Duchenne muscular dystrophy is inherited as an X-linked recessive disorder. Women are very rarely affected (1 in 50 000 000) when both parents are carriers. Up to 30% of patients have the condition as a result of a new mutation.

6.13   D: Non-dysjunction

Non-dysjunction in meiosis causes the genotype 47XXY, the additional X chromosome coming from either parent. There is an association with increased maternal age.

6.14   A: Autosomal dominant

Huntington's is inherited as an autosomal dominant trait but does not usually present until middle age, by which time most patients have already had children. There is a 50% risk of children being affected.

THEME: DISORDERS OF X AND Y CHROMOSOMES

6.15   G: Turner syndrome mosaic

Around 16% of patients with Turner syndrome are mosaics. They have pure gonadal dysgenesis but, apart from lack of secondary sexual characteristics, are phenotypically normal.

6.16   B: Klinefelter syndrome

Klinefelter syndrome has the genotype 47XXY and occurs in 1 in 1000 male births. It is caused by non-dysjunction during meiosis and is associated with developmental delay, tall stature, infertility and gynaecomastia. These patients have an increased risk of breast cancer.

6.17   F: Turner syndrome

Turner syndrome affects 1 in 2500 female births and causes a characteristic presentation of small stature, delayed puberty, webbed neck, low IQ (average is 95), lymphoedema and shield chest. There is also an association with hypertension.

6.18   D: Testicular feminisation syndrome

Patients with testicular feminisation syndrome are genetically male with the genotype 46XY but have absent testosterone receptors. The condition affects 1 in 62 000 male births. Phenotypically female, the testes are usually present in the inguinal canal and are removed due to the increased risk of malignancy. Patients are treated as female, but are infertile.

THEME: DIAGNOSTIC TESTS IN GENETICS

6.19   G: Heel-prick test

Shortly after birth a heel-prick blood sample is taken to test for TSH levels and a Guthrie test for phenylketonuria. In some areas, blood is also tested for Immunoreactive trypsin, a marker for cystic fibrosis.

6.20   B: Carrier testing

Individuals of Ashkenazi Jewish extraction are tested for serum enzyme levels to detect carriers.

6.21   F: Guthrie test

Early diagnosis of phenylketonuria allows implementation of affected homozygotes allowing normal neurological development.

6.22   J: Ultrasound

An anomaly scan at 18–20 weeks allows the prenatal diagnosis of congenital heart disease, allowing treatment in the immediate postnatal period or, in some cases, the prenatal period.

6.23   D: Fetoscopy

Fetoscopy allows cordocentesis for haemoglobinopathies at 16–20 weeks, as well as biopsies of skin and liver biopsy where relevant.

THEME: CANCER GENETICS

6.24　A:　Acoustic neuroma

Neurofibromatosis is associated with acoustic neuromas, which usually present with sensorineural hearing loss or unilateral tinnitus.

6.25　E:　Glioma

Tuberous sclerosis is an autosomal dominant inherited condition characterised by ash-leaf macules appearing on the skin in early childhood, followed by the development of red angiofibromatous papules on the face. The condition is also associated with seizures, interstitial lung disease and gliomas.

6.26　B:　Acute lymphoblastic leukaemia

People with Down syndrome have an increased risk of acute lymphocytic leukaemia, while lymphoma is common in people with X-linked agammaglobulinaemia and ataxia telangiectasia.

6.27　C:　Colonic cancer

Colonic cancer is seen at an early age (twenties) in patients with the autosomal dominant condition, familial adenomatous polyposis and these patients should all have regular colonoscopic screening from a young age.

6.28　K:　Small-cell lung cancer

Multiple endocrine neoplasia is associated with pancreatic and pituitary tumours, peptic ulcer disease, phaeochromocytoma and medullary carcinoma of the thyroid. It has autosomal dominant inheritance and is inherited as a mutation in a tumour suppressor gene, so patients are born as heterozygotes for that gene. Subsequent mutation of the other allele during the patient's lifetime then results in the development of cancer in that organ.

THEME: ANTENATAL TESTING

6.29 **L:** Screening

6.30 **G:** 10–13 weeks

6.31 **D:** 0.5–1%

6.32 **C:** 0.25%–0.5%

6.33 **L:** Screening

Investigation	Screening or diagnostic test?	Gestation	Risk of adverse effects
Nuchal translucency	Screening	10–12 weeks	0
Chorionic villus sampling	Diagnostic	10–13 weeks	0.5–1%
Amniocentesis	Diagnostic	15–18 weeks	0.25–0.5%
Triple test	Screening	15–20 weeks	0
Anomaly scan	Screening	18–20 weeks	0

6.34 **B:** The risk of affected offspring is 50%

This picture shows *café-au-lait* patches and neurofibromas, so the patient has neurofibromatosis, which is inherited as an autosomal dominant trait. Offspring therefore have a 50% risk of being affected, but if they are not affected they will not be carriers. The condition is associated with brain tumours, including acoustic neuromas.

6.35   A: The conditions is inherited as an autosomal dominant trait

The condition is expressed in 3 consecutive generations and is therefore most likely to be a dominant trait. It affects men and women and therefore is unlikely to be an X linked trait, which tend to only affect males, while women are usually carriers or free of the trait. Affected males with X linked traits cannot pass the condition to sons, while all daughters of affected males will be carriers. There are very few conditions associated with the Y chromosome and these would obviously only affect males.

6.36   A: It is currently legal to select embryos for implantation so that their cells can be used for treating siblings with genetic diseases

Stem cells have the potential to treat a combination of genetic and degenerative diseases and might also solve many of the problems associated with organ transplantation, with tailored organs not requiring immunosupression. At present, stem cells for research come predominantly from surplus embryos from IVF treatment, which are destroyed after stem cell harvesting. Legislation is currently being debated (March 2008 is last entry) to allow the creation of human–animal hybrids to increase the supply of cells. Furthermore, stem cells from skin have been reprogrammed to behave like embryonic stem cells. The Human Fertilisation and Embryology Authority authorised pre-implantation selection of compatible embryos in 2004, to allow the use of stem cells in siblings. Experimental Parkinson's treatments based on fetal stem cells from aborted fetuses have been tried in the past without success, but cloned stem cells have been shown to be effective in experiments in mice.

CHAPTER 7
HAEMATOLOGY
SINGLE BEST ANSWER QUESTIONS

7.1 A child has just registered with your practice because his family has moved to the area. He has recently been diagnosed with hereditary spherocytosis. Which one of the following statements about this condition is true?

☐ A It is an X-linked recessive condition

☐ B It is associated with aplastic crises

☐ C It is usually diagnosed incidentally in adulthood on routine blood testing

☐ D Patients should be treated with B12 supplementation

☐ E There are usually no clinical signs

7.2 You start a new job in a practice with a large Afro-Caribbean population, many of whom are affected by sickle-cell anaemia. Which one of the following statements about this condition is true?

☐ A Infarction of the bone marrow causes severe pain

☐ B Osteomyelitis is rarely seen in patients with sickle-cell disease

☐ C Sickle-cell crises should usually be treated with paracetamol or non-steroidal drugs rather than with opiates because of the risk of addiction

☐ D The condition is exclusively seen in Afro-Caribbean populations

☐ E The condition is inherited as an autosomal dominant trait

7.3 A 19-year-old man comes to see you after being diagnosed by the haematology department with leukaemia. Which one of the following statements about acute leukaemia is true?

☐ A 70% of adults under the age of 50 with acute myeloid leukaemia (AML) are treated successfully

☐ B Acute lymphoblastic leukaemia (ALL) is invariably associated with a white cell count (WCC) > 20 × 10⁹/l

☐ C ALL is usually diagnosed as an incidental finding on a routine full blood count (FBC)

☐ D AML is usually seen in children

☐ E Platelets are unaffected in acute leukaemia

7.4 Which of the following statements about bleeding disorders is true? Select one option only.

☐ A A platelet count below 50 × 10⁹/l is likely to result in bleeding and admission should be arranged

☐ B Aspirin use causes thrombocytopenia

☐ C Coagulation disorders are invariably hereditary and present from birth

☐ D Factor XI deficiency is the commonest inherited clotting disorder

☐ E Platelet disorders usually present with purpura or bleeding gums

7.5 Which of the following statements about warfarin is true? Select one option only.

☐ A Co-amoxiclav affects the international normalised ratio (INR) by inhibition of cytochrome p450 metabolism

☐ B Patients should be advised to moderate tomato consumption

☐ C Warfarin does not interact with amiodarone

☐ D Warfarin inhibits platelet function

☐ E Warfarin interacts with co-codamol but not with co-proxamol

7.6 A 62-year-old man presents with a 6-month history of back pain and weight loss. He is a lifelong non-smoker and has no gastrointestinal symptoms. Examination is unremarkable, with no hepatosplenomegaly and no lymphadenopathy, but blood tests show an erythrocyte sedimentation rate (ESR) of 92 mm/hour, raised calcium and creatinine levels, and a haemoglobin of 9.8 g/dl with normal white cells and platelets. The film has been reported as showing rouleaux. Which one of the following is the most likely diagnosis?

- [ ] A   Acute myeloid leukaemia (AML)
- [ ] B   Chronic lymphocytic leukaemia (CLL)
- [ ] C   Chronic myeloid leukaemia (CML)
- [ ] D   Multiple myeloma
- [ ] E   Myelodysplasia

7.7 A 78-year-old woman complains of several months of increasing fatigue and, more recently, bleeding gums. She has had no weight loss and no other symptoms. She takes no regular medication. Examination shows her to be pale, with no hepatosplenomegaly or lymphadenopathy. Blood tests show normal renal function and liver function and normal calcium and ESR, but an FBC shows: neutrophil count 0.4×10^9/l, platelets 18×10^9/l and reticulocyte count < 1%. Which one of the following statements is true regarding this situation?

- [ ] A   This lady has aplastic anaemia
- [ ] B   This lady has chronic lymphocytic leukaemia
- [ ] C   This lady has iron deficiency
- [ ] D   This lady has myeloma
- [ ] E   This presentation is typical of myelofibrosis

EXTENDED MATCHING QUESTIONS

THEME: ANAEMIA

Options

A   Alcoholism

B   Anaemia of chronic disease

C   B12 deficiency

D   Folate deficiency

E   Glucose-6-phosphate dehydrogenase deficiency

F   Hereditary spherocytosis

G   Iron-deficiency anaemia

H   Sickle-cell anaemia

I   Thalassaemia major

J   Thalassaemia trait

For each of the clinical scenarios below, select the most appropriate diagnosis from the list above. Each option can be used once, more than once or not at all.

☐ **7.8**   A 47-year-old, perimenopausal woman complains of fatigue and shortness of breath on exertion. On examination, she has glossitis and angular stomatitis and she complains of brittle nails which you find are spoon-shaped.

☐ **7.9**   A 36-year-old man with long-standing Crohn's disease complains of fatigue. A routine FBC shows a macrocytosis and a haemoglobin level of 10.5 g/dl. Intrinsic factor antibodies are negative.

☐ **7.10**   A 25-year-old woman from Iran is given nitrofurantoin for a urinary tract infection. Three weeks later she presents with fatigue and shortness of breath. Urine testing reveals haemoglobinuria and an FBC shows a haemoglobin level of 7.6 g/dl with reticulocytosis.

☐ **7.11** A 67-year-old woman with long-standing hypothyroidism and vitiligo has a routine FBC which shows a macrocytic anaemia. Further blood tests are positive for parietal cell autoantibodies and intrinsic factor antibodies.

☐ **7.12** A 32-year-old woman has an FBC done as part of preconceptual counselling. She is noted to have a mild microcytic hypochromic anaemia with normal ferritin levels.

THEME: CLOTTING DISORDERS

Options

A Antiphospholipid syndrome

B Autoimmune thrombocytopenia

C Disseminated intravascular coagulopathy

D Factor V Leiden

E Haemophilia

F Idiopathic thrombocytopenia

G Thrombocythaemia

H Vitamin K deficiency

I von Willebrand's disease

For each scenario described below, select the most appropriate diagnosis from the list above. Each option can be used once, more than once or not at all.

☐ **7.13** A 4-day-old breastfed baby whose mother has noticed bleeding from his umbilical stump.

☐ **7.14** A 36-year-old woman with recurrent miscarriages who has been treated by her GP for suspected rheumatoid arthritis for 10 years.

☐ **7.15** A 4-year-old girl is brought in by her parents with recurrent bruising. She has previously been fit and well and apart from multiple bruises on her arms and legs, seems well.

☐ **7.16** A 14-year-old boy comes to see you after a traumatic dental extraction that resulted in a significant amount of bleeding. On reflection, his mother reports that he does seem to bruise more than his peers and also comments that his father and paternal uncle have had similar experiences at the dentist.

☐ **7.17** A 23-year-old girl experiences pain, swelling and erythema of her right calf after a flight to Hong Kong. Her only medication is the contraceptive pill and she does not smoke. On further questioning, she reports that her mother had a similar experience some years before.

ALGORITHM QUESTIONS

THEME: INVESTIGATION OF MICROCYTIC ANAEMIA

7.18–7.22

Options

A   α-Thalassaemia trait

B   β-Thalassaemia trait

C   Ferritin

D HbA_2

E   Low

F   No

G   Normal

H   Oral iron

I   Raised

J   Sickle-cell trait

K   Transfusion

L   Yes

The following flow chart has been designed to simplify the investigation of microcytic anaemia (Hb = haemoglobin). From the list of options above, select the most appropriate choice for each numbered step in the flow chart. Each option can be used once, more than once or not at all.

PICTURE QUESTION

7.23 A 62-year-old man comes to see you 24 hours after being discharged from hospital where he had been admitted for a possible MI. He complains that shortly after discharge he started to get blood blisters in his mouth (shown below).

What is the likely diagnosis?

- [ ] A   Aphthous ulceration
- [ ] B   Behçet syndrome
- [ ] C   Immune thrombocytopenia
- [ ] D   Lichen planus
- [ ] E   Trauma

DATA INTERPRETATION QUESTION

7.24 A 53-year-old man with a history of treated hypertension has routine blood tests carried out as part of a 'well man' check. He smokes 10 cigarettes a day and drinks 10–15 units of alcohol a week. His blood results are shown below:

	Result (normal range)
Haemoglobin	20.7 g/dl (12.0–18.0 g/dl)
Platelets	196×10^9/l (150–450×10^9/l)
WCC	2.43×10^9/l (0.9–4.5×10^9/l)
Neutrophils	5.58×10^9/l (1.9–9.0×10^9/l)
Haematocrit	0.58 (0.4–0.5)
Mean corpuscular volume (MCV)	90 fl (80–99 fl)
Mean corpuscular haemoglobin (MCH)	31.7 pg (27–32 pg)

Which one of the following Is the most likely diagnosis?

- [ ] A Acute myeloid leukaemia
- [ ] B B12 deficiency
- [ ] C Chronic lymphocytic leukaemia
- [ ] D Essential thrombocythaemia
- [ ] E Polycythaemia rubra vera

HOT TOPICS/EVIDENCE BASED PRACTICE

7.25 Which one of the following statements about antenatal screening for haemoglobinopathies is true?

☐   A   Antenatal thalassaemia screening is carried out using haemoglobin electrophoresis

☐   B   Currently only 5% of patients are screened for haemoglobinopathies by 10 weeks

☐   C   In high-prevalence areas 95% of women are screened for haemoglobinopathies before 10 weeks' gestation

☐   D   Only pregnant women from high-risk ethnic groups should be offered screening in the first trimester

☐   E   Routine antenatal screening on the NHS is only available in PCTs with high prevalence

ANSWERS

7.1   B: It is associated with aplastic crises

Hereditary spherocytosis is an autosomal recessive condition that affects 1 in 5000 live births. It usually presents in childhood as jaundice or with aplastic crises, usually triggered by parvovirus infections. Most children receive folic acid supplementation. Splenomegaly is common. It is rarely diagnosed in adulthood.

7.2   A: Infarction of the bone marrow causes severe pain

Sickle-cell anaemia affects 1 in 4 West Africans and 1 in 10 Afro-Caribbeans. It is inherited as an autosomal recessive trait and is also carried in Mediterranean and Middle Eastern populations. Homozygotes suffer from infarction of bone marrow and haemolysis during times of low oxygen levels (eg with infections), causing a haemolytic anaemia and extreme bone pain, often requiring opiates. Infection of infarcted bone marrow is common.

7.3   A: 70% of adults under the age of 50 with acute myeloid leukaemia (AML) are treated successfully

In ALL, 50% of patients have a normal WCC but typically have blasts present on the film and a normocytic anaemia. AML is rarely seen in children, whereas ALL is usually seen in children and young adults. The prognosis in AML is better for the under-50s, those with a WCC $< 50 \times 10^9/l$ and those without extramedullary disease at presentation. ALL usually presents with signs of marrow failure or bone pain. Platelets are usually reduced and a diagnosis of leukaemia should always be considered in children with apparent thrombocytopenia.

7.4   E: Platelet disorders usually present with purpura or bleeding gums

Bleeding is rare with a platelet count $> 30 \times 10^9/l$. Aspirin causes platelet dysfunction but not thrombocytopenia. Coagulopathies have numerous causes, including vitamin K deficiency, warfarin and sepsis. Identification of and treatment of underlying causes is critical. Haemophilia A (deficiency of factor VIII) causes 90% of inherited coagulopathy.

7.5   B: Patients should be advised to moderate tomato consumption

Amiodarone inhibits cytochrome p450 metabolism and thus potentiates the effect of warfarin. Warfarin is a vitamin K antagonist, so reduces the levels of protein C and coagulation factors II, VII, IX and X, and excessive consumption of vitamin K (eg in tomatoes) will reverse the effect of warfarin. Dextropropoxyphene interacts with warfarin and co-proxamol should not be prescribed to patients on warfarin. Broad-spectrum antibiotics inhibit bacterial vitamin K production in the gut and therefore enhance the anticoagulant effect of warfarin.

7.6   D: Multiple myeloma

Myeloma often presents with bone pain and examination findings are usually rare. At presentation, many patients will have biochemical evidence of nephropathy and bone destruction, and hyperviscosity is often seen, with a raised ESR and rouleaux formation. Bence Jones protein is characteristically raised. AML and ALL tend to present with signs of bone marrow failure and extramedullary infiltration (eg meningeal signs in AML). CLL presents as a routine finding on an FBC in most cases while CML is usually assosciated with signs of bleeding and hepatosplenomegaly. Myelodysplasia generally presents with fatigue.

7.7   A: This lady has aplastic anaemia

Myelofibrosis typically presents over a longer period of time and is associated with hepatosplenomegaly due to extramedullary haematopoiesis. Aplastic anaemia is idiopathic in at least 70% of cases and has a poor prognosis, with < 50% of patients surviving 6 months.

THEME: ANAEMIA

7.8   G: Iron-deficiency anaemia

Iron deficiency can be caused by blood loss through heavy menstrual bleeding or parasitic infection, or by poor iron intake. An FBC will usually show a microcytosis.

7.9   D: Folate deficiency

Folate deficiency can be due to poor intake or to malabsorption (eg coeliac disease, Crohn's disease). Bloods show a macrocytic anaemia and low folate levels. Treatment is with folate supplementation.

7.10   E: Glucose-6-phosphate dehydrogenase (G6PD) deficiency

G6PD deficiency affects up to 25% of people from southern Africa and the Middle East. Haemolysis can follow infection, fava bean ingestion, drugs (eg dapsone, quinine, antibiotics). Hospital admission is required to avoid renal damage and correct the haemolysis.

7.11   C: B12 deficiency

B12 is found in animal foods, including milk and eggs, but not in vegetables, so vegans are at risk of deficiency. Other causes of B12 deficiency include malabsorption (eg after gastrectomy) and autoantibodies. There is a strong association with vitiligo and Hashimoto's thyroiditis. Treatment is with 3-monthly B12 injections.

7.12   J: Thalassaemia trait

Thalassaemia trait is usually symptomless and is really only of significance if both partners in a relationship are affected.

THEME: CLOTTING DISORDERS

7.13   H: Vitamin K deficiency

Vitamin K deficiency in babies is seen in exclusively breastfed babies who have not received vitamin K and manifests as bleeding, usually between the 2nd and 4th days of life. The cause is a combination of low natural levels at birth coupled with lack of bacterial vitamin K synthesis in the gut and immature liver function. Breast milk is low in vitamin K, whereas formula milk has vitamin K added.

7.14   A: Antiphospholipid syndrome

Antiphospholipid syndrome can be primary or secondary to connective tissue disease, most commonly SLE. It causes recurrent fetal loss, thrombocytopenia and recurrent ischaemic events. It is characterised by the presence of high titres of IgG antiphospholipid antibodies and is thought to be due to a coagulopathy rather than to a vasculitis.

7.15   F: Idiopathic thrombocytopenia

Idiopathic thrombocytopenia is the most likely diagnosis in children, although child abuse and leukaemia should be excluded. In adults taking medication, autoimmune thrombocytopenia is more likely.

7.16   I: von Willebrand's disease

Von Willebrand's disease is inherited as an autosomal dominant trait and is characterised by excessive bleeding after dental extractions and prolonged bleeding time. The bleeding is usually much less severe than in haemophilia and can usually be controlled with tranexamic acid.

7.17   D: Factor V Leiden

Factor V Leiden is a variant of factor V that predisposes to venous thromboembolism. Patients with a suspicious family history should be tested before prescribing the combined oral contraceptive pill.

THEME: INVESTIGATION OF MICROCYTIC ANAEMIA

7.18   C: Ferritin

7.19   G: Normal

7.20   E: Low

7.21   B: β-Thalassaemia trait

7.22   A: α-Thalassaemia trait

7.23   C: Immune thrombocytopenia

Immune thrombocytopenia is typically caused by heparin, sulphonamides, chloramphenicol, sulfasalazine, quinine and quinidine. It typically comes on 2–3 days after taking a drug that has been taken in the past, or 7 days after taking a new drug. It is reported to occur in up to 25% of patients on heparin. The platelet count typically rises 7–10 days after stopping the medication.

7.24   E: Polycythaemia rubra vera

The raised haematocrit and haemoglobin, with normal MCH and MCV suggest the diagnosis is polycythaemia. These results, with a normal plasma volume and raised red cell mass suggests true polycythaemia, rather than dehydration. Secondary causes include hypoxia, smoking and chronic lung disease. Patients should have a bone marrow biopsy to exclude myeloproliferative disease. Treatment is usually regular venesection to keep the haematocrit below 0.45.

7.25   B: Currently only 5% of patients are screened for haemoglobinopathies by 10 weeks

The NHS Sickle Cell and Thalassaemia Screening Programme is designed to offer thalassaemia screening using routine blood indices to all pregnant women before their 10th week of pregnancy, and to offer sickle-cell screening with haemoglobin electrophoresis where local prevalence dictates. Other trusts with lower prevalence are required to offer laboratory testing for patients based on an assessment of risk determined by a question about family origin. A paper in the *British Journal of General Practice* (*BJGP* 2008; 58: 154–9) found that less than 5% of women had been screened by 10 weeks, the target date set to allow the possibility of elective termination if thalassaemia is diagnosed.

CHAPTER 8
IMMUNOLOGY
SINGLE BEST ANSWER QUESTIONS

8.1 You are updating the protocols for pneumococcal vaccination in the practice. Which one of the following patient groups needs a booster vaccination after routine primary immunisation?

- [ ] A Patients with asthma
- [ ] B Patients with chronic kidney disease
- [ ] C Patients with chronic obstructive pulmonary disease
- [ ] D Patients with diabetes
- [ ] E Patients with stable ischaemic heart disease

8.2 The father of a 2-year-old girl with biliary atresia comes to see you. He has just been told that she will need another liver transplant and would like to know if he can be a living donor. Which one of the following statements is true regarding this situation?

- [ ] A 1-year survival after liver transplantation is 50% in children
- [ ] B Immunosupression is usually only required for 6–12 months after a transplant
- [ ] C Prednisolone is the most commonly used immunosuppressant
- [ ] D Transplantation can only occur if the donor and recipient are HLA-compatible
- [ ] E The donor must be tested for hepatitis B and C

8.3 **Which one of the following statements is true in relation to allergy testing?**

☐ A Allergy is associated with the presence of IgA antibodies

☐ B Negative radioallergosorbent testing (RAST) excludes significant allergy

☐ C RAST testing involves placing a small amount of allergen on the skin and observing the reaction

☐ D RAST detects the presence of allergen-specific IgE

☐ E RAST will provide an indication of the severity of any likely reaction if a patient is exposed to a particular antigen

8.4 **Regarding the drug management of allergic rhinitis, which one of the following statements is true?**

☐ A Anticholinergics are effective for rhinorrhoea

☐ B Antileukotrienes are effective for ocular but not nasal symptoms

☐ C Nasal steroids are effective for nasal symptoms, but not for ocular symptoms

☐ D Oral antihistamines are the most effective treatment for nasal symptoms

☐ E Treatment of asthma has no effect on allergic rhinitis

8.5 **Which of the following statements about drug treatment in allergy is true? Select one option only.**

☐ A Cromoglicate inhibits mast-cell degranulation

☐ B Loratadine is not associated with sedation

☐ C Mometasone is a mild steroid that can be safely used long-term

☐ D Oral prednisolone should not be stopped abruptly if the course is longer than 1 week due to suppression of the adrenal glands

☐ E Use of steroid inhalers in children has not been shown to be associated with long-term side-effects

EXTENDED MATCHING QUESTIONS

THEME: VACCINES

Options

A Inactivated

B Immunoglobulins

C Live attenuated

D Recombinant antigen

E Toxoid

For each of the vaccine types given below, select the most appropriate option to describe its mode of action from the list above. Each option may be used once, more than once or not at all.

☐ **8.6** Pertussis.

☐ **8.7** Measles, mumps and rubella (MMR).

☐ **8.8** Tetanus.

☐ **8.9** Hepatitis B.

☐ **8.10** Salk polio vaccine.

THEME: ALLERGY TESTING

Options

A Exclusion diet

B IgE levels

C None of these options

D Patch testing

E RAST testing

F Skin-prick testing

G Symptom diary

For each of the situations described below, select the most appropriate investigation from the list above. Each option may be used once, more than once or not at all.

8.11 A 35-year-old marketing executive complains of abdominal bloating and cramps after eating certain foodstuffs.

8.12 A 48-year-old woman who complains of 5 years of fatigue and myalgia, which she feels are due to mercury in her dental fillings.

8.13 A 13-year-old boy complains of rhinitis and wheeze for most days of the year, which are worse when he visits his father's house and better when he goes on holiday.

8.14 A 36-year-old paramedic complains of recurrent dermatitis affecting his hands when he is at work, which rapidly improves on holiday.

8.15 Associated with a risk of anaphylaxis.

ALGORITHM QUESTIONS

THEME: ALLERGY MANAGEMENT IN PRIMARY CARE

8.16–8.20

Options

A Admit

B Beta-2 agonist

C Beta blockade

D Depo-Medrone

E Intramuscular adrenaline (epinephrine)

F Intravenous adrenaline (epinephrine)

G Oral antihistamine

H Oral prednisolone

For each of the numbered gaps in the following allergy management flow chart, select the most appropriate option from the list above. Each option can be used once, more than once or not at all.

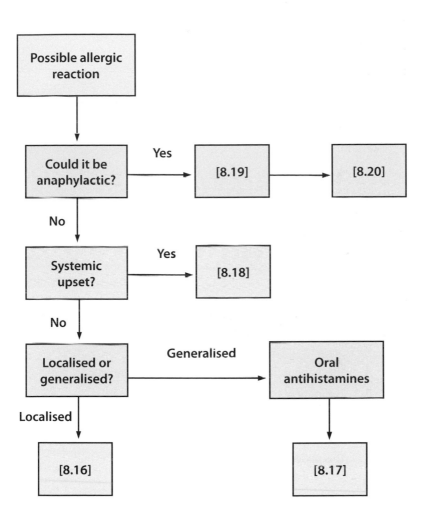

PICTURE QUESTION

8.21 Consider the picture below:

Which one of the following statements about this situation is true?

- ☐ A This patient has experienced a fixed drug reaction
- ☐ B This patient has had patch testing performed
- ☐ C This patient has had skin-prick testing
- ☐ D This patient is suffering from bullous pemphigoid
- ☐ E This patient is suffering from erythema multiforme

DATA INTERPRETATION QUESTION

8.22 A 24-year-old woman is 12 weeks pregnant. She works as a preschool teacher and one of the children has recently been diagnosed with suspected chickenpox. She feels as if she has a temperature but has no rash. She is not sure if she has had chickenpox in the past, and her mother cannot recall this either. Blood tests are carried out which show the following results:

Varicella IgG	Elevated
Varicella IgM	Normal
Measles IgG	Normal
Measles IgM	Normal

Which one of the following statements about this patient's varicella status is correct?

- ☐ A She has been infected with varicella in the past and is now immune
- ☐ B She has not been exposed in the past to chickenpox
- ☐ C She has recently been infected with chickenpox
- ☐ D She is measles-immune
- ☐ E The results are most likely to be due to childhood vaccination

HOT TOPICS/EVIDENCE BASED PRACTICE

8.23 Which one of the following statements about the use of immunotherapy in allergic conditions is true?

- ☐ A Grazax is effective in patients with allergic rhinitis due to house dust mite only where RAST tests are positive

- ☐ B Sublingual immunotherapy can be used on an as-needed basis

- ☐ C Sublingual immunotherapy is effective in patients with allergic rhinitis only

- ☐ D Sublingual immunotherapy results in angioedema in 15% of patients

- ☐ E Use of sublingual grass allergen tablets results in a significant reduction in medication use

ANSWERS

8.1   B: Patients with chronic kidney disease

Patients with chronic kidney disease, hyposplenism or asplenia should have booster doses of pneumococcal vaccine and Haemophilus vaccine every 5 years. Children vaccinated routinely should also have a booster dose at 13 months.

8.2   E: The donor must be tested for hepatitis B and C

Around 25% of children die on the waiting list for a donor. HLA matching is not necessary for liver transplants. Immunosuppression is required for life, but the regime can often be reduced with time. Ciclosporin and tacrolimus are the most commonly used agents. The presence of antibodies to hepatitis B and C will usually rule out a potential donor. One-year survival is 60% for adults and 80% for children. Overall survival figures are best for paracetamol poisoning and fulminant hepatitis A, and worst for hepatitis C.

8.3   D: RAST detects the presence of allergen-specific IgE

RAST testing detects specific IgE antibodies against allergens. It is useful for confirmation of provocation of allergy by individual allergens. It is expensive and the magnitude of reaction does not always correlate with symptoms. It is useful in anaphylaxis (eg bee venom), food allergies (but not food intolerance) and occupational allergens (eg latex allergy). It is a blood test, unlike patch testing, in which a small amount of allergen is placed on the skin and the reaction observed.

8.4   A: Anticholinergics are effective for rhinorrhoea

The ARIA (Allergic Rhinitis and its Impact on Asthma) guidelines for the treatment of allergic rhinitis suggest that oral antihistamines are effective for sneezing, rhinorrhea and eye symptoms but not for nasal obstruction. Intraocular antihistamines are effective only for eye symptoms. Corticosteroids are the most effective treatment for all symptoms, although they are not as effective for eye symptoms as intraocular antihistamines. Decongestants are effective only for nasal obstruction, while anticholinergics are effective only for rhinorrhoea. Anti-leukotriene antagonists are moderately effective for all symptoms except nasal itch.

Treatment of asthma will often improve symptoms of allergic rhinitis and vice versa.

8.5   A: Cromoglicate inhibits mast-cell degranulation

Sodium cromoglicate is useful in reducing sneezing but not nasal obstruction. It is also useful as eye drops for relieving itchy eyes. Non-sedating antihistamines cause sedation in 1–5% of patients. Mometasone is a potent steroid that is not suitable for long-term skin use but can be used in the nasal preparation for long periods. Prednisolone can be taken orally for up to 3 weeks without tapering. There are many reports of Cushing syndrome and osteoporosis in patients using high-dose steroid inhalers (>2000 micrograms/day).

THEME: VACCINES

8.6   A: Inactivated

The pertussis vaccine, either on its own or as part of a combination vaccine, contains inactivated *Bordetella pertussis*.

8.7   C: Live attenuated

MMR is a live attenuated vaccine.

8.8   E: Toxoid

Tetanus vaccine is a toxoid and is either given alone or in combination.

8.9   D: Recombinant antigen

Hepatitis B vaccine is a recombinant vaccine containing HBsAg cultured from yeast cells.

8.10   A: Inactivated

Inactivated polio vaccines are now the norm, and oral live vaccine is no longer used routinely in the UK. The current vaccine in use contains three strains of poliovirus.

THEME: ALLERGY TESTING

8.11   A: Exclusion diet

Food intolerance is distinct from food allergy and can have a metabolic basis (eg lactase deficiency). Symptoms are distinct from food allergy, an IgE-mediated reaction characterised by nausea, vomiting, diarrhoea, urticaria and angioedema. Food intolerance can be diagnosed by exclusion diet but ideally this should be under the supervision of a dietician if there are multiple potential causes, to avoid malnutrition.

8.12   C: None of these options

These symptoms are not suggestive of allergy or intolerance. She should be questioned about other somatic symptoms and a diagnosis of depression considered. She would be best advised to seek dental advice regarding her fillings.

8.13   E: RAST testing

RAST testing will help to identify allergic reactions, which would allow some lifestyle modification, for example if cats or dogs are involved. If allergy to house dust mite is detected this is often difficult to manage because of the prevalence of this allergen and the limited evidence for efficacy of house dust mite elimination.

8.14   D: Patch testing

Patch testing will identify most T cell-mediated delayed hypersensitivity contact allergens. Around 20–30 suspect allergens are tested as a batch and the responses used to identify which the culprits are. Appropriate precautions, eg hypoallergenic gloves or soaps, can then be taken.

8.15   F: Skin-prick testing

Skin-prick testing is generally safe for aero-allergens such as moulds or house dust mite, but should only be carried out in hospital for food allergies and venom, because of the risk of anaphylaxis.

THEME: ALLERGY MANAGEMENT IN PRIMARY CARE

8.16   G: Oral antihistamine

8.17   H: Oral prednisolone

8.18   H: Oral prednisolone

8.19   E: Intramuscular adrenaline (epinephrine)

8.20   A: Admit

8.21   B: This patient has had patch testing performed

This patient has had patch testing, which is suitable for occupational allergies (eg contact dermatitis). Aero-allergens are better tested with skin-prick testing.

8.22   A: She has been infected with varicella in the past and is now immune

IgM is the first antibody to be produced in infection; IgG is produced later. Recent infection therefore results in raised virus-specific IgM, while historical infection results in raised IgG with normal IgM.

8.23   E: Use of sublingual grass allergen tablets results in a significant reduction in medication use

Grazax, a purified grass allergen extract in tablet form, is taken up to 16 weeks before the start of the allergy season in patients with proven IgE-mediated grass pollen sensitivity (either through RAST testing or skin-prick testing). It is well tolerated and results in a 30% reduction in symptoms and a 38% reduction in medication use. Serious side-effects have not been reported in trials (*J Allergy Clin Immunol* 2006; 118(2): 434–40). Meta-analysis has shown that immunotherapy also reduces symptoms and medication use in paediatric asthma patients (*Chest* 2007; 133: 599–609).

CHAPTER 9
INFECTION
SINGLE BEST ANSWER QUESTIONS

9.1 A 47-year-old man who works in a water treatment plant complains of flu-like symptoms of headache, myalgia and fever. He has been taking over-the-counter medication for this but after 6 days he becomes concerned because his skin looks yellow. On examination he has widespread lymphadenopathy, an enlarged liver and is jaundiced. Reviewing his medical notes you see that he has been vaccinated against hepatitis A and hepatitis B and has no other risk factors. What is the single most likely diagnosis?

☐ A *Campylobacter*

☐ C Escherichia coli O157

☐ B Epstein–Barr virus

☐ D Leptospirosis

☐ E Shigellosis

9.2   A 26-year-old man asks for a human immunodeficiency virus (HIV) test. He has no particular risk factors but would like to be tested to make sure he is healthy. Before the test you counsel him regarding the nature of the disease, the implications of testing and likely outcomes if he is positive. Which one of the following statements is correct regarding this information?

- [ ] A   Antenatal screening in England has shown that 1 in 200 pregnant women in some inner-city areas are infected with HIV
- [ ] B   At-risk groups in the UK are almost exclusively homosexual and bisexual men, their partners and those involved in the sex industry
- [ ] C   HIV is rare throughout the UK, with a prevalence of 1 in 500 000
- [ ] D   People infected with HIV have a significantly higher death rate than the general population in spite of antiretroviral treatment
- [ ] E   The prognosis for people with HIV is the same regardless of route of transmission

9.3   Your next patient is a 12-year-old girl who has come with her mother. The girl is due to have her human papillomavirus (HPV) vaccination at school soon. Her mother is very uneasy about this and asks your advice on whether it is worth having. Which one of the following statements is true regarding this issue?

- [ ] A   A single dose is given at age 13
- [ ] B   The HPV vaccine will prevent her getting genital warts and cervical cancer
- [ ] C   The vaccine is associated with potentially serious adverse reactions
- [ ] D   Vaccination does not need to start until a girl becomes sexually active
- [ ] E   Where three doses of vaccine are given it is > 97% effective

9.4 According to current guidelines, what are the recommendations for antimalarial chemoprophylaxis for pregnant women travelling to malarial areas? Select one option only.

☐ A Doxycycline is safe in all trimesters of pregnancy

☐ B Mefloquine is thought to be safe in treatment doses in the second and third trimesters

☐ C Pregnant women are less at risk of developing malaria, so chemoprophylaxis should be avoided

☐ D Pregnant women taking chloroquine should receive supplementation with 5 mg folic acid daily

☐ E Women who have taken mefloquine prior to or during the first trimester should consider a termination

9.5 A 42-year-old man with rheumatoid arthritis was bitten by a dog yesterday. He now has an infected wound on his hand. Which one of the following is the most appropriate management option?

☐ A Copious irrigation, leave any foreign body and refer to a specialist, administer flucloxacillin or erythromycin and a tetanus vaccination, review in 24–48 hours

☐ B Copious irrigation, remove any foreign body and leave the wound open, administer co-amoxiclav and a tetanus vaccination, review in 24–48 hours

☐ C Copious irrigation, remove any foreign body, close the wound, administer co-amoxiclav and a tetanus vaccination, review in 24–48 hours

☐ D Copious irrigation, remove any foreign body, close the wound, administer flucloxacillin or erythromycin and a tetanus vaccination, review in 24–48 hours

☐ E Copious irrigation, remove any foreign body, leave the wound open, administer flucloxacillin or erythromycin only if there are signs of infection, give a tetanus vaccination, review in 24–48 hours

9.6 Which types of human papillomavirus (HPV) are known to cause the majority of cervical cancers in women? Select one option only.

- [ ] A HPV 6 and HPV 11
- [ ] B HPV 15 and HPV 17
- [ ] C HPV 15 and HPV 18
- [ ] D HPV 16 and HPV 18
- [ ] E HPV 31 and HPV 45

9.7 A 19-year-old woman presents with a burning sensation when passing urine and a yellow, bloodstained vaginal discharge. She admits to having had unprotected sexual intercourse 4 days ago. What is the single most likely diagnosis?

- [ ] A Bacterial vaginosis
- [ ] B *Chlamydia*
- [ ] C Gonorrhoea
- [ ] D Syphilis
- [ ] E Trichomoniasis

9.8 What are the current guidelines for the management of head lice in schools and other childcare settings? Select one option only.

- [ ] A All close contacts should be treated to prevent spread
- [ ] B Any child with head lice should be excluded from school until adequately treated
- [ ] C If chemical insecticides are being used, one application should be sufficient
- [ ] D Regular detection by combing should be carried out by parents
- [ ] E Treatment is recommended when hatched eggs or nits have definitely been seen

9.9 Which of the following vaccines contain live organisms? Select one option only

☐ A DTaP

☐ B Hib

☐ C Influenza

☐ D MMR

☐ E Pneumococcal vaccine

9.10 A 4-year-old girl is brought in by her mother with a 3-day history of cough, runny nose and watery eyes. Today, mum has noticed red spots with white centres inside the girl's cheeks. Which one of the following is the single most likely diagnosis?

☐ A Measles

☐ B Rhinovirus

☐ C Rubella

☐ D Scarlet fever

☐ E Varicella

9.11 Which of the following statements about conjunctivitis is true? Select one option only.

☐ A Adenoviral conjunctivitis is rarely bilateral

☐ B Children should be excluded from nursery until the eyes are no longer weeping or until they have had 24 hours of eye drops

☐ C In the UK it is a notifiable disease in neonates aged under 1 month

☐ D It should always be treated with antibiotic eye drops

☐ E Patients with simple bacterial conjunctivitis should be reviewed if is no better after 48 hours

EXTENDED MATCHING QUESTIONS

THEME: GASTROINTESTINAL INFECTIONS

Options

A *Giardia*

B *Listeria*

C Norovirus

D Rotavirus

E Typhoid

For each patient described below, select the single most appropriate diagnosis from the list above. Each option can be used once, more than once or not at all.

☐ **9.12** A 9-month-old girl presents with a 4-day history of diarrhoea, vomiting and dehydration.

☐ **9.13** A 24-year-old teacher presents with a fever and diarrhoea and vomiting for the last 24 hours.

☐ **9.14** A 32-year-old farmer has a 7-day history of mild, flu-like symptoms and mild gastroenteritis.

☐ **9.15** A 50-year-old man returned home from a riverboat trip in India 8 days ago and presents with abdominal cramps and severe diarrhoea.

☐ **9.16** A 59-year-old Kenyan woman is visiting the UK for the first time and has a 2-week history of fever, headache, stomach pains, anorexia and nausea.

THEME: ANTIBIOTICS

Options

A   Admit for intravenous antibiotics

B   Amoxicillin

C   Co-amoxiclav

D   Flucloxacillin

E   Fucidic acid cream

F   Metronidazole

G   No treatment necessary

H   Trimethoprim for 3 days

I   Trimethoprim for 7 days

For each of the following scenarios select the most appropriate antibiotic from the list of options. Each option can be used once, more than once or not at all.

☐ **9.17** An 8-year-old girl presents to the out-of-hours service with a 24-hour history of fever and a painful left ear; tonight, mum has noticed a small amount of bloody discharge on her pillow.

☐ **9.18** A 4-year-old boy has had a yellow, crusted lesion on his chin for a few days and has now developed a similar one on his right arm.

☐ **9.19** A woman with dysuria and frequency is currently 32 weeks pregnant.

☐ **9.20** A 64-year-old man comes to consult following a cat scratch to his face. On examination, he is afebrile with cellulitis around the scratch.

☐ **9.21** High vaginal swab results for a 38-year-old lady show bacterial vaginosis.

ALGORITHM QUESTIONS

THEME: THE ACUTE MANAGEMENT OF URINARY TRACT INFECTION IN CHILDREN

9.22–9.30

Options

A 5–7 days

B 7 days

C 7–10 days

D 10 days

E A once daily dose

F Await culture result before treating

G Consider referral

H Continue antibiotics for a further 5 days

I Low resistance pattern

J Intravenous antibiotics for 2–4 days

K Intravenous antibiotics for 5 days

L Oral antibiotics for 3 days

M Oral antibiotics for 5 days

N Reassess

O Refer immediately

P Send urine for culture

For each numbered question, select the correct option to complete the algorithm from the list above. Each answer can be used once, more than once or not at all.

PICTURE QUESTIONS

9.31 A 39-year-old man complains of a sore insect bite. He thinks he was bitten 2–3 days ago while camping in the New Forest and the bite has been very itchy. The bite is shown below.

What is the most appropriate treatment?

☐ A   Oral ampicillin

☐ B   Oral doxycycline

☐ C   Oral flucloxacillin

☐ D   Oral loratadine

☐ E   Topical Betnovate

9.32 This 38-year-old soldier returned from a period in Iraq 2 weeks ago. He has developed a lesion on his skin which started as an erythematous papule:

What is the single most likely diagnosis from the list below?

- ☐ A Cutaneous leishmaniasis
- ☐ B Cutaneous tuberculosis
- ☐ C Leprosy
- ☐ D Syphilis
- ☐ E Systemic lupus erythematosus

DATA INTERPRETATION QUESTION

9.33 **A 9-month-old girl presents with a fever and vomiting. A urine sample was sent to the laboratory and you receive the following result:**

White cells	> 100 cells per μl
Red blood cells	> 100 cells per μl
Organisms	3+
Epithelial cells	1+
Culture	*Escherichia coli* > 10^8

Which of the following would be the single most appropriate initial management for this child?

☐ A   Refer immediately for an urgent ultrasound scan of the kidneys

☐ B   Repeat the urine sample to ensure that it is not a contaminated specimen

☐ C   Start antibiotics, continue with a prophylactic dose and review in 2 months

☐ D   Start antibiotics immediately and refer for urgent paediatric assessment

☐ E   Start antibiotics immediately and repeat the urine sample in 7–10 days to confirm that the infection has cleared

ANSWERS

9.1   D: Leptospirosis

Leptospirosis can be spread by a number of different rodents but is usually associated with rats. People who work in environments with large numbers of rats are most at risk (eg sewage workers). Infection causes an initial flu-like illness, after which a proportion of patients go on to develop jaundice, renal failure and meningism. Most patients make an uneventful recovery. Diagnosis is by complement fixation of urine culture for leptospira. Penicillin or tetracycline is usually effective treatment.

9.2   A: Antenatal screening in the UK has shown that 1 in 200 pregnant women in some inner-city areas are infected with HIV

Routine screening of blood during pregnancy has shown levels from 1 in 500 to 1 in 200 in areas of London, while it is estimated that in parts of Edinburgh and Glasgow prevalence may be as high as 1 in 20 in areas of high intravenous drug abuse. At-risk groups in the UK include an increasing number of heterosexual men. In sub-Saharan Africa and Latin America heterosexuals make up the biggest number of cases, while in Zaire it is estimated that 90–100% of the army are HIV positive. In the first 5 years of antiretroviral treatment, the death rate is the same as the in general population, except for intravenous drug users who have higher death rates.

9.3   E: Where three doses of vaccine are given it is > 97% effective

The HPV vaccination programme aims to prevent infection with the strains of HPV (16, 18) which are associated with genital warts and cervical cancer in the UK. These vaccines are given in three doses from age 13 and provide 97–99% coverage. There have been no reports of serious adverse reactions. The vaccine covers some wart viruses but not all, so patients can still develop genital warts. There are currently two vaccines available in the UK, Gardasil and Cervarix. Gardasil also provides coverage against HPV 6 and HPV 11, so is likely to provide additional cover against warts. Vaccination should start before sexual activity begins to ensure adequate protection before first exposure.

9.4   B: Mefloquine is thought to be safe in treatment doses in the second and third trimesters

There is no strong association between mefloquine in treatment doses and stillbirths or miscarriages in the second and third trimesters, although lack of data on its use in the first trimester has encouraged caution. Pregnant women have an increased risk of developing severe malaria and have a higher risk of fatality. Doxycycline is contraindicated in pregnancy and those taking proguanil should also take folic acid. Women who have taken mefloquine prior to or during the first trimester should be advised that this is not an indication to terminate the pregnancy.

9.5   B: Copious irrigation, remove any foreign body and leave the wound open, administer co-amoxiclav and a tetanus vaccination, review in 24–48 hours

A clinical review looking at the management of dog bites was published in the *BMJ* in 2007. Copious irrigation with tap water or normal saline is essential. Any foreign body (eg teeth) should be removed, with debridement where necessary. Closure of the wound should be delayed where possible. Antibiotics should be administered according to the risk of infection. Prophylactic antibiotics are indicated for all high-risk wounds and patients. Bites to the hands, wrists and genitalia are considered high-risk as are patients with rheumatoid arthritis. Co-amoxiclav is the antibiotic of choice as it covers all commonly expected organisms. For those with a true penicillin allergy, tetracycline or doxycycline plus metronidazole or a combination with clindamycin should be used. Flucloxacillin or erythromycin alone should not be used for prophylaxis as they do not cover the virulent *Pasteurella multocida*, commonly found in dog bites. Tetanus immunoglobulin and toxoid should be given to all patients with a history of two or fewer immunisations.

9.6   D: HPV 16 and HPV 18

Cervical cancer is the second most common cancer in females worldwide. HPV 16 and HPV 18 are responsible for approximately 70% of all cervical cancers.

9.7   C: Gonorrhoea

The early signs of gonorrhoea can be mild and are often missed, but symptoms in women can include a painful and burning sensation when passing urine and a yellow, bloodstained vaginal discharge. Symptoms usually appear 2–10 days after becoming infected. *Chlamydia* infection usually presents 1–3 weeks after becoming infected. Symptoms include bleeding between periods, an unusual vaginal discharge and lower abdominal pain. Around 70% of women have no symptoms at all. The symptoms of syphilis are generally non-specific and it usually presents with a painless but infectious sore anywhere on the body which resolves spontaneously in 2–6 weeks. Bacterial vaginosis presents with a typical grey–yellow, fishy, offensive discharge and it is not a sexually transmitted infection. Trichomoniasis presents with a typical yellow–green, frothy discharge and is less common than other sexually transmitted infections.

9.8   D: Regular detection by combing should be carried out by parents

Plastic combs have been designed to be used with conditioner and studies have shown 38–57% cure rates after 14 days of treatment. Children should no longer be excluded from school if they have head lice. Treatment is only recommended where live lice have definitely been seen; hatched eggs or nits are not evidence of infestation. Close contacts should be checked and only treated if live lice have been seen. If chemical insecticides are being used, at least two applications are needed, 7 days apart, to kill the lice that emerge from eggs after the first treatment.

9.9   D: MMR

The MMR vaccine contains attenuated (modified) live organisms. DTaP, Hib, influenza, pneumococcal and rabies vaccines do not contain live organisms and so cannot cause the illness which they immunise against.

9.10   A: Measles

Tiny, bluish-white spots with surrounding erythema seen on the buccal mucosa of the cheek, known as 'Koplik's spots', are pathognomonic of early-stage measles. The first symptoms of measles include cough, coryza, conjunctivitis, fever and malaise. A florid erythematous maculopapular rash, which starts at the head appears 3–4 days later. Koplik's spots can appear 1–2 days before the rash.

9.11   C: Conjunctivitis is a notifiable disease in neonates aged under 1 month

Ophthalmia neonatorum, conjunctivitis in the first 28 days of life, is a notifiable disease under the Public Health Regulations Act 1988. A seminal randomised controlled trial (RCT) published in the *Lancet* in 2005 comparing placebo with chloramphenicol drops in children with conjunctivitis concluded that we should stop prescribing antibiotic drops for conjunctivitis in children and instead advise them to keep the eye clean and return for review if no better after 1 week. The HPA's guidance on infection control in schools and other childcare settings does not recommend any time away for children with conjunctivitis. Simple bacterial conjunctivitis is usually self-limiting, lasting 10–14 days. Review if no better at 1 week to exclude corneal involvement or other complications is recommended. Adenoviral conjunctivitis is highly contagious, so often rapidly becomes bilateral.

THEME: GASTROINTESTINAL INFECTIONS

9.12   D: Rotavirus

Rotavirus is the most common cause of gastroenteritis in infants. It can cause severe vomiting, diarrhoea and stomach cramps. These symptoms usually last for 3–8 days. Once someone has had rotavirus they usually develop immunity, so it is rare in adults.

9.13   C: Norovirus

Norovirus is the most common cause of gastroenteritis in England and Wales. It can occur at any age because immunity is not long-lasting. It tends to be seasonal and is more common in the winter months. Outbreaks of norovirus are seen particularly in semi-closed environments such as hospitals, nursing homes and schools.

9.14   B: *Listeria*

Listeria is a rare but potentially life-threatening infection. Healthy adults usually experience a mild infection with flu-like symptoms or gastroenteritis. Pregnant women, the elderly and the immunosuppressed are more susceptible to *Listeria*.

9.15   A: *Giardia*

Giardia grows in the intestines of infected humans or animals and causes diarrhoeal disease in humans. It is transmitted by direct contact with infected humans or animals or by consumption of water, food or drinks contaminated by the faeces of infected humans or animals. People can be infected by swimming in contaminated water, for example in rivers or lakes. Many cases are associated with foreign travel.

9.16   E: Typhoid

Typhoid varies in severity but nearly all patients experience fever and headache. The incubation period is usually 7–14 days. Symptoms include sustained fever, headache, anorexia, nausea and stomach pains. Some patients develop a rash. It is almost exclusively acquired abroad through ingestion of heavily contaminated food or water.

THEME: ANTIBIOTICS

9.17   B: Amoxicillin

This girl has otitis media with a perforated eardrum. Most GPs would prescribe antibiotics once a perforation occurs. However, most cases of uncomplicated otitis media are viral and 80% resolve without antibiotics.

9.18   D: Flucloxacillin

This is impetigo which has spread. Because of increasing resistance, current advice is for topical treatment to be reserved for very localised lesions.

9.19   I: Trimethoprim for 7 days

Current guidelines for urinary tract infections in pregnancy suggest that trimethoprim is unlikely to cause problems in the fetus in the third trimester, so first-line antibiotics for urinary tract infections in pregnancy are trimethoprim or nitrofurantoin; second-line antibiotics are cefalexin or amoxicillin. All these antibiotics should be given for 7 days in pregnancy.

9.20   C: Co-amoxiclav

Co-amoxiclav is used for facial cellulitis, and is the drug of choice for animal scratches and bites. Flucloxacillin or erythromycin (if penicillin-allergic) can be used for cellulitis elsewhere unless the infection is due to an animal scratch or bite. A febrile or ill patient should be admitted for intravenous antibiotics.

9.21   F: Metronidazole

Bacterial vaginosis can be treated with oral or vaginal metronidazole or vaginal clindamycin cream.

THEME: THE ACUTE MANAGEMENT OF URINARY TRACT INFECTION IN CHILDREN

9.22   O: Refer immediately

9.23   I: Low resistance pattern

9.24   G: Consider referral

9.25   C: 7–10 days

9.26   J: Intravenous antibiotics for 2–4 days

9.27   D: 10 days

9.28   L: Oral antibiotics for 3 days

9.29   P: Send urine for culture

9.30   N: Reassess

9.31   C: Oral flucloxacillin

This lesion is a secondarily infected insect bite. When these bites are very itchy, patients often scratch and introduce staphylococcal infection. Patients who have been in areas where deer are found can contract Lyme disease from tick bites, but these usually present with annular erythema rather than pus at the bite site. Non-infected bites can be treated with antihistamines or in severe cases with topical steroids. Lyme disease is treated with doxycycline in adults or a macrolide antibiotic in children.

9.32   A: Cutaneous leishmaniasis

Leishmaniasis is a parasitic disease spread by infected female sandflies and is mainly seen in the tropics and subtropics. It can be visceral, cutaneous or mucocutaneous. Visceral leishmaniasis is serious and can be fatal. Cutaneous leishmaniasis presents with one or more skin lesions that start as red papules and develop into ulcers. These can change in shape and appearance over time. There can be associated lymphadanopathy. With no treatment these ulcers will heal themselves, usually within 10 months, but can leave depigmented scars or go on to cause mucocutaneous leishmaniasis, which is very disfiguring. It is therefore advisable to treat after seeking advice from the local centre for disease control.

9.33   D: Start antibiotics immediately and refer for urgent
paediatric assessment

This result indicates a genuine bacterial infection. The risk of ascending infection and renal damage is high from birth to 6 years of age. Infection at this age suggests a structural renal abnormality.

CHAPTER 10
MENTAL HEALTH AND
LEARNING DISABILITY
SINGLE BEST ANSWER QUESTIONS

10.1 You see a 21-year-old patient who has recently been discharged from a mental health unit after a psychotic incident. His mother thinks it has been caused by smoking cannabis. Which one of the following statements regarding this association is true?

    ☐ A   Cannabis use moderates pre-existing psychotic symptoms

    ☐ B   Patients with recent psychosis are twice as likely to have used cannabis as patients without psychosis

    ☐ C   Skunk is associated with psychosis, but cannabis is not

    ☐ D   There is no evidence of long-term harm from cannabis use

    ☐ E   There is unequivocal proof that smoking cannabis causes psychosis

10.2 **Which one of the following statements about the risk factors for schizophrenia is true?**

☐ A Development of schizophrenia is not associated with physical health

☐ B Genetic factors account for 90% of the risk of developing schizophrenia

☐ C Patients with premorbid schizoid personality traits are more likely to develop schizophrenia

☐ D Studies have failed to show any genetic factors in schizophrenia

☐ E There are no known biochemical triggers for the development of schizophrenia

10.3 **You work in an area with a number of care homes and are approached to give a talk on the Mental Capacity Act, 2005, which has recently come into force. Which one of the following statements is true regarding this legislation and its impact on everyday practice?**

☐ A It allows for the establishment of a Lasting Power of Attorney (LPA), which allows both financial and treatment decisions to be made on behalf of patients

☐ B It can be used to make treatment decisions on behalf of severely brain-damaged children

☐ C Next of kin are automatically nominated to make decisions in the event of incapacity

☐ D The Act specifies that advance directives are legally binding, whether verbal or written, as long as they are witnessed

☐ E Where a decision about place of residence needs to be made and there is no close relative to make it, the decision can be made by the treating doctor

10.4 Which of the following is the most appropriate first-line management for mild depression? Select one option only.

☐ A Citalopram

☐ B Cognitive behavioural therapy (CBT)

☐ C Fluoxetine

☐ D Paroxetine

☐ E Psychodynamic psychotherapy

10.5 Which one of the following is a risk factor for the development of depression?

☐ A Antisocial personality traits

☐ B Anxious/avoidant personality traits

☐ C High incidence of expressed emotion

☐ D Male sex

☐ E Paranoid personality traits

10.6 Mania is associated with which of the following? Select one option only.

☐ A Increased sleep

☐ B Increased frequency of pregnancy in women

☐ C Mild overspending

☐ D Reduced productivity

☐ E Symptom duration of not less than 2 weeks

10.7 **Which one of the following symptoms is a first-rank symptom of schizophrenia?**

☐ A Delusional perception

☐ B Incongruent affect

☐ C Loosening of associations

☐ D Second-person auditory hallucinations

☐ E Splitting

10.8 **Which one of the following statements about physical health in mental illness is true?**

☐ A Physical health improves during manic periods in patients with bipolar disorder

☐ B Physical health is at risk in patients with mental health problems

☐ C Physical health is significantly better in obsessive–compulsive disorder (OCD) when compared with the general population

☐ D Physical health is unaffected by depression

☐ E Physical health is unaffected by schizophrenia

10.9 **Which one of the following is suggestive of alcohol dependency?**

☐ A Binge drinking

☐ B Drinking alone

☐ C Family history of alcohol dependency

☐ D Salience of drinking habits

☐ E The drinking of clear spirits only

10.10 Which one of the following statements about delirium is correct?

☐ A Delirium is best treated with antipsychotics

☐ B Delirium is categorised as an organic disorder

☐ C Delirium is typified by auditory hallucinations

☐ D Delirium only occurs in the elderly

☐ E Delirium only occurs in those with a pre-existing psychiatric diagnosis

10.11 Which one of the following is a feature of dementia?

☐ A Impairment of consciousness

☐ B Impairment of intellectual functioning

☐ C Preservation of personality

☐ D Spontaneous recovery

☐ F Onset in childhood

10.12 Which one of the following statements about obsessive-compulsive disorder (OCD) is true?

☐ A OCD involves unpleasant thoughts that the individual does not recognise as being their own

☐ B OCD is commonly associated with anxiety and depression

☐ C OCD is commonly associated with mania

☐ D OCD raises the risk of suicide in sufferers

☐ E The onset of OCD tends to be earlier in men than in women

10.13 **Which one of the following statements about childhood autism is true?**

- [ ] A   Involves a preference for consistency and routine
- [ ] B   Involves the normal early development of social interactions
- [ ] C   Is a subtype of psychosis
- [ ] D   Is associated with a reciprocal 'social smile'
- [ ] E   Is not associated with self-harm

10.14 **Which one of the following statements about encopresis is true?**

- [ ] A   It cannot be diagnosed before the age of 4 years
- [ ] B   It involves the voluntary passage of faeces
- [ ] C   It is a particularly common problem in lower socio-economic groups
- [ ] D   It is best managed with a coercive approach to potty training
- [ ] E   It is more common in females

10.15 **Which one of the following statements about suicide is true?**

- [ ] A   Rates are highest over the Christmas and New Year holiday period
- [ ] B   Suicide by dangerous methods is more common in women
- [ ] C   Suicide is more common in men
- [ ] D   The incidence is 1/100 000 per year
- [ ] E   The risk of suicide is raised in schizophrenia when accompanied by akathisia

EXTENDED MATCHING QUESTIONS

THEME: SIDE-EFFECTS OF ANTIDEPRESSANTS

Options

A   Amisulpiride

B   Citalopram

C   Fluoxetine

D   Lamotrigine

E   Mirtazepine

F   St John's wort

G   Tryptophan

H   Venlafaxine

For each of the descriptions of side-effects below, select the most likely drug from the list above. Each option can be used once, more than once or not at all.

☐ **10.16** Sedation and weight gain are common side-effects.

☐ **10.17** This antidepressant can cause a rise in anxiety levels during initial titration.

☐ **10.18** Blood pressure should be monitored during initiation of this antidepressant.

☐ **10.19** Extrapyramidal side-effects can occur with this antidepressant.

☐ **10.20** Caution should be exercised when choosing an antidepressant in a patient who is self-medicating with this.

THEME: SECTIONS OF THE MENTAL HEALTH ACT 1983

Options

A 2

B 3

C 4

D 5(2)

E 5(4)

F 17

G 48

H 49

I 117

J 135(2)

For each of the following statements about sections of the Mental Health Act 1983, select the most appropriate choice from the list above. Each option can be used once, more than once or not at all.

☐ **10.21** Allows detention for up to 28 days for observation and assessment.

☐ **10.22** Executed by the police.

☐ **10.23** Allows detention for up to 6 months for assessment and treatment.

☐ **10.24** Allows short-term leave from hospital for patients otherwise detained under section.

☐ **10.25** This detaining section is related to the criminal justice system and forensic psychiatry.

THEME: LEARNING DISABILITY

Options

A Mild learning disability

B Moderate learning disability

C No learning disability ·

D Profound learning disability

E Severe learning disability

F Suggestive of Down syndrome

For each of the intelligence quotient (IQ) scores below, select the most appropriate statement from the list above. Each option can be used once, more than once or not at all.

☐ **10.26 IQ: 100**

☐ **10.27 IQ: 38**

☐ **10.28 IQ: 16**

☐ **10.29 IQ: 63**

☐ **10.30 IQ: 28**

THEME: PERVASIVE DEVELOPMENTAL DISORDERS

Options

A   Acquired aphasia with epilepsy

B   Asperger's syndrome

C   Atypical autism

D   Autistic psychopathy

E   Childhood autism

F   Early-onset schizophrenia

G   Elective mutism

H   Heller's syndrome

I   Rett's syndrome

J   Selective mutism

For each of the statements below regarding pervasive developmental disorders, select the most appropriate diagnosis from the list above. Each option may be used once, more than once or not at all.

☐ **10.31** A pervasive developmental disorder, evident before the age of 3 years, that is characterised by abnormal or impaired development of communication and social interaction and the adoption of restricted, often repetitive behaviour.

☐ **10.32** A pervasive developmental disorder, not evident before the age of 3 years, that is characterised by abnormal or impaired development in one or two of the following areas – communication, social interaction and the adoption of restricted, repetitive behaviour.

☐ **10.33** A pervasive developmental disorder of unknown cause and only seen in girls. There is apparently normal or near-normal development, followed by complete or partial loss of acquired hand skills and speech. Hyperventilation and hand-wringing movements are also characteristic.

☐ **10.34** A pervasive developmental disorder, evident before the age of 3 years, that is characterised by abnormal or impaired development of communication and social interaction and the adoption of restricted, often repetitive behaviour, but with no general delay or retardation in language or cognitive development.

☐ **10.35** Also known as 'childhood disintegrative disorder'. Developmental milestones that have been reached in multiple areas of functioning by the age of 2 years are lost, with an associated abnormality in social functioning.

CHAPTER 10 QUESTIONS

ALGORITHM QUESTIONS

THEME: MENTAL HEALTH ACT ASSESSMENT IN THE COMMUNITY

10.36–10.40

Options

A   1

B   2

C   3

D   4

E   135(2)

F   136

G   A clinical psychologist

H   A community psychiatric nurse

I   A consultant psychiatrist

J   A lay person

K   An approved social worker

L   Section 12

The following algorithm describes the process for detention under the Mental Health Act 1983. Using the list of options above, select the most appropriate option for each stage in the flow chart. Each option can be used once, more than once or not at all.

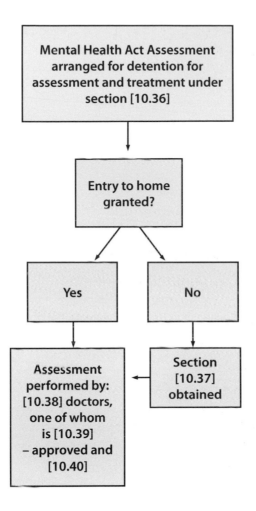

THEME: THE TREATMENT OF SCHIZOPHRENIA

10.41–10.46

Options

A   2–4-week trial

B   6–8-week trial

C   Add an antidepressant

D   Atypical antipsychotic

E   Clozapine

F   CBT

G   Depot antipsychotic

H   Generic counselling

I   Olanzapine

J   Try a different atypical antipsychotic

K   Typical antipsychotic

Complete the following algorithm for the treatment of schizophrenia using the list of options above. Each option can be used once, more than once or not at all.

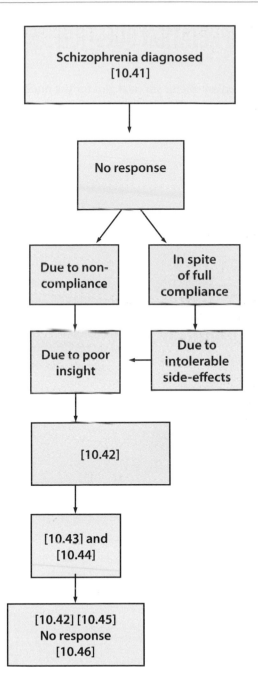

DATA INTERPRETATION QUESTION

10.47 This is a Kaplan–Meier survival plot for the number of patients maintaining remission after a severe depressive episode treated with antidepressants compared with placebo.

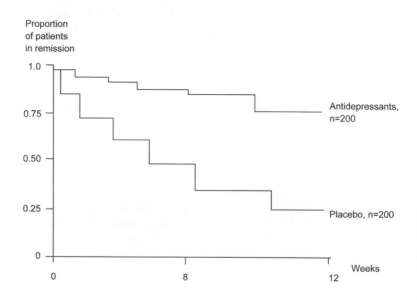

CHAPTER 10 QUESTIONS

Which of the following best describes the data as it is represented?

☐ A   All patients taking antidepressants maintain their initial improvement after 12 weeks of treatment

☐ B   Approximately 150 patients taking antidepressants remain in remission at the end of the treatment represented by the graph

☐ C   Approximately 75% of patients in the placebo arm remain in remission at the end of the treatment represented by the graph

☐ D   Patients taking placebo show a similar rate of relapse after 12 weeks of treatment

☐ E   Placebo and antidepressants are equivocal for maintaining long-term remission

CHAPTER 10 QUESTIONS

HOT TOPICS/EVIDENCE BASED PRACTICE

10.48 According to the NICE guidance, *Management of depression in primary and secondary care*, which one of the following statements is most accurate?

☐ A 'Doing nothing' is an appropriate course of action in an initial presentation of mild depression

☐ B CBT is more effective than antidepressants in the treatment of an initial presentation of a severe depressive episode

☐ C SSRIs are the first choice in the management of mild depressive episodes

☐ D Tricyclic antidepressants are more effective than SSRIs

☐ E Venlafaxine can be appropriately introduced by any GP for patients who have failed to respond to other agents

ANSWERS

10.1   B: Patients with recent psychosis are twice as likely to have used cannabis as patients without psychosis

There is clear evidence of a link between cannabis use and psychosis, although it is not clear whether this is causal or represents self-medication of pre-existing low-grade symptoms. A prospective study of cannabis use in Swedish conscripts showed that regular cannabis use before the age of 18 was associated with a sevenfold increase in risk of developing psychosis in the next 15 years. Cannabis use has increased from 10% of people ever having used it in the late 1960s to 50% in the 21st century but the incidence of psychosis has not increased this much, suggesting any influence is likely to be multifactorial. Stronger strains of cannabis such as skunk seem to be more likely to produce mental health problems, but these are seen with all types of cannabis.

10.2   C: Patients with premorbid schizoid personality traits are more likely to develop schizophrenia

There are numerous associations with the development of schizophrenia. Premorbid schizoid personality traits (fanaticism, hypochondriasis, excessive shyness, eccentricity) and a positive family history are both associated with increased risk of developing schizophrenia, as is drug use (both cannabis and LSD/amphetamines). Twin studies show a 10–15% concordance for dizygotic twins and 30–60% concordance for monozygotic twins. Life events such as bereavement or losing a job, or brain injury (eg after a head injury) can be associated with the onset of schizophrenia.

10.3   A: It allows for the establishment of a Lasting Power of Attorney (LPA), which allows both financial and treatment decisions to be made on behalf of patients

The Act includes provision for an LPA, which, unlike an Enduring Power of Attorney (EPA), allows for both welfare decisions (eg where to live, payment of bills) and health decisions (eg treatment) to be made by the nominated person. These must be pre-arranged when the patient has capacity and registered with the Office of the Public Guardian. The Act applies only to those aged over 16, and advance directives are covered only if they are written, if they do not have an appointed attorney at the time that they come into force, and if the patient does not have capacity at the time this comes to be enforced.

10.4   B: Cognitive behavioural therapy (CBT)

Antidepressants would not ordinarily be chosen as first-line therapy for an individual suffering from a mild depressive episode. For such an episode the best evidence exists for CBT, although availability in some areas can be a problem. There might be instances where psychodynamic therapy may be of benefit, for example where the major precipitating event for psychological distress appears to be difficulties in relating to others.

10.5   B: Anxious/avoidant personality traits

Anxious/avoidant personality traits are a risk factor for depression. These will often need exploring in CBT in order to prevent subsequent episodes occurring, either in isolation or in combination with antidepressant medication. Paranoid and antisocial personality traits might actually protect against depression. Depression is more common in women, with lifetime prevalence between 4.9% and 8.7%, compared with 2.3–4.4% in men (Epidemiological Catchment Area Study). High incidence of expressed emotion is a risk factor for schizophrenia.

10.6   B: Increased frequency of pregnancy in women

Sexual indiscretions are common in manic episodes, with the result that patients can be at greater risk of unplanned pregnancy and sexually transmitted infections. Counselling of this risk is important and the use of an oral contraceptive might be advisable, but be cautious of drug interactions with mood stabilisers.

10.7   A: Delusional perception

Delusional perception occurs in two stages. First, the individual experiences a normal perception (eg 'The traffic lights turned red.'), which is then followed by a delusional interpretation (eg 'That is when I realised they thought I was the devil and wanted to kill me.'). Other Schneiderian first-rank symptoms include auditory hallucinations (in the third person, as a running commentary or perceived as emanating from parts of the body), delusions of passivity (including thought insertion, broadcasting and withdrawal and passivity of impulses) and somatic passivity. Loosening of associations (a thought disorder), splitting and incongruent affect are symptoms of psychosis that Bleuler, not Schneider, felt to be important in schizophrenia – they are not first-rank symptoms.

10.8   B: Physical health is at risk in patients with mental health problems

Physical health is often a significant concern in mental disorder. For example, schizophrenia is associated with a lower life expectancy, and this is unrelated to the effects of antipsychotic medication. This is generally well known, but depression is also associated with significant comorbidity and health risks, including a greater risk of MI. OCD does not protect physical health, but is the only mental disorder that is thought to protect against suicide.

CHAPTER 10 ANSWERS

10.9   D: Salience of drinking habits

Binge drinking is an increasing problem in the UK, especially in younger age groups and including under-age drinkers. While it is not without health consequences, it is not specifically associated with the factors that Edwards and Gross (1976) classically described as being associated with alcohol dependence syndrome. These include reinstatement after abstinence, salience of drinking habits, relief drinking to avoid withdrawal, increasing tolerance to the effects of alcohol, a compulsion to drink and the experience of withdrawal symptoms.

10.10   B: Delirium Is categorised as an organic disorder

Delirium is listed under 'Organic mental disorders' in ICD-10. It is also commonly referred to as an 'acute confusional state'. It is a non-specific syndrome charcterised by concurrent disturbances of consciousness, perception, cognition, behaviour, emotion and the sleep–wake cycle. Although its frequency rises with age, it is not unique to the elderly. The highest frequency is seen in terminally ill patients (American Psychiatric Association, 1999). Disorientation in time and place is almost universal. Patients have a marked difficulty in sustaining concentration. These two points often make the assessment challenging. It is best treated by the management of the underlying cause, which can be as simple as a urinary tract infection or a recent change in medication. Low-dose antipsychotics and benzodiazepines can be used to treat the disorder symptomatically. Visual hallucinations are typical and the presence of these should always alert one to the possibility of an organic cause.

10.11   B: Impairment of intellectual functioning

Dementia is the global impairment of intellectual functioning without impairment of consciousness. Features can include initial amnesia for recent events, catastrophic reactions and personality deterioration. Spontaneous recovery is not associated with dementia, where a progressive deterioration is seen.

10.12   E: The onset of OCD tends to be earlier in men than in women

OCD comprises the experience of intrusive obsessional thoughts and the compulsion to do something in response. It is commonly associated with depression (30%), anxiety and depersonalisation. The obsessional thoughts experienced are recognised as being the individual's own, are unpleasant, and at least one must still be resisted in order for the diagnosis to be made. The mean age of onset is 20 years but it often occurs earlier in men, who can experience it in their early teens. The best treatment is through gradual exposure to environmental cues combined with response prevention, although in practice (serotonergic) antidepressant therapy is also required.

10.13   A: Involves a preference for consistency and routine

Autism is typified by abnormalities of language and social interaction, which are marked and early. There is a strong preference for routine and alterations to routines already established will often be met with an abnormal behavioural response, which can include forms of self-injurious behaviour. Children with autism develop unusual preoccupations with objects and this will extend to toys, which will typically be played with in a way that suggests interest in function rather than fantasy. Compulsions are common and there can be poor speech comprehension. There is a lack of normal attachment behaviour, including reciprocal smiling (a 'social smile'), which is often deeply distressing for parents.

10.14   A: It cannot be diagnosed before the age of 4 years

Encopresis is the involuntary passage of fully formed faeces and is not a diagnosis that can be made before the age of 4. It is an uncommon disorder but much more common in young boys. Coercive potty training is likely to worsen the condition. Organic disorders such as Hirschsprung's disease must be excluded before psychiatric management is considered. The treatment of choice includes behavioural management, such as the use of a star chart, along with parental counselling or family therapy to help modify hostile attitudes.

10.15   C: Suicide is more common in men

Suicide has an incidence in the UK of approximately 1/10 000 per year. The risk is raised in all mental disorders with the exception of OCD and in schizophrenia the risk is higher in those that experience akathisia as a side-effect of antipsychotic medication. The rates are highest during the summer and the spring in both hemispheres. It is more common in men, who are also more likely to choose dangerous or violent methods such as shooting. Jumping from structures is more commonly a method used in young people than the elderly. Remember that an individual does not need to suffer from a mental disorder to commit suicide and that socio-political solutions are often more important than psychiatric ones.

THEME: SIDE-EFFECTS OF ANTIDEPRESSANTS

10.16   E: Mirtazepine

10.17   B: Citalopram

10.18   H: Venlafaxine

10.19   C: Fluoxetine

10.20   F: St John's wort

Mirtazepine's action at the histamine receptor is greater than at the noradrenergic receptor at the starting dose (15 mg). This is outweighed at higher doses so that the initial sedation experienced by most patients generally subsides. This can be usefully taken advantage of in patients with insomnia and a predominantly anxious presentation. Anxiety is a common side-effect on starting citalopram, which might require symptomatic treatment, but patients should be advised that this is likely to pass after the first week or two. St John's wort is available over the counter. It is an enzyme inducer and possesses serotoninergic activity, which, when combined with selective serotonin reuptake inhibitors (SSRIs) or other serotoninergic drugs can give rise to the serotonin syndrome.

THEME: SECTIONS OF THE MENTAL HEALTH ACT 1983

10.21 A: 2

10.22 J: 135(2)

10.23 B: 3

10.24 F: 17

10.25 G: 48

Section 2 of the Mental Health Act is for the compulsory detention of individuals for 28 days for assessment and observation and is not renewable. Section 3 is for the assessment and treatment of mental disorder and lasts for up to 6 months, at which point it can be renewed. Section 135 is used to gain entry to private property in order to remove a person to a designated place of safety for further assessment. Section 136 enables a police officer to remove someone from a public place and take them to a place of safety should they be found acting in a bizarre way that is thought could be due to the effects of mental disorder. Like section 135, this is not an admission section, but one which allows assessment to take place at the place of safety, as to whether a section 2 or other admission section should be implemented. Section 17 pertains to leave granted at the responsible medical officer's discretion for patients detained under the Mental Health Act. Section 48 gives the Home Office the power to make a direction for the transfer of individuals not yet convicted to hospital for further assessment and treatment. Section 49 can be used to place a further restriction on this, preventing discharge without permission from the Home Office.

THEME: LEARNING DISABILITY

10.26 C: No learning disability

10.27 B: Moderate learning disability

10.28 D: Profound learning disability

10.29 A: Mild learning disability

10.30 E: Severe learning disability

The IQ ranges for the determination of the severity of learning disability are: mild 50–69, moderate 35–49, severe 20–34, profound < 20. Lower IQ has an association with lower social class of parents. With increasing severity there are an increasing number of organic causes associated with learning difficulty, the vast majority of which are detectable in utero or during the perinatal and postnatal period. The cause (eg Down syndrome) cannot be elucidated by IQ measurement, however.

THEME: PERVASIVE DEVELOPMENTAL DISORDERS

10.31 E: Childhood autism

10.32 C: Atypical autism

10.33 I: Rett's syndrome

10.34 J: Selective mutism

10.35 H: Heller's syndrome

THEME: MENTAL HEALTH ACT ASSESSMENT IN THE COMMUNITY

10.36 **C:** 3

10.37 **E:** 135(2)

10.38 **B:** 2

10.39 **L:** Section 12

10.40 **K:** An approved social worker

The Mental Health Act is currently in the process of being revised to allow indefinite detention for people with personality disorders but for the time being the above rules apply.

THEME: THE TREATMENT OF SCHIZOPHRENIA

10.41 **D:** Atypical antipsychotic

10.42 **J:** Try a different atypical antipsychotic

10.43 **F:** CBT

10.44 **G:** Depot antipsychotic

10.45 **B:** 6–8-week trial

10.46 **E:** Clozapine

10.47   B: Approximately 150 patients taking antidepressants remain in remission at the end of the treatment represented by the graph

This graph shows the number of patients maintaining improvement on antidepressants compared with placebo after 12 weeks of initial treatment. It shows that after this 12 week treatment period only 25% maintain their improvement on placebo, whereas approximately 75% (ie 150 patients) of those on antidepressants maintain their treatment response.

10.48   A: 'Doing nothing' is an appropriate course of action in an initial presentation of mild depression

'Watchful waiting' is often the most appropriate course of action in such a presentation. The natural history of low mood dictates that over the following 2 weeks it might resolve (in which case the diagnosis of an adjustment disorder might be considered), stay the same or worsen. SSRIs are as effective as tricyclic antidepressants with a more favourable side-effect profile and should be considered as first-line therapy for moderate and severe episodes treated in primary care. Venlafaxine should only be initiated by specialist mental health medical practitioners, including GPs with a Special Interest in Mental Health. For those presenting with severe depression, a combination of CBT and an SSRI should be considered as this is considered more cost-effective. There is no evidence to suggest that CBT alone is a superior management strategy.

CHAPTER 11
MUSCULOSKELETAL
SINGLE BEST ANSWER QUESTIONS

11.1   A 67-year-old woman with long-standing rheumatoid arthritis has recently started taking etanercept. She feels this is working very well but has developed an acutely swollen, red knee. She comes to see you and asks if she can have this aspirated and steroid injected, which has always worked well in the past for exacerbations of her arthritis. Which one of the following would be an appropriate action in this situation?

- [ ]   A   Aspirate the joint and inject with steroid
- [ ]   B   Increase the dose of etanercept
- [ ]   C   Prescribe oral non-steroidal anti-inflammatories
- [ ]   D   Prescribe oral steroids
- [ ]   E   Stop the etanercept, check blood for inflammatory markers and send aspirate for microscopy

11.2 A 34-year-old IT worker comes to you with a 6-month history of back pain, with no recent history of trauma and no red flag symptoms. He has presented in the past with intermittent episodes of back stiffness and occasional neck ache and was treated for plantar fasciitis last year. On examination he has no neurological signs but does have reduced range of movement in his cervical spine, particularly for extension. Which one of the following options is the most likely diagnosis?

- ☐ A   Ankylosing spondylitis
- ☐ B   Mechanical back pain
- ☐ C   Osteoarthritis
- ☐ D   Rheumatoid arthritis
- ☐ E   Wedge fracture

11.3 An overweight 64-year-old 'lady who lunches' presents with a 2-day history of an acutely painful, tender right knee associated with erythema and a fever. She is usually well and suffers only from hypertension, for which she takes bendroflumethiazide. On examination you notice that she has palmar erythema. What is the single most likely underlying diagnosis?

- ☐ A   Gout
- ☐ B   Haemarthrosis
- ☐ C   Osteoarthritis
- ☐ D   Rheumatoid arthritis
- ☐ E   Septic arthritis

11.4 A sprightly 72-year-old man, who is a keen gardener, presents with a 1-week history of a pain around his hip which he tells you he feels most prominently in his right buttock, especially when he is gardening and when he turns on that side in bed. He is normally well and rarely comes to the surgery. He denies trauma, although he has spent the past few weeks digging his new allotment. On examination, leg lengths are equal and straight-leg raising is normal. He is markedly tender over the right hip but he has a normal range of movement in the hip. There is no rash. What is the single most likely diagnosis?

- [ ] A Myeloma
- [ ] B Osteoarthritis of hip
- [ ] C Osteoarthritis of lumbar spine
- [ ] D Sciatica
- [ ] E Trochanteric bursitis

11.5 A 53-year-old schoolteacher presents with a history of gradually increasing deformity of the small joints of both her hands, associated with stiffness and swelling. She has found it increasingly difficult to carry textbooks and is often clumsy with coffee cups and pens. She also tells you she feels tired all the time. There is no relevant medical history and no family history of note. Her metacarpophalangeal joints are red and swollen. What is the single most likely diagnosis?

- [ ] A Gout
- [ ] B Osteoarthritis
- [ ] C Pseudogout
- [ ] D Rheumatoid arthritis
- [ ] E Systemic lupus erythematosus

11.6 Which one of the following ligaments is the most commonly torn knee ligament following an injury involving valgus displacement and external rotation? Select one option only.

☐ A Anterior cruciate

☐ B Lateral collateral

☐ C Medial collateral

☐ D Patellar

☐ E Posterior cruciate

11.7 Using the Ottawa rules in a patient with ankle pain following an injury, what findings would indicate the need for an X-ray? Select one option only.

☐ A Bone tenderness 4 cm above the lateral malleolus

☐ B Bone tenderness at the head of the fifth metatarsal

☐ C Bone tenderness over the cuboid bone

☐ D Patient unable to weight-bear at the time of injury but now managing despite some pain

☐ E Tenderness and swelling inferior to the lateral malleolus

11.8 A 36-year-old woman has a 2-month history of pain in her right hip radiating to her groin. She has a good range of movement in the hip and no focal tenderness. Which one of the following is the single most likely diagnosis?

☐ A Osteoarthritis

☐ B Polymyalgia rheumatica

☐ C Sacroiliitis

☐ D Sciatica

☐ E Tronchanteric bursitis

EXTENDED MATCHING QUESTIONS

THEME: SOFT-TISSUE RHEUMATISM

Options

A	De Quervain's tenosynovitis	**F**	Osgood–Schlatter disease
B	Dorsal tenosynovitis	**G**	Polymyalgia rheumatica
C	Fibromyalgia	**H**	Tennis elbow
D	Flexor tenosynovitis	**I**	Trigger finger
E	Golfer's elbow	**J**	Trochanteric bursitis

For each of the scenarios below, select the most appropriate diagnosis from the list above. Each option may be used once, more than once or not at all.

☐ **11.9** A 53-year-old woman complains of pain in her back, neck and abdomen over a period of several months. This seems to be worse in cold weather and she reports being very tender, particularly over her bony prominences. She gets headaches and sleeps badly. Examination is unremarkable apart from generalised tenderness. Blood tests are normal.

☐ **11.10** A 34-year-old baker complains of pain in the medial part of his elbow. On examination he is tender over the medial epicondyle, with pain on resisted pronation.

☐ **11.11** A 44-year-old electrician complains of recurrent pain in the elbow. On examination he is tender over the lateral epicondyle and the pain is made worse on resisted wrist extension.

☐ **11.12** A 45-year-old housewife complains of pain and reduced movement of her thumb after spending the afternoon pruning roses. On examination there is pain on resisted abduction of the thumb and pain and tenderness on the radial side of the thumb proximal to the thumb base.

THEME: ARTHROPATHIES

Options

A   Calcium pyrophosphate deposition disease

B   Gout

C   Osteoarthritis flare

D   Osteomyelitis

E   Psoriatic arthritis

F   Reactive arthritis

G   Reiter syndrome

H   Rheumatoid arthritis

I   Septic arthritis

J   Sjögren syndrome

K   Systemic lupus erythematosis

For each of the scenarios described below, select the single most appropriate diagnosis from the list of options above. Each option can be used once, more than once or not at all.

☐ **11.13** A 44-year-old ex-professional footballer asks for an out-of-hours visit. He is complaining of severe pain in his ankle for 24 hours, 'worse than when I broke my leg'. He feels feverish and his ankle is hot and red. The doctor admits him to hospital. Blood tests show the CRP, ESR and WCC all to be significantly raised; the uric acid level is low. Microscopy under polarised light shows negatively birefringent crystals.

☐ **11.14** An elderly man with osteoarthritis and haemochromatosis develops an acutely painful, swollen knee. The GP aspirates the joint, which is reported by the lab as 'Clear with low viscosity, WCC $10\,000 \times 10^6$/l; crystals – brick-shaped and positively birefringent'.

☐ **11.15** A young man in his twenties developed severe pain and swelling in his right knee. The knee was hot to touch. His eye was red and painful, with an irregular pupil. He had recently returned from travelling in India, where he had unprotected intercourse with a prostitute. The fluid aspirated was negative on microscopy and culture.

☐ **11.16** A 67-year-old lady with long-standing arthritis complains of a dry mouth and sore, dry eyes. She has also been treated for suspected atrophic vaginitis in the past.

☐ **11.17** A 44-year-old man complains of increasingly painful arthropathy. He uses over-the-counter moisturisers for what he describes as 'a little bit of eczema' on his ankles. On examination, he has pitting of his fingernails and tender joints.

CHAPTER 11 QUESTIONS

THEME: INFLAMMATORY DISEASE

Options

A Dermatomyositis

B Fibromyalgia

C Giant-cell arteritis

D Motor neurone disease

E Polymyalgia rheumatica

F Polymyositis

G Rheumatoid arthritis

H Sjögen syndrome

I Systemic lupus erythematosus

J Wegener's granulomatosis

For each of the scenarios described below, select the single most appropriate diagnosis from the list of options above. Each option can be used once, more than once or not at all.

☐ **11.18** A 77-year-old man presents to his GP complaining of malaise, fever and generalised weakness. The doctor notices a purplish-red rash on his face. Examination reveals generalised muscle weakness. The ESR and creatine kinase are found to be markedly raised.

☐ **11.19** The staff at a rest home becomes increasing concerned about a woman in her eighties who is usually very sprightly. She appears very depressed and tired and complains bitterly of pain and stiffness in her arms and legs, particularly in the morning, and severe temporal headache. Blood tests reveal a normocytic normochromic anaemia and an ESR of 100.

11.20 A woman in her early forties developed a florid erythematous facial rash following a holiday in the Canaries. She also had a fever and complained of muscle and joint aches and swelling. This was put down to a virus and to too much sun. Her symptoms got steadily worse over the next few weeks and she eventually saw her GP who did some bloods. These showed a normocytic normochromic anaemia, an ESR of 60, and positive antinuclear antibody and rheumatoid factor. Complement levels (C3 and C4) were reduced and the double-stranded DNA was raised.

11.21 A relatively fit 50-year-old man developed breathlessness, haemoptysis, fever, weight loss and malaise. He had been troubled with rhinorrhoea and chronic sinusitis. Initial blood tests showed a high ESR and CRP and a normocytic normochromic anaemia with normal eosinophil levels. The creatinine was normal, but dipstick examination of his urine showed blood ++. A chest X-ray reveals multiple nodules.

11.22 Since the death of her husband, an elderly woman has frequently complained to her GP of fatigue, myalgia, arthralgia, sore eyes and a dry mouth. She also suffers from Raynaud's phenomenon. He treats her for depression but she gets no better. Subsequent blood tests show a normocytic normochromic anaemia and a raised ESR; rheumatoid factor and Ro/SSA and La/SSB antibodies are positive.

ALGORITHM QUESTIONS

THEME: MANAGEMENT OF OSTEOARTHRITIS OF THE KNEE

11.23–11.28

Options

A Chondroitin

B Exercise

C Glucosamine

D Intra-articular hyalurinic acid injections

E NSAID

F Opioids

G Paracetamol

H Refer for surgery

I Sibutramine

J Weight loss

In conjunction with the local physiotherapy service, your practice has developed a flow chart to standardise the management of osteoarthritis of the knee. Complete the following flow chart with the most appropriate item from the list of options given above. Each option can be used once, more than once or not at all.

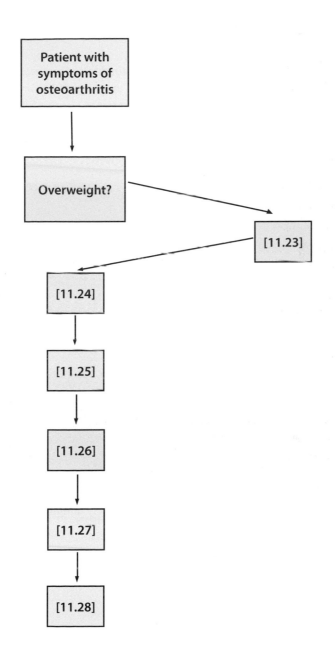

PICTURE QUESTION

11.29 A 67-year-old man with a history of prostate cancer treated with Zoladex complains of persistent pain in his right hip for the last few weeks. He thinks this might have started after he fell over while playing golf. On examination, he has a reduced range of movement in his hip and you arrange an X-ray at the local cottage hospital. The X-ray is shown below.

Which one of the following is the most likely diagnosis?

☐   A   Constipation

☐   B   Fractured neck of femur

☐   C   Fractured pubic ramus

☐   D   Osteoarthritis of the hip

☐   E   Perthes' disease

DATA INTERPRETATION QUESTIONS

11.30 What is the most likely diagnosis in a patient with the following immunology results?

ANA positive (speckled)

High titre of nuclear RNP and Sm autoantibodies

No antibodies to Ro(SSA), La (SSB), Jo-1 (RNA synthetase), PM-1 (nucleolar protein), double-stranded DNA, Scl-70 (topoisomerase) and centromere

- ☐ A Mixed connective tissue disorder (MCTD)
- ☐ B Polymositis/dermatomyositis
- ☐ C Sjögren syndrome
- ☐ D Systemic sclerosis/CREST
- ☐ E Systemic lupus erythematosus (SLE)

11.31 What is the most likely metabolic bone disease in a patient with the following results?

Serum levels of calcium, phosphate, vitamin D and parathyroid hormone (PTH) all normal

Markedly raised levels of alkaline phosphatase

- ☐ A Osteomalacia
- ☐ B Osteoporosis
- ☐ C Paget's disease
- ☐ D Primary hyperparathyroidism
- ☐ E Renal disease

HOT TOPICS/EVIDENCE BASED PRACTICE

11.32 Which of the following statements about new developments in the management of shoulder pain is true? Select one option only.

- [ ] A   Adhesive capsulitis usually settles after 6 months
- [ ] B   All patients with shoulder pain seen in primary care should have an X-ray performed
- [ ] C   In the management of rotator cuff disorders, short-term outcomes are superior for physiotherapy compared with steroid injection
- [ ] D   Red flag symptoms include unexplained wasting and sensory loss
- [ ] E   Steroid injections should not be repeated due to the risk of cartilage damage

MUSCULOSKELETAL ANSWERS

ANSWERS

11.1   E: Stop the etanercept, check blood for inflammatory markers and send aspirate for microscopy

Anti-tumour necrosis factor (anti-TNF) treatments are associated with septic arthritis and can mask the severity of this complication. In any patient on anti-TNF treatment where infection is suspected, the treatment should be stopped and the infection investigated and treated. Prior to starting treatment with an anti-TNF you should ensure that vaccinations are up to date and patients should be warned of the possibility of infection and advised what to do if they develop symptoms and/or signs of infection. There should be a low threshold for admission in these patients.

11.2   A: Ankylosing spondylitis

Ankylosing spondylitis has a prevalence of approximately 1 in 2200 and affects men twice as frequently as women. It tends to present in young men with morning back pain and stiffness. As progressive spinal fusion occurs there can be reduced spinal movement, with kyphosis and sacroiliac joint pain. It is associated with plantar fasciitis, lung fibrosis, inflammatory bowel disease and amyloidosis. X-ray of the spine might show a 'bamboo spine', with vertebral fusion. The disease is associated with HLA-B27 positivity.

11.3   A: Gout

Gout is more common in men but does also occur in women, and the clues here are that this lady is overweight, drinks alcohol (hence the palmar erythema) and is on a diuretic. The hint about her lifestyle suggests that she enjoys rich foods – purine-based foods such as certain fish and meats can predispose to gout. Although gout commonly occurs in the big toe, it can occur at any joint and usually results in a severely painful, tender and erythematous joint. In this instance it would be sensible to aspirate some fluid from the knee if there is an effusion and to send the sample for microscopy, culture and sensitivity as septic arthritis is a differential diagnosis. Microscopy reveals sodium monourate crystals. Treatment is with rest and NSAIDs. Modification of risk factors is important in preventing recurrence, as is allopurinol treatment.

11.4   E: Trochanteric bursitis

Trochanteric bursitis is the most likely diagnosis, given the information provided in the history. One would expect to find tenderness on palpation of the affected side but a full range of movement. The pain is often felt deep in the buttock. Repeated trauma can result in inflammation of the bursa. Treatment options include NSAIDs and physiotherapy; corticosteroid injections can be useful for chronic episodes.

11.5   D: Rheumatoid arthritis

This is a classic presentation of rheumatoid arthritis in a middle-aged woman – symptoms affecting the small joints of her hands symmetrically, with pain, stiffness, swelling and loss of function. This can be associated with tiredness, malaise and other non-articular features, such as fever, weight loss, pleural effusion, mouth ulcers and dry eyes. Gout usually affects only one joint and pseudogout more typically affects the knee. This lady needs to be referred to a rheumatologist because early treatment with disease-modifying drugs can alter the progression of the disease and help to minimise the progression to involvement of larger joints.

11.6   C: Medial collateral

The medial collateral ligament is the ligament that is most likely to be damaged following a twisting or wrenching injury with valgus stress and external rotation. More severe stress can also damage the anterior cruciate ligament.

11.7   A: Bone tenderness 4 cm above the lateral malleolus

X-ray if there is pain in the malleolar area or midfoot and bone tenderness in one or more of the following:

- Lower 6 cm of the distal fibula above the lateral malleolous

- Distal tibia above the medial malleolus

- The navicular bone

- The fifth metatarsal base.

Also X-ray if the patient is unable to weight-bear at the time of the injury and subsequently.

11.8   D: Sciatica

Sciatica can cause symptoms which are very similar to osteoarthritis of the hip and in cases of doubt a diagnostic injection of anaesthetic may be used to differentiate these conditions.

CHAPTER 11 ANSWERS

THEME: SOFT-TISSUE RHEUMATISM

11.9   C: Fibromyalgia

Fibromyalgia is usually diagnosed on the basis of the history and lack of any evidence of other causes of symptoms. The American College of Rheumatology diagnostic criteria state that pain should be present in all four quarters of the body and should be present in at least 11 of 18 trigger points. Graded exercise and low-dose amitriptyline are helpful.

11.10   E: Golfer's elbow

Golfer's elbow is caused by inflammation over the flexor origin at the medial epicondyle. Treatment involves rest and support. If this doesn't help (together with the avoidance of exacerbating factors), steroid injections might help.

11.11   H: Tennis elbow

Tennis elbow is more common than golfer's elbow. It is caused by inflammation of the common extensor origin. The principles of treatment are the same as for golfer's elbow.

11.12   A: De Quervain's tenosynovitis

De Quervain's tenosynovitis is caused by inflammation of the extensor pollicis brevis and abductor pollicis longus tendons resulting from repetitive activity. It usually settles with rest and sometimes steroid injection, but surgery might be needed if it becomes chronic.

THEME: ARTHROPATHIES

11.13   B: Gout

This is a typical description of gout. The main differential diagnosis is cellulitis but this is not usually so tender.

11.14   A: Calcium pyrophosphate deposition disease (pseudogout)

This typically affects the knee. Differentiation from gout is usually on the basis of microscopy of fluid from the effusion.

11.15   G: Reiter syndrome

Arthritis, urethritis and iritis are classically reported as sequelae to unprotected sexual intercourse, but many cases are due to gastrointestinal infections (eg shigellosis).

11.16   J: Sjögren syndrome

Keratoconjunctivitis sicca is caused by infiltration of mucus-secreting tissues in the eyes, mouth and genital tract. It can be seen as a primary or a secondary condition, and is usually treated with lubricants. Schirmer's test is diagnostic.

11.17   E: Psoriatic arthritis

Psoriatic arthritis is not always associated with skin lesions but there is usually pitting of the fingernails.

THEME: INFLAMMATORY DISEASE

11.18   A: Dermatomyositis

Dermatomyositis is typically associated with a heliotrope rash, myalgia and weakness. Blood tests show raised creatine kinase and raised ESR or plasma viscosity.

11.19   C: Giant-cell arteritis

The association of headache, temporal tenderness or visual symptoms with a history of polymyalgia rheumatica should prompt immediate action to exclude giant-cell arteritis, which can rapidly lead to blindness if left untreated.

11.20   I: Systemic lupus erythematosus (SLE)

This is a typical history of SLE, with a butterfly rash affecting the face. This is a complex multisystem disease and patients should be referred early.

11.21   J: Wegener's granulomatosis

Wegener's granulomatosis should be considered in patients presenting with nasal symptoms and signs of systemic disease. It can cause septal perforation and should be considered in patients with multisystem disease.

11.22   H: Sjögen syndrome

Sjögren syndrome causes dry mucous membranes. Schirmer's test involves placing a piece of blotting paper between the eye and lower eyelid and can be used to diagnose the condition (although the diagnosis is usually obvious from the history). Treatment is aimed at the underlying disease where possible but usually consists of symptomatic measures, eg artificial tears.

THEME: MANAGEMENT OF OSTEOARTHRITIS OF THE KNEE

11.23   J: Weight loss

11.24   B: Exercise

11.25   G: Paracetamol

11.26   E: NSAID

11.27   F: Opioids

11.28   H: Refer for surgery

11.29   B: Fractured neck of femur

This X-ray shows a right-sided fractured neck of femur. In the context of minor trauma there should be a high degree of suspicion that this is a pathological fracture. In this case it was due to bony metastases and he received radiotherapy to the hip after a surgical repair of the fracture.

11.30   A: Mixed connective tissue disorder (MCTD)

MCTD has some features of SLE, scleroderma and polymyositis. A negative profile for all components of ANA except anti-RNP antibody is quite specific for MTCD. Sm antibodies are also seen in SLE but titres are high in MTCD. SLE is associated with antibody to double-stranded DNA. Anti-Jo-1 and anti-PM-1 antibodies are seen in polymyositis/dermatomyositis. Anti-centromere antibody is seen in CREST (**c**alcinosis, **R**aynaud's disease, (o)**e**sophageal dysmotility, **s**clerodactyly and **t**elangiectasia) and anti-Scl-70 is seen in systemic sclerosis. Sjögren syndrome is commonly associated with anti-Ro and ant-La antibodies but these can be also seen in SLE.

11.31   C: Paget's disease

Paget's disease is characterised by excessive and disorganised resorption and formation of bone. This is reflected by high levels of alkaline phosphatase. Osteomalacia often shows low calcium, phosphate and vitamin D levels. Alkaline phosphatase and PTH levels can be raised in osteomalacia but the best marker of disease is the serum vitamin D level. In osteoporosis there are usually normal levels of all these minerals and hormones.

11.32   D: Red flag symptoms include unexplained wasting and sensory loss

Adhesive capsulitis usually resolves after 18–24 months. Red flag symptoms include systemic signs of infection, bony abnormality (eg undisplaced fracture), history of cancer and neurological signs. Systematic reviews suggest equivalent short-term benefit for steroids and physiotherapy. Steroid injections can be repeated up to three times, but should not be used in the presence of a large tear.

CHAPTER 12
NEUROLOGY
SINGLE BEST ANSWER QUESTIONS

12.1 A 23-year-old girl presents with recurrent twitching of her face and abdomen, which started after one of her friends gave her a pill for travel sickness. On examination, she has repetitive twitching movements of her face and both arms and abdomen, every 20–30 seconds. Examination is otherwise normal. Which of the following is the most likely diagnosis? Select one option only.

- [ ] A Jacksonian epilepsy
- [ ] B Multiple sclerosis
- [ ] C Non-organic symptoms
- [ ] D Tardive dyskinesia
- [ ] E Temporal lobe epilepsy

12.2 Which one of the following statements about drug treatment of Alzheimer's disease is true?

- [ ] A Cholinesterase inhibitors are available only in oral formulation
- [ ] B Cholinesterase inhibitors have been shown to reverse cognitive impairment in patients with Alzheimer's disease
- [ ] C Cholinesterase inhibitors can be initiated in primary care
- [ ] D Long-acting benzodiazepines are useful in prevention of irritability and aggression
- [ ] E Regular exercise has been shown to maintain performance in activities of daily living

12.3 A 53-year-old woman complains that for several months her family have commented that her eyelids seem to droop. Over this time she has also started to notice double vision at times and finds that she gets tired easily. Further questioning reveals that she finds particular difficulty with lifting her arms above her head. On examination there is a slight ptosis but no ophthalmoplegia. Power in her arms is slightly reduced for extension, but tone, coordination and reflexes are all normal. What is the most likely diagnosis?

- ☐ A Motor neurone disease
- ☐ B Multiple sclerosis
- ☐ C Myalgic encephalitis
- ☐ D Myasthenia gravis
- ☐ E Polymyalgia rheumatica

12.4 A 40-year-old man complains of numbness and paraesthesia of the left thumb, index and middle fingers and half of the ring finger over a period of several weeks. Initially the symptoms were only present at night, but now he is starting to get symptoms in the daytime and is getting pain in the shoulder. On examination he has wasting and weakened abduction of the thumb, but no fasciculation. He has diet-controlled diabetes but no other history of note. What is the most likely diagnosis?

- ☐ A Carpal tunnel syndrome
- ☐ B Cervical radiculopathy
- ☐ C Diabetic neuropathy
- ☐ D Motor neurone disease
- ☐ E Multiple sclerosis

12.5 Which of the following statements about the drug management of Parkinson's disease is true? Select one option only.

☐ A All patients should be referred for consideration of deep brain stimulation surgery

☐ B Combination of levodopa and a dopa-decarboxylase inhibitor is associated with less nausea and vomiting than levodopa alone

☐ C Patients with tremor only should be treated with propranolol

☐ D Ropinirole is associated with significant motor complications and should not be used as a first-line treatment

☐ E Selegiline is often used in combination with levodopa

12.6 One of your patients has just been diagnosed with motor neurone disease and comes to see you to discuss the diagnosis. Which one of the following statements about the management of this condition is true?

☐ A All patients should have a tracheostomy performed to prevent aspiration

☐ B Baclofen does not help in the treatment of spasticity

☐ C NICE guidance does not support the use of riluzole in motor neurone disease

☐ D Riluzole has been shown to bring about remission in 25% of patients

☐ E Riluzole increases the period of time to need for ventilation but does not improve prognosis

12.7 **Which of the following statements about the initial management of suspected meningitis is correct? Select one option only.**

- [ ] A A stat dose of ciprofloxacin is effective prophylaxis in close contacts
- [ ] B Cefotaxime can be used safely in patients known to have anaphylaxis with penicillin
- [ ] C Dexamethasone should be given with the first dose of antibiotics
- [ ] D Intravenous amoxicillin is the first-line empirical treatment for suspected meningitis
- [ ] E Treatment should be guided by the results of blood culture

12.8 **Which of the following statements about trigeminal neuralgia is true? Select one option only.**

- [ ] A Amitriptyline is the most effective treatment
- [ ] B It always affects the mandibular branch of the trigeminal nerve
- [ ] C It can be associated with a facial nerve palsy
- [ ] D It is typically relapsing and remitting
- [ ] E Paroxysms of pain usually last at least 30 minutes

12.9 **A 48-year-old primary school teacher complains of pins and needles in his feet 3 weeks after an episode of gastroenteritis. He has also noticed weakness in his legs and on examination he has absent ankle tendon and patellar tendon reflexes but normal biceps tendon reflexes. His plantar response is normal. The sensation in his feet is normal. Which of the following is the single most likely diagnosis?**

- [ ] A Chronic inflammatory demyelinating polyneuropathy
- [ ] B Guillain–Barré syndrome
- [ ] C Motor neurone disease
- [ ] D Multiple sclerosis
- [ ] E Reiter's syndrome

EXTENDED MATCHING QUESTIONS

THEME: NEUROLOGICAL DISORDERS

Options

A	Lewy body dementia	F	Myasthenia gravis
B	Motor neurone disease	G	New-variant Creutzfeld–Jakob disease
C	Multiple sclerosis		
D	Muscular dystrophy	H	Parkinson's disease
E	Myalgic encephalitis		

For each of the scenarios below, select the most appropriate diagnosis from the list above. Each option may be used once, more than once or not at all.

☐ **12.10** Predominantly affects younger patients, causes psychiatric symptoms, followed by cerebellar ataxia and myoclonus, then progressive dementia.

☐ **12.11** A 72-year-old man complains of loss of strength in his right hand that has developed over a period of several weeks. On examination he has some wasting of his thenar eminence and fasciculation.

☐ **12.12** A 23-year-old woman wakes up with double vision on looking to the left. On examination she has a unilateral lateral rectus palsy. She has no other symptoms or signs. Three months ago she was seen with paraesthesia in her left leg, which had no apparent cause and which resolved over a period of 2 weeks.

☐ **12.13** A 79-year-old man is brought to see you by his daughter after suffering a number of falls recently. He has a shuffling gait and on examination has a resting tremor, with hypertonia in his arms.

THEME: HEADACHE

Options

A   Analgesic overuse headache

B   Brain tumour

C   Chronic paroxysmal hemicrania

D   Chronic sinusitis

E   Cluster headache

F   Giant-cell arteritis

G   Migraine

H   Postcoital cephalgia

I   Subarachnoid haemorrhage

J   Temporal lobe epilepsy

K   Tension-type headache

L   Transient global amnesia

M   Transient ischaemic attack

For each of the descriptions below, select the most appropriate diagnosis from the list above. Each option can be used once, more than once or not at all.

☐ **12.14 A 67-year-old man with a history of several weeks of malaise, now complaining of headache and scalp tenderness in the sides of his head, together with pain in his scalp on eating.**

☐ **12.15 A 44-year-old man complains of daily headaches that are centred around his right eye over the past 2 months. These are severe and are not improving despite taking paracetamol and ibuprofen every day. They are associated with nasal congestion and epiphora.**

☐ **12.16** A 67-year-old man is brought in by his wife with a 3-hour history of complete amnesia, which seemed to come on after sexual intercourse. He reports no headache and has no other symptoms. Physical examination is normal except for the amnesia.

☐ **12.17** A 73-year-old woman presents with 2 months of headaches, worse in the morning, that usually improve by mid-afternoon. They are getting gradually worse, and seem particularly bad when she bends over. She feels nauseous with them and experiences visual disturbances at times.

☐ **12.18** A 23-year-old woman who takes the combined oral contraceptive pill complains of severe headache with flashing lights and loss of vision in one eye. She reports that she felt 'out of sorts' immediately before with hypersensitivity to lights and sound started.

THEME: PERIPHERAL NERVE DISORDERS

Options

A   Carpal tunnel syndrome

B   Charcot–Marie–Tooth disease

C   Diabetic neuropathy

D   Drug-induced peripheral neuropathy

E   Polio

F   Vitamin B deficiency

For each of the scenarios below, select the most likely cause from the list above. Each option may be used once, more than once or not at all.

☐ **12.19** A 29-year-old woman complains of progressive problems with walking. She had pes cavus diagnosed in childhood. On examination her legs have a champagne-bottle appearance. Reflexes are reduced on both sides. She reports other affected family members.

☐ **12.20** A 73-year-old man complains of pins and needles and numbness in both feet. He takes amiodarone and warfarin for atrial fibrillation but is otherwise well.

☐ **12.21** A 21-year-old woman with a long history of anorexia complains of paraesthesia and numbness of her feet. Blood tests are taken and these show a macrocytic anaemia.

THEME: NEUROLOGICAL INVESTIGATIONS

Options

A Computed tomography (CT)

B Doppler scanning

C Electroencephalography (EEG)

D Lumbar puncture

E Magnetic resonance angiography (MRA)

F Magnetic resonance imaging (MRI)

G Myelogram

H Nerve conduction studies

I Positron-emission tomography

For each clinical scenario below, select the most appropriate investigation from the list above. Each option can be used once, more than once or not at all.

☐ **12.22** A 46-year-old man with unilateral tinnitus and unilateral sensorineural hearing loss.

☐ **12.23** A 39-year-old woman with intermittent paraesthesiae and weakness in her right hand, worse at night.

☐ **12.24** A 78-year-old man who complains of a 3-hour history of expressive dysphasia 2 weeks ago that has now resolved. On examination, he is in sinus rhythm with no added heart sounds. Neurological examination is unremarkable.

☐ **12.25** A 38-year-old woman complains of sudden-onset double vision. On examination, she has a VIth nerve palsy. On further questioning, she admits to having had several similar episodes in the past.

☐ **12.26** A 62-year-old woman requests screening after her sister died from a ruptured berry aneurysm. She has already lost her mother to a stroke and her older brother suffered a subarachnoid haemorrhage 2 years ago.

ALGORITHM QUESTIONS

THEME: NEW-ONSET SEIZURE

12.27–12.31

Options

A Epilepsy likely

B Epilepsy unlikely

C Incontinence

D No

E Petit mal

F Syncope likely

G Syncope unlikely

H Tongue biting

I Yes

The differentiation of epilepsy from syncope can be difficult. The following flow chart has been developed to simplify the diagnosis.

From the list of options above, select the most appropriate choice for each question in the flow chart.

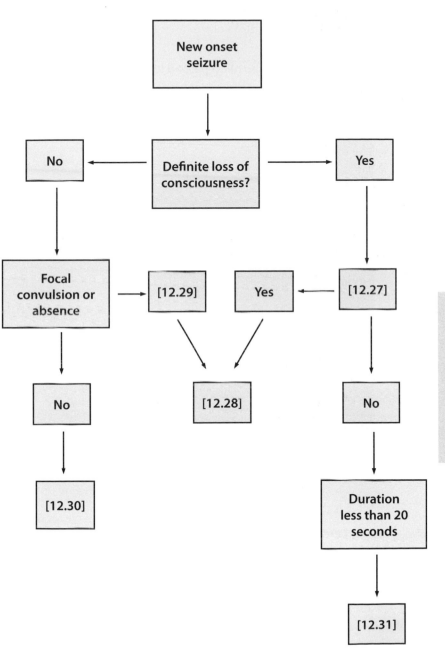

PICTURE QUESTION

12.32 A 76-year-old man who had a parotid tumour removed last year complains that he has developed a lopsided smile. He feels fine in himself. His picture is shown below.

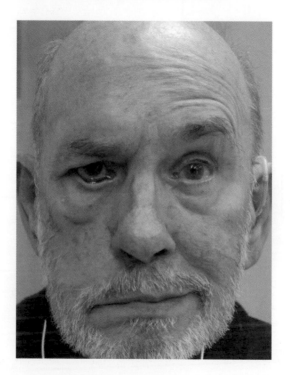

What is the most likely cause?

- [ ] A Cerebrovascular accident
- [ ] B Malignant infiltration
- [ ] C Meningioma
- [ ] D Motor neurone disease
- [ ] E Multiple sclerosis

DATA INTERPRETATION QUESTION

12.33 Consider the graph shown below, which illustrates the epidemiology of epilepsy.

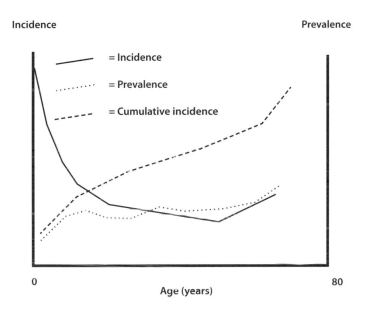

Which one of the following statements about this data is true?

☐ A The fact that the cumulative incidence is higher than the prevalence in middle to older age suggests that most people enter remission at some stage

☐ B The fall in incidence in early to middle age is due to the high mortality of childhood epilepsy

☐ C The graph shows that most patients with epilepsy suffer from the condition all of their lives

☐ D The increase in incidence in old age is due to an increase in idiopathic epilepsy

☐ E The increase in prevalence in old age is due to physiological changes affecting seizure threshold

HOT TOPICS/EVIDENCE BASED PRACTICE

12.34 Which one of the following statements regarding NICE guidance on the treatment of multiple sclerosis is true?

- ☐ A   Acute exacerbations of multiple sclerosis can be treated with cyclophosphamide in patients intolerant of steroids
- ☐ B   Hyperbaric oxygen is useful in relapsing and remitting multiple sclerosis
- ☐ C   Long-term oral prednisolone is generally well tolerated in patients with progressive multiple sclerosis
- ☐ D   Natalizumab is recommended only for the treatment of rapidly evolving, severe, relapsing–remitting multiple sclerosis
- ☐ E   The risk of relapse is increased during pregnancy

ANSWERS

12.1   D: Tardive dyskinesia

Tardive dyskinesia is characterised by repetitive facial grimaces and choreo-athetoid movements of the upper limbs and is usually seen after neuroleptic use, although it can occur after taking antiemetics or over-the-counter medications. It is more common in females and usually settles with drug withdrawal, although 40% still have symptoms after 3 years. Anticholinergics (eg Kemadrin) or benzodiazepines usually help with symptoms. Jacksonian epilepsy is a condition where seizures are initially localised but spread to become a generalised tonic–clonic seizure; temporal lobe epilepsy is characterised by unusual behaviour or hallucinations.

12.2   E: Regular exercise has been shown to maintain performance in activities of daily living

Alzheimer's disease should be treated using a multidisciplinary approach, including regular exercise and group activities, which have been shown to slow the decline in performance of activities of daily living. Cholinesterase inhibitors are useful in mild to moderate disease and NICE guidance suggests they should only be initiated by specialists. Sedatives and alcohol should be avoided because of the risk of falls and increased confusion. Cholinesterase inhibitors are available as patches, which are useful where nausea or vomiting occurs with the oral form or in more advanced cases for control of agitation.

12.3   D: Myasthenia gravis

Myasthenia gravis is caused by autoantibodies against acetylcholine receptors. The condition affects the eyes in almost all cases, causing diplopia and ptosis, can affect skeletal muscles and respiratory muscles and can cause bulbar symptoms. It has a prevalence of 20:100,000 and can be exacerbated by drugs such as phenytoin. Diagnosis is by antibody detection and administration of a short-acting acetylcholinesterase inhibitor. Newly diagnosed patients should be investigated to exclude thymoma, which is associated in some cases. Treatment is usually with oral pyridostigmine, and surgical if there is a thymoma. Short-term immunosuppression might be used for acute attacks.

12.4   A: Carpal tunnel syndrome

Carpal tunnel syndrome is caused by compression of the median nerve at the wrist. Diagnosis can be confirmed by Phalen's or Tinel's tests or by nerve conduction studies where there is doubt. Treatment is with steroid injection, although surgery is often required when there is muscle wasting.

12.5   B: Combination of levodopa and a dopa-decarboxylase inhibitor is associated with less nausea and vomiting than levodopa alone

Combining levodopa and a dopa-decarboxylase inhibitor allows smaller doses of levodopa to be used and reduces peripheral cardiovascular side-effects and vomiting. It is often particularly useful in the elderly. Ropinirole is effective in younger patients and causes fewer motor complications, but can be associated with nausea. It can be used with levodopa. Selegiline cannot be used with levodopa because of the risk of postural hypotension. Only patients with intractable symptoms should be referred for surgery.

12.6   E: Riluzole increases the period of time to need for ventilation but does not improve prognosis

Riluzole has been shown to increase the mean time to need for ventilation but does not affect the final outcome. The multidisciplinary approach involving occupational therapy and physiotherapy as well as speech and language therapy can lead to significant benefits, and symptomatic drug treatments such as benztropine for drooling and baclofen or diazepam for spasticity are very helpful. The decision to ventilate is one that must be made with the patient because this will often be seen as simply prolonging the patient's suffering.

12.7 A: A stat dose of ciprofloxacin is effective prophylaxis in close contacts

Rifampicin is traditionally used for prophylaxis but ciprofloxacin has fewer side-effects and interactions, although is it is unlicensed for this use. Intravenous or intramuscular benzylpenicillin should be used for suspected meningitis, or cefotaxime if there is a history of drug reaction with penicillin. In cases of anaphylaxis, however, chloramphenicol should be used. Amoxicillin is the treatment of choice for *Listeria* meningitis. Meningitis is a life-threatening condition and treatment should not be delayed for blood cultures. Polymerase chain reaction (PCR) testing will often confirm the diagnosis after initiation of therapy, regardless of antibiotic use.

12.8 D: It is typically relapsing and remitting

Trigeminal neuralgia is a relapsing and remitting neuralgic pain in any of the branches of the trigeminal nerve, nearly always unilateral and characterised by paroxysms lasting less than 2 minutes. Associated neurological signs suggest the presence of alternative causes such as tumour. Carbamazepine is effective in 70% of patients and gabapentin is often used as an alternative. Refractory cases can be treated with surgery.

12.9 B: Guillain–Barré syndrome

This history is typical of Guillain–Barré syndrome and ascending polyneuropathy, usually triggered by *Mycoplasma* or *Campylobacter* infection. An ascending paralysis occurs which can cause respiratory failure. Treatment is supportive, although plasmapheresis or intravenous immunoglobulin might be used. Approximately 5% of patients go on to develop a relapsing and remitting pattern of disease (chronic inflammatory demyelinating polyneuropathy or CIDP). Muscle weakness usually evolves over 3–21 days and can start proximally. Reiter's syndrome is also triggered by infection but usually causes iritis and polyarthritis in HLA-B27-positive people.

THEME: NEUROLOGICAL DISORDERS

12.10 G: New-variant Creutzfeld–Jakob disease

Creutzfeld–Jakob disease can be iatrogenic, familial or idiopathic. The new-variant form causes symptoms in younger patients, who often present initially with psychiatric symptoms. Early-onset cerebellar disease is typical and patients invariably become demented, with choreiform movements and myoclonus. Familial forms have variable presentation according to the genetic mutation.

12.11 B: Motor neurone disease

Motor neurone disease typically starts with loss of strength in the hands, with wasting and fasciculation. Most patients have a combination of upper and lower motor neurone signs. The disease is progressive and bulbar symptoms are common. There is no sensory or cognitive loss and there are no ocular symptoms, unlike myasthenia or multiple sclerosis.

12.12 C: Multiple sclerosis

Multiple sclerosis typically causes multiple neurological deficits separated in location and over time. Visual symptoms, particularly optic neuritis, are common but it can also cause upper motor neurone lesions, cerebellar lesions and vertigo. A high index of suspicion should be maintained in young patients with unexplained neurological symptoms and signs.

12.13 H: Parkinson's disease

Parkinson's disease is characterised by resting tremor, increased tone, hypokinesia and bradykinesia. Patients typically have a flat affect and are often misdiagnosed as depressed, although this is common in these patients.

THEME: HEADACHE

12.14   F: Giant-cell arteritis

Giant-cell arteritis causes a prodromal illness of malaise, anorexia and weight loss, followed by temporal headache and scalp tenderness. Jaw claudication is pathognomonic of this condition. Late features include visual loss and severe temporal tenderness.

12.15   E: Cluster headache

Cluster headache typically affects men in their forties and causes daily severe headaches, often with associated watering of the eye and nasal symptoms. They are severe and last 1–2 hours. They are often triggered by alcohol.

12.16   L: Transient global amnesia

Transient global amnesia is a syndrome of complete amnesia that often arises after vigorous exercise such as sexual intercourse or swimming, particularly in cold water. There are no other neurological symptoms and the memory gradually returns over some hours. CT or MRI might be required to differentiate between this and stroke, and there is an association with migraine. No treatment is usually necessary.

12.17   B: Brain tumour

These symptoms are consistent with raised intracranial pressure (ICP). Common chronic causes include brain tumour but, when presenting acutely, a colloid cyst or intracranial bleed should be excluded.

12.18   G: Migraine

This is a typical history of focal migraine, with a prodrome, aura and headache, followed by resolution. Treatment is aimed at avoiding provoking factors (including the pill) where appropriate and treating symptoms, often with a triptan.

THEME: PERIPHERAL NERVE DISORDERS

12.19   B: Charcot–Marie–Tooth disease

Charcot–Marie–Tooth disease is a hereditary peripheral neuropathy that usually presents with walking difficulties in the first or second decade. There are reduced reflexes and sensorimotor neuropathy and peripheral nerves can be palpably thickened. It is inherited as an autosomal dominant condition and usually causes mild disability with a normal lifespan.

12.20   D: Drug-induced peripheral neuropathy

Many drugs can cause peripheral neuropathy, but the commonest causes are amiodarone, phenytoin, isoniazid, vincristine, nitrofurantoin and gold. The neuropathy is often irreversible.

12.21   F: Vitamin B deficiency

Vitamin B12 deficiency causes peripheral neuropathy and can cause subacute combined degeneration of the cord if it is not treated. It also causes megaloblastic anaemia, glossitis, alopecia and malabsorption, and can cause optic neuritis. It is rare in developed countries in people who are otherwise healthy, but might be seen in people with malabsorption, for example patients with pernicious anaemia or patients who have had bowel resection (eg for Crohn's disease).

THEME: NEUROLOGICAL INVESTIGATIONS

12.22   F: Magnetic resonance imaging (MRI)

MRI is superior to CT for the identification of small soft-tissue lesions and is the investigation of choice for brain tumours, suspected multiple sclerosis and acoustic neuromas.

12.23   H: Nerve conduction studies

Nerve conduction studies are useful where peripheral nerve lesions are suspected.

12.24   B: Doppler scanning

In cases of suspected transient ischaemic attack (TIA), carotid Dopplers are indicated, even in the absence of a bruit on auscultation. Stenosis of >69% indicates that surgery is likely to be beneficial.

12.25   F: Magnetic resonance imaging (MRI)

This lady has symptoms suggestive of multiple sclerosis, for which she should have an MRI scan.

12.26   E: Magnetic resonance angiography (MRA)

Magnetic resonance angiography is non-invasive and provides good-quality images of the intracranial circulation. Aneurysms identified by MRA can then be dealt with by endovascular embolisation.

THEME: NEW-ONSET SEIZURE

12.27 H: Tongue biting

12.28 A: Epilepsy likely

12.29 I: Yes

12.30 B: Epilepsy unlikely

12.31 F: Syncope likely

Syncope can cause stiffening of the body, twitching of the limbs, and occasional incontinence. These symptoms are not therefore always useful in differentiating epilepsy from syncope. Attempt to identify a precipitating factor for syncope, such as standing for long periods (particularly if the ambient temperature is high), pain, strong emotion, micturition, diarrhoea or vomiting. It is uncommon for syncope to occur without some warning symptoms, usually including some combination of nausea, blurred vision, light-headedness, and a sensation of muffled hearing. Syncope is often accompanied by pallor and sweating, while cyanosis is usual in the early stages of generalised tonic–clonic seizures. The actual duration of the loss of consciousness in syncope usually amounts to a few seconds only; it can, however, be longer if the patient is supported in the upright position after fainting. The postictal phase following syncope does not involve prolonged drowsiness and confusion, and recovery is generally rapid, though the patient might feel a sense of malaise for some time. Tongue biting suggests a seizure.

12.32   B: Malignant infiltration

This gentleman has a lower motor neurone lesion, as evidenced by the fact that he cannot furrow his brow (the brow is innervated bilaterally). Causes of this include Bell's palsy, Lyme disease, herpesvirus infection (zoster or acute infection) and cholesteatoma. Trauma, Guillain–Barré syndrome, diabetes and sarcoidosis are other common causes. Lower motor neurone facial nerve palsy can be seen in patients with a history of parotid gland tumours, either due to iatrogenic damage or to tumour infiltration. Upper motor neurone causes include central nervous system tumours, multiple sclerosis, syphilis and cerebrovascular disease. Bell's palsy is a diagnosis of exclusion.

12.33   A: The fact that the cumulative incidence is higher than the prevalence in middle to older age suggests that most people enter remission at some stage

The risk of recurrence following a single seizure is approximately 50–70% but the long-term prognosis is good. Retrospective studies suggest that after 20 years, 76% of patients had at least one 5-year period of complete freedom from seizures, and 70% remained seizure-free. Approximately 50% were in remission of at least 5 years' duration and had been off all antiepileptic drugs for at least 5 years. The cumulative incidence of epilepsy is considerably higher than the prevalence, suggesting that most patients enter long term remission at some stage.

12.34   D: Natalizumab is recommended only for the treatment of rapidly evolving, severe, relapsing–remitting multiple sclerosis

NICE guidance released in August 2007 recommended that natalizumab is only used for relapsing and remitting multiple sclerosis where there is rapid evolution of disease. Cyclophosphamide, hyperbaric oxygen and long-term corticosteroids are not recommended because there is no evidence for benefit. Multiple sclerosis usually improves during pregnancy but often relapses transiently afterwards. Acute exacerations should be treated with high-dose intravenous methylprednisolone.

CHAPTER 13
OPHTHALMOLOGY
SINGLE BEST ANSWER QUESTIONS

13.1 A 20-year-old man complains of a 3-week history of persistent conjunctivitis. He has tried using over-the-counter brolene and fucidic acid eyedrops but these have not helped. Of note, he returned from a stag weekend in Amsterdam 4 weeks ago, following which he was treated for a urinary tract infection at the local walk-in centre. On examination he has a profuse, mucopurulent discharge and hyperaemia. Which one of the following is the most likely diagnosis?

- [ ] A   Allergic conjunctivitis
- [ ] B   Chlamydial infection
- [ ] C   Dry eyes
- [ ] D   Fungal conjunctivitis
- [ ] E   Herpes keratitis

13.2 A 65-year-old man comes in for a repeat prescription of eye drops. He is a known asthmatic who also smokes from time to time. He complains that since his review at the eye hospital 1 month ago, his breathlessness has been getting a lot worse. What is the single most likely explanation for these symptoms?

- ☐ A   He is on Xalatan
- ☐ B   He recently stopped timolol and started Xalatan
- ☐ C   He was changed from Xalatan to 0.5% timolol
- ☐ D   He was started on brimonidine, which exacerbates asthma
- ☐ E   He was started on pilocarpine, which is known to exacerbate heart failure

13.3 A 47-year-old short-sighted woman complains of a 1-week history of flashes of light at the edge of her vision in her left eye. Today she has noticed a dark curtain over one side of her visual field which does not go away with head movements. The single most likely diagnosis is:

- ☐ A   Migraine
- ☐ B   Retinal detachment
- ☐ C   Uveitis
- ☐ D   Vitreous haemorrhage
- ☐ E   Vitrous detachment

13.4 Which one of the following is the single most important risk factor for developing a central retinal vein occlusion (CRVO)?

- ☐ A   Diabetes
- ☐ B   Gout
- ☐ C   Hypertension
- ☐ D   Obesity
- ☐ E   Smoking

13.5 A 70-year-old woman complains of several weeks of generalised aches and pains and difficulty getting out of a chair. Over the last 24 hours she has become aware of loss of vision in her left eye, with pain in her jaw on chewing. On examination, she has a visual acuity of 6/60 and a left relative afferent pupillary defect. Her left disc appears pale and swollen. The single best option in the management of this patient is:

☐ A A 7-day course of 15 mg prednisolone and then review
☐ B Conservative management as the vision has already been lost
☐ C Refer to neurology with an MRI scan
☐ D Start 80 mg of prednisolone and refer to ophthalmology
☐ E Urgent temporal artery biopsy

13.6 An 80-year-old man complains of sudden-onset double vision. He is otherwise extremely well, is not known to have high BP or high cholesterol, but he does smoke. On examination, he appears to have restricted lateral gaze in the left eye. His double vision is horizontal and worse on looking to the left and into the distance. His pupils react normally and there is no headache or ptosis. Which one of the following statements about his management is correct?

☐ A Advise him to attend his optometrist, who will prescribe glasses with prisms
☐ B Do nothing – it is likely that this will resolve in a few weeks
☐ C Start aspirin and investigate for cardiovascular risk
☐ D Start aspirin, investigate for cardiovascular risk and refer to ophthalmology
☐ E Urgent referral to neurosurgery

13.7 A 50-year-old man has recently moved to your area. He complains that his vision is getting worse and that he has difficulty getting around, especially at night. He was diagnosed with retinitis pigmentosa several years ago. On examination, he wears very thick glasses and his visual acuity is 6/9 in both eyes (ie he is able to read most of the Snellen chart). Which one of the following management options is most appropriate?

☐   A   Reassure him that his vision is within the normal range

☐   B   Refer to ophthalmology for an assessment

☐   C   Register him as partially sight-impaired

☐   D   Register him as severely sight-impaired

☐   E   Tell him to go to his optometrist for some new glasses

13.8 A 68-year-old man presents to your clinic with a painful red eye. He had cataract surgery 2 days ago and aside from some mild grittiness, his eye was comfortable. Since then his eye has become very red and painful and he is no longer able to see properly. The single most likely diagnosis is:

☐   A   Acute angle-closure glaucoma due to the drops used to dilate the pupil prior to the surgery

☐   B   Endophthalmitis

☐   C   Postoperative iritis

☐   D   Severe allergy to the anaesthetic injection

☐   E   Severe conjunctivitis

EXTENDED MATCHING QUESTIONS

THEME: VISUAL FIELDS

Options

For each of the following patients, select the most likely visual field defect from the options above. Each option can be used once, more than once or not at all.

- [ ] **13.9** An elderly lady who has had a stroke.

- [ ] **13.10** A homeless, alcoholic smoker.

- [ ] **13.11** A man with acromegaly.

- [ ] **13.12** A diabetic who has had panretinal photocoagulation.

- [ ] **13.13** A patient with glaucoma.

THEME: PATIENTS PRESENTING WITH PTOSIS

Options

A   Bilateral ptosis in a patient with excessive skin around the eyes

B   Bilateral ptosis in a patient with frontal balding and a prolonged handshake

C   Bilateral ptosis, worse at the end of the day, with associated intermittent diplopia

D   Unilateral ptosis with the eye deviated down and out, with a large pupil

E   Unilateral ptosis with a history of orbital cellulitis

F   Unilateral ptosis with a small pupil, anhidrosis and enophthalmos

---

For each of the diagnoses below, select the most likely findings from the list of options above. Each option can be used once, more than once or not at all.

☐   **13.14**   Third nerve palsy.

☐   **13.15**   Myotonic dystrophy.

☐   **13.16**   Myasthenia gravis.

☐   **13.17**   Levator disinsertion.

☐   **13.18**   Horner syndrome.

PICTURE QUESTIONS

13.19 A myopic man complains of seeing flashing lights and floaters. The appearance of his fundus is shown below:

Which one of the following statements about this patient is correct?

☐ A   Being short-sighted usually reduces the risk of this condition

☐ B   He has a retinal tear that can be treated with laser in the out-patient department

☐ C   He has already lost vision and therefore surgery is not urgent

☐ D   He will need an urgent operation to prevent irreversible visual loss

☐ E   He will need surgery within 1 week

13.20 Study the photo below.

Which one of the following is the correct diagnosis?

- ☐ A   Glaucomatous cupping
- ☐ B   Optic atrophy
- ☐ C   Macular hole
- ☐ D   Normal fundus
- ☐ E   Silver wiring

13.21 A patient presents to you with visual problems in one eye. Examination reveals the appearance shown below:

The single most likely clinical history that would match this appearance is:

- [ ] A   A 20-year-old poorly controlled diabetic man who complains of floaters

- [ ] B   A 30-year-old woman with a history of migraine

- [ ] C   A 70-year-old man who has previously had a stroke and complains of intermittent loss of vision in one eye lasting a few seconds

- [ ] D   A 75-year-old woman with myalgia and weight loss who has noticed pain in her temples when combing her hair and pain on chewing

- [ ] E   A very short-sighted patient who has similar disc appearances on both sides

13.22 A 70-year-old lady complains of a gradual deterioration in vision in both eyes. Her visual acuity is 6/9 and 6/12. She has been told by her optician that she has macular degeneration and has heard of new treatments available for this condition. She would like your advice regarding treatment. Examination findings are shown below:

Which one of the following statements is correct regarding this clinical situation?

- [ ] A   She has evidence of diabetic maculopathy and needs to have her diabetes managed
- [ ] B   She requires an urgent referral to ophthalmology for intravitreal Lucentis
- [ ] C   She would be a suitable candidate for laser treatment
- [ ] D   She would be a suitable candidate for photodynamic therapy
- [ ] E   You should advise her to stop smoking and ensure a diet high in fresh fruit and vegetables

13.23 You see a young diabetic patient in your clinic. He is in his early twenties and has very poorly controlled type 1 diabetes. He doesn't like taking his insulin and he drinks and smokes to excess. His BP is slightly elevated. Fundoscopic findings are shown below:

Which one of the following statements is true regarding his visual prognosis?

- [ ] A   Following laser treatment his vision should remain stable
- [ ] B   He is at risk of visual loss due to retinal detachment
- [ ] C   He needs surgery to maintain his vision
- [ ] D   Regardless of the amount of laser treatment given, he is likely to be registered blind in 5 years
- [ ] E   With adequate laser and optimisation of diabetic control and risk factors, his vision can be maintained

DATA INTERPRETATION QUESTION

13.24 A patient complains of dry, gritty eyes. She has not been feeling well over the past few weeks and has lost weight. She also reports some mild breathlessness and complains of a dry cough. More recently she has developed floaters in her vision and some discomfort when looking at the light. You arrange blood tests, the results of which are shown below:

Haemoglobin	12.3 g/dl
WCC	9.0×10^9/l
Platelets	222×10^9/l
Urea	10.0 mmol/l
Creatinine	165 µmol/l
Calcium	2.9 mmol/l
Phosphate	1.8 mmol/l
Serum ACE	432 U/l (40–135)
ESR	70 mm/hr
HLA-B27	Negative

The single most likely diagnosis is:

☐ A   Ankylosing spondylitis
☐ B   Behçet syndrome
☐ C   Retinal detachment
☐ D   Sarcoidosis
☐ E   Systemic lupus erythematosis

HOT TOPICS/EVIDENCE BASED PRACTICE

13.25 A 79-year-old woman complains of relatively sudden deterioration of vision in her left eye. She has very poor vision in her right eye because of macular degeneration. She states that over the past 2 weeks when she looks at straight edges they appear bent. Also, when looking at a fence or a brick wall, all the straight lines appear wavy. Which one of the following statements about this condition is correct?

☐ A She has developed wet macular degeneration in her left eye and needs laser treatment

☐ B She has dry macular degeneration in her left eye and needs to start taking oral anti-VEGF tablets

☐ C She has macular degeneration in her left eye. There is no treatment other than recommending vitamins and stopping smoking

☐ D She has wet macular degeneration and is eligible for intravitreal anti-VEGF therapy on the NHS

☐ E She has wet macular degeneration and needs surgery

ANSWERS

13.1   B: Chlamydial infection

This patient is at risk of sexually transmitted infections. *Chlamydia* is a relatively common cause of persistent conjunctivitis and is diagnosed on a conjunctival swab. The patient will need systemic treatment and referral to a genitourinary medicine (GUM) clinic. Gonorrhoea can also affect the eye, causing a severe conjunctivitis. There is classically a profuse, frothy discharge and an intensely red eye. This can progress rapidly and can lead to corneal perforation if not managed promptly. It is treated with intramuscular penicillin and is regarded as an ophthalmological emergency. It is possible that the patient has dry eyes, but if this is due to a long-haul flight, it should resolve shortly after arrival. Allergic conjunctivitis is usually bilateral, with a history of atopy or an exacerbating factor.

13.2   C: He was changed from Xalatan to 0.5% timolol

Timolol is commonly prescribed in drops used to treat glaucoma. It is a β blocker used either on its own or in combination with other drugs and is given topically. Although the dose is low, systemic absorption does occur and can exacerbate underlying medical conditions such as asthma, hypotension and bradycardia.

13.3   B: Retinal detachment

Although all of the options can cause 'flashes and floaters', the complaint of a dark, constant, peripheral shadow demands an exclusion of retinal detachment. Myopic (short-sighted) people are more at risk because of their relatively large eyes. The treatment of retinal detachment is surgical. In the early stages vision can be maintained at normal levels but if the detachment is left and the macula detaches (a macula–off retinal detachment) the visual prognosis is poor.

13.4   C: Hypertension

Patients who develop a central retinal vein occlusion are likely to be followed-up by the eye hospital as a minority of patients will develop neovascularisation at the iris and drainage angle of the eye which can develop into painful rubeotic glaucoma. Patients who develop this condition (or who are at risk of it) will require laser treatment. It is important to address any blood pressure problem because this is the main risk factor in predisposing patients to CRVO; diabetes and smoking are also important risk factors, though mainly via their effect on systemic cardiovascular disease. Without adequate blood pressure control, patients are at increased risk of further vascular events in the affected eye or indeed in the contralateral eye. It is important to note that there is no current treatment for CRVO other than preventing the complications of rubeosis. Aspirin is often advised. This is not to treat the eye, but rather for secondary prevention of cardiovascular events in the affected individual.

13.5   D: Start 80 mg of prednisolone and refer to ophthalmology

Giant-cell arteritis is an emergency. The patient has a high risk of blindness. In a patient such as the one in the question, the risk is to the other eye, which can rapidly become affected if the condition is not treated. Characteristically, patients have a prodrome of temporal artery tenderness, jaw claudication, malaise, weight loss and fatigue and might have already been diagnosed with polymyalgia rheumatica. Classically, the ESR is very elevated, and is accompanied by a rise in the C-reactive protein (CRP). This is by no means always the case, however, and giant-cell arteritis can still occur in the absence of a very high ESR. Treatment comprises high-dose steroids, which are very slowly tapered down. The patient is often on a maintenance dose of about 5 mg for several years. In order to confirm the diagnosis, a temporal artery biopsy is performed by the ophthalmologist.

13.6   D: Start aspirin, investigate for cardiovascular risk and refer to ophthalmology

The patient has developed a left VIth nerve palsy. The most common reason for this to occur in a patient of this age is microvascular disease due to high BP/cholesterol/diabetes/smoking. He will need assessment for cardiovascular risk factors and secondary prevention as appropriate. Referral to ophthalmology is necessary to:

- Confirm the diagnosis and exclude involvement of other cranial nerves (including the optic disc)

- Obtain an orthoptic assessment in order to quantify the diplopia and prescribe the correct prisms

- Arrange relevant investigations and follow-up.

It is also possible to develop cranial nerve palsies in association with giant-cell arteritis and so if there is any suspicion of polymyalgia rheumatica, this diagnosis should be considered.

13.7   B: Refer to ophthalmology for an assessment

Retinitis pigmentosa is a condition which results in photoreceptor and retinal pigment epithelium degeneration. Both rods and cones are affected. Patients typically develop impaired night vision and constricted visual fields. This then progresses to a reduction in visual acuity. Patients with retinitis pigmentosa can also develop cataracts and macular oedema (fluid at the macula), which contribute to the deterioration of vision. Referral is advisable to treat exacerbating factors such as cataract, potentially register them as partially sighted and arrange assessment by the low visual aids service. As the GP, you will be informed of registration as partially sighted and the patient will be put in touch with social services.

13.8   B: Endophthalmitis

This is an emergency and the patient needs urgent referral to ophthalmology. This condition, where there is intraocular infection, can rapidly progress to irreversible blindness and retinal detachment. The classic presentation is one of a painful red eye developing a few days after surgery. There might be a hypopyon (pus in the anterior chamber) and slit-lamp examination will reveal significant intraocular inflammation. Deterioration to irreversible blindness or retinal detachment is rapid and prognosis is poor, even with prompt treatment. Management includes intravitreal sampling and injection of antibiotics. Vitrectomy might be necessary to clear debris. If retinal detachment occurs due to necrosis of the retina, further vitreoretinal surgery is indicated.

THEME: VISUAL FIELDS

13.9   B

Stroke usually causes a homonymous hemianopia.

13.10   E

Tobacco typically causes a caecocentral scotoma.

13.11   C

Optic chiasm compression (eg from a pituitary tumour) causes a bitemporal hemianopia.

13.12   G

Photocoagulation involves burning the peripheral visual field and results in constricted visual fields.

13.13   F

Glaucoma causes bilateral arcuate scotomata and delayed diagnosis can result in irreversible tunnel vision.

THEME: PATIENTS PRESENTING WITH PTOSIS

13.14   D: Unilateral ptosis with the eye deviated down and out, with a large pupil

13.15   B: Bilateral ptosis in patient with frontal balding and a prolonged handshake

13.16   C: Bilateral ptosis, worse at the end of the day, with associated intermittent diplopia

13.17   E: Unilateral ptosis with a history of orbital cellulitis (note the history might not be recent)

13.18   F: Unilateral ptosis with a small pupil, anhidrosis and enophthalmos

13.19   D: He will need an urgent operation to prevent irreversible visual loss

The photograph shows a large retinal tear and a peripheral retinal detachment. Small tears alone can be treated with laser in order to prevent retinal detachment but once the retina has detached, surgery is necessary. The detachment is peripheral and the subretinal fluid has not reached the macula. This means that the patient's vision may be saved with urgent surgery to reattach the retina. Once the macula has detached, vision becomes poor – typically 6/60 or worse. Surgery can restore vision to some degree but not usually to previous levels. Myopic individuals are at higher risk of detachment because their eyes are relatively large.

13.20 D: Normal fundus

It is very easy to be tricked into interpreting a normal eye as being abnormal. Disc appearances and fundus markings differ between individuals, especially among different races. In optic atrophy there is usually a strikingly pale disc and this is caused by damage to or ischaemia of the optic nerve head. Glaucomatous discs have a large cup to disc ratio and the rim of the optic disc is thin compared with the disc as a whole (a normal ratio is up to 0.5). Macular holes usually cause a gradual reduction in visual acuity, although where a hole forms following trauma the visual deterioration is more rapid. Slit-lamp examination will reveal a hole in the retina at the macula. Direct ophthalmoscopy may reveal an abnormal foveal reflex. Silver wiring occurs in hypertension. In a young patient, there is a higher reflectivity of the fundus than in an older patient. The fundus and vessels can appear shiny. This is not to be confused with the silver wiring seen in hypertension.

13.21 D: A 75-year-old lady with myalgia and weight loss who has noticed pain in her temples when combing her hair and pain on chewing

Anterior ischaemic optic neuritis can be arteritic or non-arteritic. The history provided suggests giant-cell arteritis as an arteritic cause. The main risk is to the other eye. Visual prognosis in the affected eye is poor.

Eye examination in migraine is normal. A young lady with raised intracranial pressure and headaches might have swollen optic discs. Amaurosis fugax can precede a central retinal artery occlusion (CRAO), but CRAO typically causes a pale fundus with a cherry-red spot at the macula – the disc is not typically swollen or haemorrhagic. There are no new vessels to be seen, so diabetic retinopathy is unlikely. Patients who are very short-sighted (myopic) can have abnormal-looking discs but it is usually long-sighted patients (hypermetropes) who have crowded discs which are sometimes confused with early papilloedema (the extent of disc swelling and the presence of haemorrhages exclude this diagnosis in this picture).

13.22   E: You should advise her to stop smoking and ensure a diet high in fresh fruit and vegetables

The photo shows areas of drusen, pigment changes and atrophy consistent with dry macular degeneration. Dry macular degeneration is more common than wet macular degeneration and there is no treatment for this, with slowly progressive loss of central vision. Abstinence from smoking and a diet rich in fresh fruit and vegetables can help slow the progression of the disease.

Wet macular degeneration is characterised by fluid leakage and subretinal oedema, resulting in visual distortion. Intravitreal Lucentis, an anti-VEGF drug, restores vision and prevents scarring. Photodynamic therapy destroys abnormal blood vessels near the macula. This treatment is aimed at preventing deterioration in vision, although the treatment itself causes significant scarring. It can be difficult to detect wet changes without a slit-lamp examination and therefore ophthalmology referral might be indicated. Most importantly, the patient should be aware that if she starts to experience distortion of her vision, this could herald the development of wet changes and an urgent referral to ophthalmology would then be appropriate.

13.23   E: With adequate laser and optimisation of diabetic control and risk factors, his vision can be maintained

This photograph shows proliferative diabetic retinopathy with extensive neovascularisation at the optic disc. There are multiple dot and blot haemorrhages, microaneurysms and hard exudates. This patient is at high risk of visual loss due to vitreous haemorrhage and maculopathy. Urgent panretinal laser is indicated. It is likely that several sessions of laser will be needed to bring about regression and involution of the abnormal blood vessels. Management of the patient's risk factors is most important, including the psychological side of his condition. Surgery might be necessary if vitreous haemorrhage does not clear after several months, or if there is a progressive tractional retinal detachment. This type of detachment is different from that due to a retinal tear as it can remain stable for a long time, requiring monitoring only.

13.24   D: Sarcoidosis

Sarcoidosis is a multisystem disease characterised by non-caseating granulomas on biopsy. Note the raised serum ACE and calcium, both characteristic of this condition (although not always present). In this patient renal function is impaired and the dry cough suggests pulmonary involvement. Sarcoid can affect the eyes, where it can result in impaired lacrimal gland function and intermediate uveitis, as in this patient. In a patient presenting like this, further investigations will be necessary, including imaging. It can be difficult to exclude malignancy and a biopsy, either renal or bronchial, is often indicated. Treatment is likely to consist of steroids in the first instance, followed by a second-line immunosuppressant such as Cellcept. This will require long-term monitoring of blood results and can be carried out in primary- or secondary-care settings.

13.25   D: She has wet macular degeneration and Is eligible for intravitreal anti-VEGF therapy on the NHS

There are two main types of macular degeneration, wet and dry. Intravitreal injections of Lucentis (anti-VEGF) at 4–6-weekly intervals in patients with recently diagnosed wet macular degeneration can bring about dramatic improvement in vision. Referral to an ophthalmologist is indicated so that the patient can be fully assessed for eligibility for these drugs. There is no treatment for dry macular degeneration, although stopping smoking and ensuring a diet rich in fresh fruit and vegetables is recommended.

CHAPTER 13 ANSWERS

CHAPTER 14
PAEDIATRICS
SINGLE BEST ANSWER QUESTIONS

14.1 A 3-month-old baby boy is brought to see you by his mother. She came home from work after leaving him in the care of her older daughter and found that he had suffered a nosebleed. Her daughter does not recall this happening and says that he has been fine all morning. He was born at term after a normal delivery and is formula-fed. On examination the child appears well but there is some dried blood in each nostril. There are no other signs of bleeding. Which one of the following would be the most appropriate action in this situation?

- [ ] A   Admit under the on-call paediatrician
- [ ] B   Give vitamin K
- [ ] C   Prescribe topical antibiotics to use while the nose heals
- [ ] D   Reassure his mother that the bleeding is likely to be due to a cold and should settle
- [ ] E   Report the family to social services

14.2 A 3-year-old child has had a fever, sore throat and reluctance to eat for the last 48 hours. On examination you note vesicles on the buccal mucosa and tongue. Examining his body you also find tender papules on the hands and feet. What is the most likely cause of these symptoms?

- ☐ A Coxsackievirus infection
- ☐ B Henoch–Schönlein purpura
- ☐ C Idiopathic thrombocytopenic purpura
- ☐ D Parvovirus B19 infection
- ☐ E Rotavirus infection

14.3 While carrying out a routine baby check on a 6-week-old baby you note that there seems to be an absent red reflex in both eyes. The eyes look otherwise normal and the rest of the examination is unremarkable. The mother says that her pregnancy was unremarkable other than a flu-like illness in the second trimester. Which one of the following would be an appropriate action in this instance?

- ☐ A Admit under the on-call paediatrician
- ☐ B Inform the health visitor
- ☐ C Reassure mother that this is unlikely to be significant
- ☐ D Refer to ophthalmology routinely
- ☐ E Refer to orthoptic clinic

14.4 You receive a telephone call from one of your patients whose son has been admitted to hospital with suspected Kawasaki disease. She has been doing some research on the Internet and has heard that it has fatal complications. She asks if this is true. Which one of the following statements is true in this situation?

☐ A 70% of patients develop cardiac complications

☐ B Aspirin should not be used due to the risk of Reye syndrome

☐ C Kawasaki disease can cause myocardial infarction

☐ D Mortality is approximately 20%

☐ E Nephrotic syndrome is frequently seen in these patients

14.5 Regarding the management of attention deficit hyperactivity disorder (ADHD), which one of the following statements is true?

☐ A Cognitive behavioural therapy (CBT) has no role in the management of ADHD

☐ B Methylphenidate can cause growth retardation

☐ C Methylphenidate is the treatment of choice in preschool children

☐ D Patients on drug treatment for ADHD should have a treatment holiday periodically to assess their ongoing need for treatment

☐ E Patients taking methylphenidate need monthly blood counts

14.6 A 10-year-old boy is brought to see you with a viral upper respiratory tract infection. On examination, you hear a heart murmur that has not been noted previously. Which one of the following would reassure you that this is an innocent murmur?

☐ A The murmur is grade 4/6

☐ B The murmur is short and diastolic in nature

☐ C The murmur is short and systolic in nature

☐ D The murmur radiates to the back

☐ E You listen again in 2 weeks and the murmur is still present

14.7 A 12-year-old girl is brought in to see you by her parents after an episode of deliberate self-harm the previous weekend. Her parents are obviously distraught and are terrified that she will do this again and be more successful next time. Which one of the following is a risk factor for successful suicide attempt following deliberate self-harm?

- [ ] A   Drug or alcohol abuse
- [ ] B   Early presentation following an episode of deliberate self-harm
- [ ] C   High performance at school
- [ ] D   Isolated episode of deliberate self-harm
- [ ] E   Spontaneous act of deliberate self-harm

14.8 Following a practice significant event, you decide to actively screen for patients with eating disorders. Which one of the following patients has a possible eating disorder?

- [ ] A   A 10-year-old girl who has started her periods a year earlier than her peers
- [ ] B   A 13-year-old girl with type 1 diabetes who is poorly compliant
- [ ] C   A 14-year-old boy who has lost 10 kg since becoming a vegan
- [ ] D   A 15-year-old girl with a BMI of 31 kg/m² who asks for help losing weight
- [ ] E   A 16-year-old girl with a BMI of 26 kg/m²

14.9 A 9-month-old boy has suffered from chronic constipation since birth. His mother had been told by his health visitor that this would improve with weaning but she finds he is no better. He opens his bowels every few days and his mother tells you that it is usually liquid. When you examine him his abdomen is distended, although his mother says he has always been like that. What is the most likely diagnosis in this case?

- [ ] A Anal fissure
- [ ] B Hirschsprung's disease
- [ ] C Hypothyroidism
- [ ] D Lactose intolerance
- [ ] E Simple constipation

14.10 An 18-month-old baby has been discharged after a febrile seizure. Which of the following statements about this condition is true? Select one option only.

- [ ] A 60% of children have recurrent febrile seizures during subsequent illnesses
- [ ] B A prolonged seizure is a risk factor for further prolonged attacks
- [ ] C In most cases the seizure lasts 10–15 minutes
- [ ] D Rigorous attempts should be made to reduce the temperature with ibuprofen and/or paracetamol
- [ ] E Seizures do not occur until the fever is apparent

14.11 A 4-year-old boy with no history of note comes to see you with a 24-hour history of pain in his right hip and refusal to weight-bear. His temperature is 38°C. When you examine him he will not move his hip but there are no signs if bruising and no rash. The single most likely diagnosis is:

- [ ] A   Henoch–Schönlein purpura
- [ ] B   Juvenile rheumatoid arthritis
- [ ] C   Perthes' disease
- [ ] D   Septic arthritis
- [ ] E   Slipped upper femoral epiphysis

14.12 A 7-year-old boy has a 4-week history of intermittent leg pains. They occur at night, and wake him from sleep. The pain is relieved when his mother rubs his legs. The boy is otherwise well and examination is normal. What is the single most likely diagnosis?

- [ ] A   Acute lymphoblastic leukaemia
- [ ] B   Growing pains
- [ ] C   Henoch–Schönlein purpura
- [ ] D   Juvenile chronic arthritis
- [ ] E   Perthes' disease

14.13 A mother is concerned that her 3-week-old baby 'makes a funny noise with his breathing'. A soft inspiratory stridor is heard. You suspect that he may have laryngomalacia. Which one of the following statements would support your diagnosis?

- [ ] A   The child has a barking cough
- [ ] B   The child has signs of respiratory distress
- [ ] C   The child is struggling to feed
- [ ] D   The stridor is intermittent and positional
- [ ] E   The stridor worsens over time

14.14 A mother is concerned that her 12-week-old baby does not respond to sound. From your records you see that the baby passed her neonatal hearing screening at birth and that there were no concerns at the 8-week check. On examination, the child is developing well, thriving, and appears to respond to sound during the consultation. The mother is not convinced and is still very concerned. The single best course of action is:

- [ ] A Arrange for a colleague at your practice to give a second opinion
- [ ] B Arrange to follow up the child yourself in 1 month
- [ ] C Ask the health visitor to visit mum at home
- [ ] D Reassure mum that all is well
- [ ] E Refer to paediatric audiology for assessment

14.15 A health visitor asks you to see a 9-month-old child regarding his development. Which one of the following statements about him would be of concern?

- [ ] A He does not say 'mama' or 'dada'
- [ ] B He first smiled at 8 weeks of age
- [ ] C He has never crawled
- [ ] D He is unable to pull himself up to stand
- [ ] E He shows a preference for using his right hand

14.16 A student midwife asks you to tell her what the current advice for minimising the risk of infant cot death is. Which one of the following would be included in your answer?

- [ ] A Babies should sleep in the same room as their parents for the first year of life
- [ ] B Place the baby on their front to sleep
- [ ] C The ideal room temperature for a baby is 20-24 °C
- [ ] D The use of dummies is not recommended
- [ ] E You should not smoke in the same room as the baby

CHAPTER 14 QUESTIONS

14.17 A 2-week-old breastfed baby is brought to see you by his mother. She is concerned that he has not opened his bowels for 5 days. The baby is well and examination is normal. Which is the single most appropriate statement?

☐ A A history of passage of meconium within the first 24 hours rules out Hirschprung's disease

☐ B It might be normal for this infant not to open his bowels for up to 7 days

☐ C Macrogol laxative would be an appropriate treatment

☐ D Prune juice would be an appropriate treatment

☐ E The baby needs to be referred urgently to hospital

14.18 A 9-year-old boy has been given a diagnosis of Henoch–Schönlein purpura and has now had the rash for 2 weeks. Regarding his outpatient follow-up, which one of the following statements is most appropriate?

☐ A The boy needs no further paediatric follow-up

☐ B The boy needs to be followed up by the paediatric team until his rash has resolved

☐ C The boy needs to be seen by an ophthalmologist and a paediatrician within 2 weeks

☐ D The boy should be followed up by the paediatric team for at least 6 months after the rash has resolved

☐ E The boy needs no follow-up now that he has had the rash for 2 weeks

14.19 An 18-month-old girl is brought to see you following a seizure. The mother describes how the little girl was hit by her older brother. She became still and very pale, stiffened, and fell to the floor. She was unresponsive for 20 seconds, with her eyes rolled up and with jerking of all four limbs. She did not wet herself or bite her tongue. She has no previous history of note and seems well now. The single most likely diagnosis is:

- [ ] A   Breath-holding
- [ ] B   Febrile convulsion
- [ ] C   Grand mal epilepsy
- [ ] D   Reflex anoxic seizure
- [ ] E   Simple faint

14.20 A 14-month-old child is brought to see you out of hours with croup. It is 2 am. The child started with symptoms 2 hours ago. He has a barking cough and stridor at rest. He has no other signs of respiratory distress. The single most appropriate course of action would be:

- [ ] A   Explain the diagnosis to parents and send him home with advice to return if he gets worse
- [ ] B   Give oral dexamethasone and send him home with advice to return if he gets worse
- [ ] C   Give oral dexamethasone and send him home with a further dose to be given in a further 12 hours
- [ ] D   Give oxygen and send to hospital in an ambulance
- [ ] E   Refer for paediatric assessment

14.21 A 12-month-old boy is brought to the surgery for his first measles mumps and rubella (MMR) vaccination. Which one of the following would be a contraindication to his receiving the vaccine today?

- [ ] A After his third meningococcal C vaccination he developed an area of localised erythema and induration at the site of injection
- [ ] B He has an egg allergy
- [ ] C He has an upper respiratory tract infection; his temperature is 38 °C
- [ ] D He is HIV-positive
- [ ] E His brother developed a measles-like rash and neck swelling after the MMR vaccine

14.22 You have been informed by the local hospital that a 4-year-old patient from your practice has been admitted with definite meningococcal sepsis. There have not been any previous cases. You need to organise appropriate prophylaxis. Which of the following is the single most appropriate group to treat?

- [ ] A All family members
- [ ] B All family members and friends who have played with the child in the last 48 hours
- [ ] C All family members and children at the same nursery
- [ ] D All household members
- [ ] E All household members and children at the same nursery

EXTENDED MATCHING QUESTIONS

THEME: BRUISING

Options

A	Blood culture	**F**	Skeletal survey
B	Clotting	**G**	Urea and electrolytes
C	Full blood count	**H**	Urine dipstick
D	Lumbar puncture	**I**	Urine toxicology
E	No investigation	**J**	von Willebrand factor

From the options given above, choose the single most appropriate investigation for each of the following clinical scenarios. Each option can be used once, more than once or not at all.

☐ **14.23** A 7-year-old boy develops a non-blanching rash on his legs. He is well in himself but complains of pain in his ankles.

☐ **14.24** A 15-month-old girl attends the surgery for immunisation. The practice nurse notices that she has three small bruises across her forehead and bruised knees. Her mother says that she has just started walking.

☐ **14.25** A 4-month-old baby attends the surgery for immunisation. The practice nurse notices that he has a large bruise on one thigh. His mother had not noticed it.

☐ **14.26** An 8-week-old Afro-Caribbean child is brought to the surgery for immunisation. The practice nurse notices a large blue bruise over his buttocks and extending up his back. His mother thinks that this has always been there.

☐ **14.27** An 8-year-old girl develops some non-blanching spots on her legs. She has recently been unwell with an upper respiratory tract infection. She noticed that her gums bled when she brushed her teeth this morning and has a large bruise on her arm, which she knocked this morning. She has no other symptoms and feels well.

THEME: VOMITING

Options

A   Cow's milk protein intolerance

B   Gastroenteritis

C   Gastro-oesophageal reflux

D   Hiatus hernia

E   Hirschprung's disease

F   Lactose intolerance

G   Overfeeding

H   Posseting

I   Pyloric stenosis

J   Reduced gastric motility

For each of the following clinical situations, choose the single most likely diagnosis from the list of options given above. Each option can be used once, more than once or not at all.

☐ **14.28 A 1-week-old baby is brought by his mother. He was born at home. Mum is concerned that he is vomiting and not feeding well. On questioning, his mother tells you that she cannot remember her child opening his bowels. On examination, the child appears grey, his abdomen is distended and firm. He vomits forcefully when you palpate his abdomen.**

☐ **14.29 A 6-week-old baby is brought to see you with increasing vomiting. His mother reports that he feeds very well and is always hungry. Initially he vomited small amounts after some feeds. Over the last week, he has had large vomits after every feed. On examination, the baby is alert and hungry but appears to have lost weight.**

14.30 A 6-week-old baby has a history of vomiting. His mother reports that from the age of 1 week her child has vomited after almost every feed. He is distressed when he vomits and if he is laid flat after a feed. He is thriving and examination is unremarkable.

14.31 A 6-week-old baby has a history of vomiting. His mother reports that he vomits after feeds, two or three times a day. He is described as a hungry baby. He takes 300 ml every 3 hours during the day, having seven feeds in 24 hours. His weight is above the 99th centile. Examination is otherwise unremarkable.

14.32 An 8-month-old baby has a history of vomiting. She attends nursery 3 days per week. She has a 2-day history of vomiting after some feeds and the vomiting is worsening today. She is opening her bowels regularly and had one loose stool this morning. Examination is unremarkable, although she cries throughout.

THEME: JAUNDICE

Options

A   ABO incompatibility

B   Biliary atresia

C   Breast milk jaundice

D   Galactosaemia

E   Gilbert syndrome

F   Hepatitis

G   Hypothyroidism

H   Physiological jaundice

I   Rhesus incompatibility

J   Sepsis

For each of the following clinical situations choose the single most likely diagnosis from the options given above. Each option can be used once, more than once or not at all.

☐ **14.33** A 20-day-old baby is noted to be jaundiced by the health visitor. The baby is breastfeeding well and gaining weight well and the baby's mother has no concerns. On further questioning, she tells you that the baby's urine is dark in colour and that the stools are the same colour as the baby's nappy. Examination reveals no abnormality.

☐ **14.34** A 10-day-old baby is noted to be jaundiced by the health visitor. The baby is breastfeeding well and gaining weight well. The jaundice was first noted on day 2 of life. The baby's mother is concerned that her baby has a red rash in the nappy area and some small spots on the face. Examination reveals no other abnormalities.

14.35 A 4-day-old baby is brought to your surgery by his father. He is concerned that the baby has not been feeding well for the past 24 hours. On examination, the baby is jaundiced and floppy and the heart rate is 160/minute. The father cannot give you any further history.

14.36 A 6-day-old baby is brought to your surgery by her mother. She is the third baby in the family and the mother is concerned about her baby's feeding. She describes her baby as sleepy and floppy and taking a long time to finish bottles. The mother says that the baby has been jaundiced since day 3 of life. On examination, the baby is jaundiced and floppy with a large fontanelle.

14.37 You see a 6-day-old baby who is jaundiced. The baby was noted to be jaundiced on day 2 of life. Bilirubin levels were checked in the hospital and the baby did not require any treatment. Although he took a few days to start feeding, he is now breastfeeding well. The mother feels he is slightly less jaundiced than yesterday. Other than jaundice you can find no other abnormalities on examination.

THEME: WHEEZE

Options

A Anaphylaxis

B Asthma

C Bronchiolitis

D Chronic lung disease

E Croup

F Cystic fibrosis

G Foreign body inhalation

H Primary ciliary dyskinesia

I Recurrent aspiration

J Virus-induced wheeze

For each of the following clinical situations, choose the single most likely diagnosis from the options given above. Each option can be used once, more than once or not at all.

☐ **14.38** A 2-year-old child is brought to see you with sudden onset of wheeze and shortness of breath. The symptoms started when the child was at nursery this morning. She has been otherwise well. There is no significant past medical or family history. On examination, she is distressed, with mild subcostal recession; there is an audible wheeze. On auscultation, you can hear wheeze on the right side of the chest, with good air entry throughout.

☐ **14.39** A 20-month-old boy is brought to see you with respiratory distress. He has been unwell for 2 days with a runny nose, cough and reduced feeding. He is normally fit and well. On examination, the child is coryzal and has a temp of 38.1 °C. His respiratory rate is 32/minute, with mild subcostal recession. Wheeze can be heard throughout the chest with good air entry. He has a blanching maculopapular rash on his trunk.

14.40 A white 22-month-old boy is brought to see you by his mother. They have recently moved to the area. His mother tells you that he often needs antibiotics for his chest and that this is why she has brought him in now. On examination, the child is small and thin (weight and height are on 0.4th centile) with visible Harrison's sulci. He has mild subcostal recession. Wheeze can be heard throughout the chest.

14.41 You are asked to visit a 3-year-old girl at home. She is not known to you but from her notes you see that she has diagnoses of cerebral palsy, kyphoscoliosis and severe gastro-oesophageal reflux. She is fed via a gastrostomy tube. She has symptoms of a moist cough and fever. On examination, she has a respiratory rate of 28/minute and wheeze and crepitations throughout the chest.

14.42 A 6-week-old baby is brought to see you with breathing difficulties. She was born at 33 weeks' gestation and was discharged home 2 weeks ago. She has a 24-hour history of fast, noisy breathing and reduced feeding and the mother thinks that she might have stopped breathing just now in the waiting room. On examination, there is subcostal recession and wheeze is heard bilaterally.

ALGORITHM & TABLE QUESTIONS

THEME: ASSESSMENT AND MANAGEMENT OF FEBRILE CHILDREN (1 MONTH TO 5 YEARS) IN PRIMARY CARE

14.43–14.47

Options

A Call 999 ambulance

B Capillary refill time (CRT) < 2 seconds

C CRT < 3 seconds

D Crying

E Dry mucous membranes

F Moist mucous membranes

G Reduced skin turgor

H Refer for paediatric assessment < 2 hours

I Refer for paediatric outpatient assessment

J Safety net*

* Safety net:

- Providing written or verbal information on warning symptoms and how to access further health care

- Arranging follow-up at specified time and place

- Liasing with other heath-care professionals to ensure direct access is available if required.

Using the options above, complete the following algorithm, in each case using the single most appropriate answer. Each option can be used once, more than once or not at all.

* **A**irway, **B**reathing, **C**irculation and conscious level (**D**isability) not compromised (life-threatening features).

THEME: VESICULAR RASH IN CHILDREN

14.48–14.55

Options

A Central dimple

B Contact with disease

C Crops of lesions

D Face and hands

E Limbs

F May be seriously ill

G No

H Trunk

I Yellow crusting

J Yes

Complete the table below from the list of options listed above.

	Fever	Malaise	Distribution	Pruritis?	Features
Chickenpox	Mild to moderate	Mild	Mainly truncal	Yes	[14.48] [14.49]
Dermatitis herpetiformis	No	No	[14.50]	[14.51]	Sporadic cases
Eczema herpeticum	Moderate to high	Moderate	In areas of eczema	[14.52]	[14.53]
Hand, foot and mouth disease	Mild	Mild	Palms, soles and inside mouth	No	Minor epidemics
Impetigo	No	No	Face and hands	Yes	Vesicles replaced by [14.54]
Molluscum contagiosum	Nil	Nil	Variable	No	Pearly vesicles with [14.55]

PICTURE QUESTIONS

14.56 The child in the photograph below attends the surgery. He has had a febrile illness for several days and today this rash has appeared. The child is now afebrile and well in himself.

Credit: DR H.C.ROBINSON/ SCIENCE PHOTO LIBRARY

Which is the single most appropriate advice to give the family?

☐ A The child is at high risk of renal impairment over the next few days

☐ B The child is currently infectious and should not attend nursery

☐ C The child requires oral antibiotics

☐ D The disease is self-limiting and requires no treatment

☐ E The rash is very rare and might indicate an underlying problem with immunity

14.57 This 10-year-old boy attends the surgery. He has been unwell for 4 days, with a high fever, conjunctivitis, sore throat and harsh cough. He is lethargic. The rash started yesterday behind his ears and has now spread to his body. The child is normally well but it is noted that he has never received any immunisations.

Credit: CNRI/SCIENCE PHOTO LIBRARY

What is the single most likely diagnosis?

- [ ] A Measles
- [ ] B Mumps
- [ ] C Parvovirus
- [ ] D Pertussis
- [ ] E Rubella

DATA INTERPRETATION QUESTION

14.58 A 9-week-old baby is brought to see you by his mother. She is concerned about the baby's feeding and feels that he has been unsettled and irritable for the last 5 days. He has started to vomit forcefully over the past 24 hours. You cannot find any abnormality on examination. The baby is thriving and height and weight are both on the 25th centile today. The boy's head circumference chart is shown below; the latest measurement is from today.

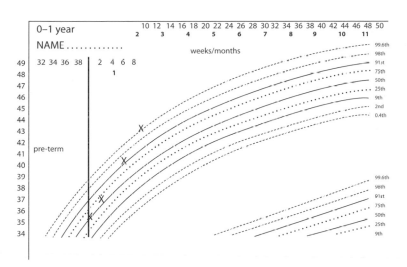

The single most appropriate action would be:

- [ ] A   Ask the health visitor to review the child's head circumference in 1 week
- [ ] B   Paediatric admission
- [ ] C   Reassure mum that all is well
- [ ] D   Review the child yourself in 1 week
- [ ] E   Routine paediatric outpatient referral

HOT TOPICS/EVIDENCE BASED PRACTICE

14.59 In 2006 a systematic review was published in the BMJ entitled 'Effectiveness of antibiotics given before admission in reducing mortality from meningococcal disease: systematic review' (Hahné et al, 2006; 332: 1299–303). Which one of the following statements regarding the findings is the most appropriate?

- [ ] A   Parenteral (intravenous or intramuscular) antibiotics should not be given as they increase mortality

- [ ] B   Parenteral antibiotics should not be given as they make diagnosis difficult

- [ ] C   Parenteral antibiotics should not be given due to the risk of anaphylaxis

- [ ] D   The paper did not provide evidence of benefit from parenteral antibiotics

- [ ] E   The paper recommended giving oral antibiotics

ANSWERS

14.1   A: Admit under the on-call paediatrician

Spontaneous nosebleeds in infants are very rare and this presentation raises concerns over clotting disorders or non-accidental injury. Assessment by a paediatrician will rule out organic causes and allow assessment of possible abuse. Vitamin K-deficient bleeding would be unusual in a bottle-fed baby.

14.2   A: Coxsackievirus infection

These are symptoms of hand, foot and mouth disease caused by a coxsackievirus. There is usually a 3-day incubation period followed by a febrile prodromal phase. The lesions typically heal in 7 days and the infection is usually followed by immunity. Transmission is by droplet spread. Henoch–Schönlein purpura lesions are purpuric and are usually seen on the legs only, although there can be renal involvement with haematuria. Idiopathic thrombocytopenic purpura (ITP) causes bruising over any part of the body, while parvovirus B19 infection causes slapped cheek syndrome. Rotavirus causes epidemics of diarrhoea.

14.3   D: Refer to ophthalmology routinely

Loss of red reflex can be a sign of congenital cataract or of retinoblastoma. Congenital cataract is more likely than retinoblastoma in bilateral cases, although this can be bilateral. Causes of congenital cataract include maternal infection (eg rubella, varicella), hypercalcaemia, Down syndrome, myotonic dystrophy and Alport syndrome. Correction at an early age is necessary to avoid amblyopia.

14.4   C: Kawasaki disease can cause myocardial infarction

Kawasaki disease is a vasculitis of unknown origin. It causes a febrile illness in children aged under 5 years that is characterised by fever, polymorphous rash, cervical lymphadenopathy, conjunctival injection and erythematous desquamation of the hands and feet. Up to a third of untreated patients will develop coronary artery stenosis and aneurysms and these can lead to myocardial infarction. Treatment is with intravenous immunoglobulin and aspirin and if aneurysms are found this treatment should be lifelong. Mortality in the UK is less than 5%.

14.5 B: Methylphenidate can cause growth retardation

Treatment of ADHD should combine psychological therapies such as CBT with drug management and the treatment plan should be tailored to the patient and their family. Drug treatment is not appropriate in preschool children. Methylphenidate can cause growth retardation and can cause abnormalities of blood count, but monthly monitoring is not necessary. Bloods should be checked after initiation of treatment but this does not have to be monthly. The blood pressure might also rise and should be checked at the same time as height and weight.

14.6 C: The murmur is short and systolic in nature

Features that indicate that a murmur is likely to be innocent are: short, soft, systolic and symptom-free. Features that should prompt further investigation are: radiation to the back, heard throughout the praecordium, louder than grade 3/6 or diastolic in nature. Children are often found to have heart murmurs during febrile illnesses. If a murmur seems innocent but persists when the child is well, this too warrants further investigation.

14.7 A: Drug or alcohol abuse

Risk factors for successful suicide after an episode of deliberate self-harm can be classified as either relating to the current episode or to the background of the patient. Factors relating to the current episode that indicate high risk include efforts to avoid being found, planning, use of a dangerous method and refusal of help. Patients who have drug and/or alcohol problems, underlying mental illness or personality disorders, patients who are socially isolated or who have had previous episodes of deliberate self-harm, and older males are higher risk. Between 1% and 2% of patients who deliberately self-harm will be dead within 12 months, and 50% of those who die from suicide have taken a non-fatal overdose previously.

14.8 C: A 14-year-old boy who has lost 10 kg since becoming a vegan

Risk factors for eating disorders include late-onset or irregular periods, seeking advice on weight loss when the BMI is normal, signs of vomiting or laxative abuse, and poor compliance with insulin treatment in diabetics and vague gastrointestinal symptoms and poor growth. At least 10% of patients with eating disorders are male, although these are often under-diagnosed. The SCOFF questionnaire might be useful:

- Do you make yourself sick when you feel uncomfortably full?
- Do you fear you have lost control over how much you eat?
- Have you lost more than 1 stone over a 3-month period?
- Do you believe yourself to be fat when others say you are thin?
- Would you say that food dominates your life?

A score of > 2 indicates a likely case of bulimia or anorexia.

14.9 B: Hirschsprung's disease

Hirschsprung's disease is caused by lack of parasympathetic innervation to a segment of bowel. It often presents as failure to pass meconium but in 6% of cases the infant will pass meconium, but go on to develop chronic constipation. Stools are often liquid and there is frequently failure to thrive. Treatment usually involves resection of the affected portion of bowel. Hypothyroidism is a cause of chronic constipation, as is cystic fibrosis, but these would normally be picked up by the neonatal screening programme. Anal fissure is associated with passage of hard stools accompanied by fresh blood and pain.

14.10   B: A prolonged seizure is a risk factor for further prolonged attacks

A clinical review of febrile seizures in children was published in the *BMJ* in 2007. Seizures can occur before the fever is apparent and can occur early or late in the course of the febrile illness. The fever is usually at least 38 °C. In 87% of cases the seizure lasts less than 10 minutes and only 30% of children have recurrent febrile seizures during subsequent illnesses. Rigorous attempts to reduce the temperature with paracetamol or ibuprofen are not recommended because there is no evidence that this decreases recurrence of seizures. Parents should be reassured. Febrile status epilepticus occurs in 5% of children and a prolonged seizure is a risk factor for further prolonged attacks.

14.11   D: Septic arthritis

The features of refusal to weight-bear and fever warrant immediate referral to rule out septic arthritis. Transient synovitis ('irritable hip') can also present in this way but is a diagnosis of exclusion. Slipped upper femoral epiphysis and Perthes' disease both affect older children. Acute myeloid leukaemia and Henoch–Schönlein purpura can both present with bone and joint pain but it would be unusual for there to be no other features.

14.12   B: Growing pains

Also known as 'nocturnal musculoskeletal pains', these are episodic muscular pains and usually last approximately 30 minutes. They commonly affect the legs and classically wake children from sleep. If there is a classic history and normal examination, reassurance, with or without simple analgesia, is all that is needed.

14.13   D: The stridor is intermittent and positional

Laryngomalacia (congenital laryngeal stridor) is a condition seen commonly in young babies. It is due to delayed maturation of the cartilage of the trachea and larynx, resulting in collapse on inspiration. It is classically more noticeable when lying supine, crying, sleeping and during intercurrent illness. Symptoms will resolve with time and no treatment is needed. Other diagnoses need to be considered if the stridor is worsening, if the child has other symptoms, respiratory distress, poor feeding or visible strawberry haemangiomas (which can also be present in the airway).

14.14   E: Refer to paediatric audiology for assessment

Parental concern regarding their child's vision or hearing should be taken seriously. The child should be formally assessed by a specialist, irrespective of past investigations or your own clinical assessment.

14.15   E: He shows a preference for using his right hand

It is abnormal to show a hand preference before 18 months of age and this can indicate an underlying neurological problem such as cerebral palsy. Other warning signs at the 8-month developmental assessment include persistence of primitive reflexes (such as moro, stepping, grasp), fisting, squint or parental concern regarding vision or hearing.

14.16   E: You should not smoke in the same room as the baby

The following advice should be given to parents:

- Babies should sleep in the same room as their parents for the first 6 months of life.

- Babies should be placed on their backs to sleep, with feet touching the end of the cot, so that they cannot slip under the covers.

- The use of pillows is not recommended.

- The ideal room temperature is 16–20 °C.

- You should not smoke in the same room as the baby.

- The use of dummies while settling the baby to sleep reduces the risk of cot death.

CHAPTER 14 ANSWERS

14.17   B: It might be normal for this infant to not open his bowels for up to 7 days

Breastfed infants tend to open their bowels more often than formula-fed babies but there is a wide normal variation. Some infants might only open their bowels once a week. If they are feeding well and are not distressed, no action is necessary. Until children are weaned at 4–6 months it is not recommended to give them prune juice or other fruit juice to treat constipation. Macrogol laxatives are not licensed for use in infants aged under 1 year. Hirschprung's disease classically presents soon after birth as a failure to pass meconium, but milder forms can present as chronic constipation years later.

14.18   D: The boy should be followed up by the paediatric team for at least 6 months after the rash has resolved

Henoch–Schönlein purpura is a vasculitic disorder of unknown aetiology. The diagnosis is made clinically on the basis of a characteristic purpuric rash on the lower limbs and buttocks. The disease can affect many systems, most typically causing abdominal pain (which can be due to intussusception) and joint pain and swelling. Rare complications include seizures and strokes. The most common serious complication is renal disease. This occurs in 60% of cases and can progress to end-stage renal failure (1–2% of cases). Renal involvement can occur up to 6 months after the rash has disappeared. All children with Henoch–Schönlein purpura therefore require paediatric follow-up involving urine dipstick and BP monitoring for at least 6 months.

14.19   D: Reflex anoxic seizure

Also known as 'white reflex asystolic attacks'. Episodes can occur from birth but are common between the ages of 6 months and 2 years. They are precipitated by shock, anxiety or minor injury. Attacks consist of pallor, loss of consciousness, stiffening, eye deviation and vagal asystole and can progress to a seizure. There is a rapid spontaneous recovery and no treatment is required. In contrast, 'blue' breath-holding episodes occur after 6 months and resolve by 3 years. Precipitated by tantrums and frustration, they consist of an obvious Valsalva manoeuvre followed by cyanosis, loss of consciousness and stiffening and rarely progress to seizures. There is rapid recovery and no treatment is required. Febrile convulsions occur between 6 months and 6 years and accompany a febrile illness. The seizure does not require investigation or treatment, but it is important to identify the nature of the underlying infection.

14.20   E: Refer for paediatric assessment

This child has acute laryngotracheobronchitis (croup). The presence of stridor at rest indicates that this child requires acute paediatric assessment and at least a period of observation in hospital. Treatment is with oral dexamethasone or nebulised budesonide. Clinical features that suggest at least moderate croup (requiring assessment and treatment in hospital) include: stridor at rest, subcostal recession, tachypnoea or altered conscious level/irritability. Cyanosis is a very late sign and is usually preceded by a period of significant respiratory distress.

14.21   C: He has an upper respiratory tract infection; his temperature is 38 °C

Acute febrile illness and severe local or systemic reaction to previous administration are contraindications to any vaccine. Live vaccines (MMR, BCG, oral polio, varicella, yellow fever) should not be given within 3 weeks of each other (although they can be given simultaneously) or to immunosuppressed patients (ie those on long-term steroids, or after chemotherapy or organ transplantation). Mild symptoms such as rashes or transient lymphadenopathy are common following live vaccines. Children with HIV are recommended to receive the standard immunisation schedule, but should not be given BCG. Egg allergy is not a contraindication to the MMR vaccine, although immunisation under observation in hospital is sometimes offered to aid vaccine uptake.

14.22   D: All household members

The following groups would be classed as close contacts and require prophylaxis:

- People in the same household

- People who have slept in the house during the 7 days prior to the onset of the illness

- People who have spent several hours a day in the house in the last 7 days

- 'Kissing contacts', ie boy/girlfriend

- Students sharing the same room or flat as the case

- Anyone who gave mouth-to-mouth resuscitation to the index case

- Those attending the same childminder as the index case in the last 7 days.

Groups not requiring prophylaxis:

- School, nursery or playgroup contacts

- Students on the same course or in the same hall of residence who are not in the above categories.

THEME: BRUISING

14.23   H: Urine dipstick

This child has symptoms of Henoch–Schönlein purpura. The diagnosis is clinical. The only initial investigation necessary is a urine dipstick to look for blood or protein in the urine.

14.24   E: No investigation

Toddlers often have multiple bruises on bony parts of the body, typically the forehead and knees. Bruising on fleshy parts of the body such as the cheeks, buttocks or thighs should raise suspicion that they could be non-accidental.

14.25   F: Skeletal survey

A bruise on a non-mobile infant is always worrying and warrants investigation for non-accidental injury. A baby who has been involved in a genuine accident would usually have been brought to medical attention by the parents.

14.26   E: No investigation

This is a description of a Mongolian blue spot. They are present at birth and are more common in people with darker skin. They can be extensive and can be mistaken for bruising if their presence has not been documented.

14.27   C: Full blood count

The most likely diagnosis is idiopathic thrombocytopenic purpura. This often presents after a viral illness with petechiae, purpura and easy bruising and sometimes with spontaneous bleeding. Treatment is symptomatic. A possible differential diagnosis is leukaemia. The first investigation in both cases is a full blood count.

THEME: VOMITING

14.28   E: Hirschprung's disease

Classically presents in the neonatal period with failure to pass meconium within 24 hours and features of obstruction. It is caused by aganglionosis of the distal bowel. If only a small segment of large bowel is affected children can present several years later with chronic constipation. Diagnosis is made by rectal biopsy.

14.29   I: Pyloric stenosis

Caused by hypertrophy of the pyloric sphincter. Classically presents at 6 weeks with a preceding history of worsening vomiting as the pylorus becomes increasingly hypertrophied with use. Babies usually feed very well and are very hungry. Weight loss can be dramatic. Management includes stopping feeds, correction of electrolyte imbalance and surgical correction. The prognosis is very good.

14.30   C: Gastro-oesophageal reflux

Common in infancy, due to relatively poor muscle tone. Symptoms improve with age. This is due to stronger muscle tone, introduction of dietary solids and a more upright posture for the baby. In severe cases there can be failure to thrive and feeding aversion because of the distress associated with feeds. There are several management options:

- Keeping the child upright (no proven benefit)

- Propping up the head of the bed (no proven benefit)

- Thickening agents (proven benefit)

- Antacids, eg Gaviscon (no proven benefit)

- Ranitidine (proven benefit)

- Omeprazole and domperidone, often used but not licensed.

14.31   G: Overfeeding

Full-term babies normally require 150 ml/kg/day of milk. Particularly hungry babies might need more than this to settle them but volumes over 200 ml/kg/day are not recommended. Overfeeding is common and often results in vomiting.

14.32   B: Gastroenteritis

Mild, self-limiting episodes of gastroenteritis are common in this age group. Infants who attend nursery have twice the number of viral infections as those that do not.

THEME: JAUNDICE

14.33   B: Biliary atresia

This is a congenital abnormality, presenting as prolonged conjugated jaundice. A history of dark urine and pale stools might also be given. This requires urgent corrective surgery. A significant number of children operated on after 6 weeks of age develop chronic hepatic failure and some require liver transplantation.

14.34   C: Breast milk jaundice

Babies who are breastfed are more likely to become jaundiced because they are taking less milk volume in the first 48 hours. The jaundice also takes longer to resolve than in formula-fed babies. This is not harmful and there is no need to stop breastfeeding.

14.35   J: Sepsis

Infection can present with jaundice in the neonatal period. Onset of jaundice in the first 24 hours of life warrants investigation for sepsis. After this time there are usually other symptoms and signs indicating infection, as in this case. In prolonged jaundice (visible after 14 days), an untreated infective cause (eg urinary tract infection) should be ruled out.

14.36   G: Hypothyroidism

Hypothyroidism can present in the neonatal period as jaundice, poor tone and poor feeding. Examination is usually otherwise normal, although a large fontanelle and umbilical hernia may be features. Urgent investigation and treatment is necessary as mental retardation develops early and is irreversible. Screening for hypothyroidism is now part of the national neonatal screening programme, but the result would not be available at this stage. If there is clinical suspicion of hypothyroidism it is important to check the baby's full thyroid function profile as the screening test only measures thyroid-stimulating hormone levels.

14.37   H: Physiological jaundice

In full-term babies, physiological jaundice is usually visible from day 2 or day 3, peaks at day 5, and has resolved by day 14. Treatment consists of ensuring adequate milk intake and ruling out any other causes (ie infection, rhesus or ABO incompatibility). If the bilirubin level is rising rapidly, phototherapy might be necessary but can usually be avoided if feeding issues are addressed early. Physiological jaundice in preterm infants starts sooner and usually lasts longer, up to 21 days.

THEME: WHEEZE

14.38   G: Foreign body inhalation

A sudden onset of respiratory distress in a child of 18 months to 3 years should raise the suspicion of an inhaled foreign body. If there is a suggestive history and/or unilateral clinical signs it is an important diagnosis to rule out. Urgent paediatric assessment is required.

14.39   J: Virus-induced wheeze

Many children aged under 3 years wheeze with viral infections. No treatment is usually necessary. A trial of salbutamol via inhaler and spacer can be given to children aged over 1 year if respiratory distress is severe or if there is a strong family history of atopy.

14.40   F: Cystic fibrosis

Recurrent lower respiratory tract infections and poor weight gain warrant further investigation. The most likely diagnosis in the white population is cystic fibrosis. Other pathologies such as immunodeficiencies, congenital lung abnormalities and rarer causes of bronchiectasis such as primary ciliary dyskinesia should be considered if cystic fibrosis tesing is negative.

14.41   I: Recurrent aspiration

Children with chronic neurological conditions often have gastro-oesophageal reflux and are at high risk of recurrent aspiration. Fundoplication and gastrostomy feeds can help. Infections need to be treated early and aggressively because this is the main cause of mortality in this group of patients.

14.42   C: Bronchiolitis

Bronchiolitis is a viral illness affecting infants aged under 1 year. It is predominantly caused by respiratory syncitial virus (RSV). Clinical features include respiratory distress, wheeze, coryzal symptoms, low-grade temperature and reduced feeding. Treatment is supportive. Those under the age of 2 months, ex-premature babies and those with existing pathology (eg cardiac disease) are at particular risk and can develop apnoeas. Paluvizumab, a monoclonal antibody against RSV, is now available, though it is very expensive. It is currently offered to premature babies with significant lung disease and to some children with cardiac problems.

THEME: ASSESSMENT AND MANAGEMENT OF FEBRILE CHILDREN (1 MONTH TO 5 YEARS) IN PRIMARY CARE

14.43   C: Capillary refill time < 3 seconds

14.44   E: Dry mucous membranes

14.45   G: Reduced skin turgor

14.46   J: Safety net

14.47   H: Refer for paediatric assessment < 2 hours

When assessing hydration status, poor feeding, reduced urine output, a slightly prolonged CRT and dry mucous membranes are all clinical signs of dehydration but do not suggest a high risk for serious illness. The NICE guidelines suggest that these children can be managed at home with 'safety netting' or be referred for same-day paediatric assessment. Paediatric assessment might be more appropriate in younger children (under 1 year), where illness has persisited for > 24 hours, if the parents are particularly anxious or in remote settings. A child with reduced skin turgor should be recognised as at high risk for serious illness and needs urgent referral for paediatric assessment. An ambulance is not necessary in the absence of any life-threatening features.

THEME: VESICULAR RASH IN CHILDREN

14.48 **B:** **Contact with disease**

14.49 **C:** **Crops of lesions**

14.50 **D:** **Face and hands**

14.51 **J:** **Yes**

14.52 **J:** **Yes**

14.53 **F:** **May be seriously ill**

14.54 **I:** **Yellow crusting**

14.55 **A:** **Central dimple**

14.56 **D:** **The disease is self-limiting and requires no treatment**

This child has fifth disease, also known as 'slapped cheek disease'. It is caused by parvovirus B19 and commonly affects children between the ages of 4 years and 12 years.

The infectious period is 4–20 days prior to the appearance of the rash. The illness usually consists of a mild febrile illness wih the development of a characteristic 'slapped cheek' rash. The child is usually very well, although the rash can be dramatic. Infection with parvovirus B19 is associated with miscarriage in woman who are less than 20 weeks pregnant, so he should be kept away from pregnant women.

14.57   A: Measles

This child has measles, which is a notifiable disease. It is highly infectious from 14 days before the rash appears to 5 days after the onset of the rash. Children are usually unwell, with a high fever. The rash usually starts on the face on day 3 or day 4 of the illness and spreads downwards. Koplik's spots are present before the onset of the rash and are consequently only seen rarely. There is no specific treatment for measles, although complications might require treatment. The illness usually lasts for 7–10 days and most children recover well. Serious complications include pneumonia, seizures, encephalitis, deafness, long-term neurological impairment and, in some cases, death.

14.58   B: Admission

This child has a rapidly increasing head circumference and symptoms of raised intracranial pressure. He needs to be seen urgently by a paediatrician. Physical signs associated with raised intracranial pressure in a baby can include dilated scalp veins, 'sun setting' eyes and a bulging fontanelle, although these are usually late signs. A child should have a paediatric assessment if their head circumference crosses two centile lines, or is greater than the 98th centile and not in proportion with height and weight measurements. Children should be seen urgently if there is a rapid change in head circumference or associated physical symptoms or signs.

14.59   D: The paper did not provide evidence of benefit from parenteral antibiotics

The paper showed:

- No benefit or harm from the use of parenteral antibiotics

- That parenteral antibiotics correlated with higher mortality rates (conclusion: they had only been given in the most severe cases)

- That oral antibiotics correlated with lower mortality rates (conclusion: they had only been given in the milder cases)

- That oral antibiotics were not recommended if meningococcal disease was suspected

- No evidence to support the theoretical risk of haemodynamic instability following parenteral antibiotics in meningococcal disease

- That the potential benefits of administering the antibiotics far outweigh the small risk of anaphylaxis

- That antibiotics given before hospital admission do not affect PCR diagnosis of meningococcal disease.

Current recommendations are that doctors in primary care who suspect meningococcal disease should administer parenteral (intramuscular) antibiotics prior to transfer to hospital.

CHAPTER 15
RENAL
SINGLE BEST ANSWER QUESTIONS

15.1 One of your patients is in her second pregnancy and has just had a growth scan at 30 weeks that has shown that her baby has polycystic kidneys. She has researched this on the Internet and is worried that her 6-year-old son will have inherited the condition. She comes to see you to discuss this situation. Which one of the following statements is true regarding this situation?

- A   Childhood polycystic kidney disease is inherited as an autosomal recessive trait
- B   Many patients with polycystic kidneys are asymptomatic
- C   She can be reassured that infantile polycystic kidney disease is always present on prenatal ultrasound and so her other child will not be affected
- D   She should be advised that her other child has a 50% chance of being affected
- E   With medical treatment from an early age most children have a normal life expectancy

15.2 A 63-year-old lady complains of fatigue following an episode of gastroenteritis last week. She has no other symptoms and no longer has diarrhoea or vomiting. Examination shows a normal blood pressure of 126/70 mmHg and pulse of 90 bpm. You arrange for some blood tests, which give the following results (NR = normal range):

Haemoglobin	13.2 g/dl (NR for women 11.5–15.5 g/dl)
Sodium	144 mmol/l (NR 136–145 mmol/l)
Potassium	5.4 mmol/l (NR 3.5–5.5 mmol/l)
Creatinine	76 µmol/l (NR 50–120 µmol/l)
Urea	9.5 mmol/l (NR 2.8 – 7.6 mmol/l)

What is the single most likely diagnosis?

- [ ] A Acute gastrointestinal bleeding
- [ ] B Acute renal failure
- [ ] C Chronic renal failure
- [ ] D Malnutrition due to gastroenteritis
- [ ] E Mild dehydration

15.3 You see a 39-year-old diabetic for his annual review. He was noted to have stage 3 chronic renal impairment 2 years ago and although his estimated glomerular filtration rate (eGFR) has been stable, his haemoglobin has dropped over that period to 10.1 g/dl. He has had a colonoscopy and gastroscopy and has been told that his anaemia is due to his chronic renal impairment. According to NICE guidelines, which one of the following statements about his management is correct?

☐ A Anaemia in chronic renal disease is usually macrocytic so folic acid should be prescribed

☐ B He should be referred for erythropoietin injections

☐ C He should have regular blood transfusions

☐ D No treatment is necessary as long as his haemoglobin is greater than 10 g/dl

☐ E Oral iron supplements should be prescribed

15.4 You are reviewing the treatment protocols for the management of chronic renal disease in your practice. One of your nurses has recently been on a course and feels that the immunisation regime is inadequate for these patients. Which one of the following statements regarding vaccination of patients with chronic renal disease is correct?

☐ A All patients with chronic kidney disease (CKD) should have 5-yearly pneumococcal and *Haemophilus* immunisations

☐ B All patients with eGFR < 60 ml/minute should be vaccinated against hepatitis B

☐ C No particular vaccinations are required in CKD

☐ D Vaccination against hepatitis A is indicated for patients with CKD stages 4 and 5

☐ E Vaccination against *Pneumococcus* confers lifelong immunity and only needs to be given once

15.5 A 67-year-old man comes to see you with his third *Proteus* urinary tract infection in 3 months. These seem to settle down with antibiotics but he does report that he gets a persistent ache in his back between attacks, and often notices blood in his urine. Clinical examination is unremarkable apart from microscopic haematuria. Urine cytology is positive for blood but shows no atypical cells. You arrange an ultrasound scan, which shows unilateral hydronephrosis. What is the single most likely diagnosis?

☐ A   Chronic renal failure

☐ B   Prostatic enlargement

☐ C   Schistosomiasis

☐ D   Ureteric calculus

☐ E   Urethral valves

15.6 If patients with type 1 diabetes mellitus develop urinary microalbuminuria, which one of the following actions is most useful in terms of prognosis?

☐ A   Ensure insulin is given as a long-acting injection each day

☐ B   Ensure insulin is given as multiple short-acting injections each day

☐ C HbA_{1c} target should be 8.5% or less

☐ D   Reduce BP to 135/75 mmHg or less using ACE inhibitors

☐ E   Reduce BP to 140/80 mmHg or less using calcium-channel blockers

15.7 A 19-year-old man has had perineal pain for the past 3 days and has developed a fever. He also describes dysuria. On rectal examination he is found to have a tender, boggy prostate gland. Which one of the following actions is the most appropriate next step?

☐ A   An HIV test should be organised as soon as possible

☐ B   A urine sample should be obtained for culture

☐ C   Antibiotics should be started only after any culture results are received

☐ D   Rectal tissue should be swabbed and sent to the laboratory

☐ E   The prostate should be massaged to obtain prostatic fluid for culture

15.8 A 55-year-old patient has long-standing treated hypertension. He has had his estimated glomerular filtration rate (eGFR) measured on an annual basis. Last year, his eGFR was estimated at 54 ml/minute/1.73m^2. This year, he has an unexplained fall in eGFR to 41 ml/minute/1.73m^2. He feels otherwise well. Which one of the following actions is the most appropriate?

☐ A   Arrange renal ultrasound and only refer to renal team if ultrasound is abnormal

☐ B   Repeat eGFR in 6 months

☐ C   Repeat eGFR in 1 year

☐ D   Routine outpatient referral to the renal team

☐ E   Urgent outpatient referral to the renal team

15.9 Considering patients with stage 4 chronic kidney disease, which of the following blood abnormalities is most likely? Select one option only.

- [ ] A Hypercalcaemia
- [ ] B Hyperphosphataemia
- [ ] C Hypokalaemia
- [ ] D Hypoparathyroidism
- [ ] E Polycythaemia

15.10 Which one of the following symptoms suggests upper urinary tract infection in women?

- [ ] A Fever
- [ ] B Haematuria
- [ ] C Pain on passing urine
- [ ] D Urinary frequency
- [ ] E Urinary urgency

15.11 A foundation-year doctor has joined the practice for a working placement. You agree to teach him about renovascular hypertension. Which one of the following statements would it be correct to include in your teaching?

☐ A   A 15% or greater rise in serum creatinine following ACE inhibition is strongly suggestive of renal artery stenosis

☐ B   An abdominal bruit is heard in approximately 80% of patients who have renal artery stenosis and hypertension

☐ C   Patients who are hypertensive despite a regular prescription for two antihypertensive medications should always be referred to the renal team

☐ D   Patients with renovascular hypertension usually develop hypokalaemia if started on an ACE inhibitor

☐ E   Renovascular disease affects more than 50% of patients in primary care who are receiving treatment for hypertension

15.12 Which one of the following microorganisms is most likely to be associated with struvite (mixed infective) renal calculi?

☐ A   *Candida albicans*

☐ B   *Enterococcus* sp.

☐ C   *Escherichia coli*

☐ D   *Proteus* sp.

☐ E   *Streptococcal sp.*

EXTENDED MATCHING QUESTIONS

THEME: LOIN PAIN

Options

A   Adrenal cortical necrosis

B   Aortic aneurysm

C   Polycystic kidneys

D   Pelviureteric junction obstruction

E   Pyelonephritis

F   Renal adenocarcinoma

G   Renal haemangioma

H   Renal vein thrombosis

I   Retroperitoneal haemorrhage

J   Ureteric calculus

For each of the scenarios below, select the most appropriate diagnosis from the list above. Each option can be used once, more than once or not at all.

☐ **15.13 A 56-year-old man on long-term warfarin therapy following prosthetic heart valve replacement complains of right-sided back pain, hip weakness and malaise for the past week. He has a pulse of 110 bpm, and a BP of 110/80 mmHg.**

☐ **15.14 A 29-year-old woman diagnosed with vesicoureteric reflux some years previously presents with loin pain, malaise and fever.**

☐ **15.15 A 48-year-old man presents with a 3-month history of intermittent haematuria and discomfort in the left loin. A mass is palpable in the left upper quadrant.**

☐ **15.16 A 30-year-old woman presents with acute right-sided loin pain which comes in waves and radiates to her groin, with vomiting. Abdominal examination is negative and urinalysis shows microscopic haematuria.**

☐ **15.17 A 67-year-old man presents with sudden-onset, severe left loin pain that is radiating to the left groin, with nausea and dizziness. He has a pulse of 136 bpm and a BP of 90/60 mmHg.**

THEME: URINARY FREQUENCY

Options

A Alcohol intoxication

B Cold weather

C Diabetes mellitus

D Diuretic therapy

E Overhydration

F Overflow incontinence

G Physical exertion

H Stress incontinence

I Urge incontinence

J Vesicovaginal fistula

For each of the scenarios below, select the most appropriate diagnosis from the list above. Each option can be used once, more than once or not at all.

☐ **15.18** A 30-year-old woman gives a history of an obstructed labour resulting in stillbirth. This was followed by urinary leak per vaginum.

☐ **15.19** An 82-year-old woman complains of leaking of urine before she is able to get to a toilet. Flow studies reveal strong detrusor contractions during filling.

☐ **15.20** A 63-year-old man suffering from progressive motor neurone disease complains of inability to initiate micturition. He has a palpable bladder.

☐ **15.21** A 50-year-old multiparous woman complains of leaking urine during coughing and laughing.

☐ **15.22** A 70-year-old man gives a history of nocturia, poor stream and dribbling and a sense of incomplete emptying.

THEME: PROSTATE CANCER THERAPY

Options

A Chemotherapy

B Hormone therapy

C Immunotherapy

D Local radiotherapy

E Monoclonal antibody therapy

F No specific therapy

G Radical prostatectomy

H Thermotherapy

I Transurethral prostatectomy

J Whole-body irradiation

For each of the scenarios below, select the most appropriate treatment option from the list above. Each option can be used once, more than once or not at all.

☐ **15.23** A 69-year-old man who underwent androgen-deprivation therapy for prostatic carcinoma 3 years ago presented with a pathological fracture of the femur. The fracture has been treated with open reduction and intermedullary nail. What adjuvant therapy would be indicated?

☐ **15.24** A 41-year-old man presenting with prostatic symptoms is found to have a small tumour on transrectal core biopsy. The serum prostate-specific antigen (PSA) is slightly elevated (5 ng/ml) and CT and bone scans show no extra-prostatic spread.

☐ **15.25** An 82-year-old man underwent transurethral prostatectomy for progressive prostatic symptoms. A well-differentiated prostatic carcinoma was found in 2/24 random prostatic chips examined.

☐ **15.26** A 76-year-old man presenting with pelvic pain is found to have prostatic cancer deposits in the pelvis and sacrum. The PSA is > 500 ng/ml.

☐ **15.27** A 70-year-old man who underwent a transurethral resection for benign prostatic hyperplasia 1 year ago has been found on random testing to have a PSA of > 20 ng/ml. Further evaluation reveals a T2 prostatic carcinoma.

ALGORITHM QUESTIONS

THEME: THE MANAGEMENT OF CHRONIC RENAL IMPAIRMENT IN PRIMARY CARE

15.28–15.32

Options

A Aim for BP < 125/75 mmHg

B Aim for BP < 130/80 mmHg

C Aim for BP < 140/80 mmHg

D Aim for BP < 150/90 mmHg

E Check phosphate levels

F Check urine for protein

G eGFR < 15 ml/minute

H eGFR < 30 ml/minute

I eGFR 30–60 ml/minute

J eGFR > 60 ml/minute

K eGFR > 90 ml/minute

L Refer to renal physician

Complete the following algorithm, which describes the management of chronic renal impairment in primary care, from the list of options above (CKD = chronic kidney disease). Each option can be used once, more than once or not at all.

PICTURE QUESTION

15.33 A 74-year-old man with no previous history of note complains of discoloured urine for the last 2 days. He has no other urinary symptoms and does not take any regular medications. His urine specimen is shown below.

Which one of the following is the most appropriate initial stage in his management?

- [ ] A   Check platelet levels and prothrombin time
- [ ] B   Refer for plain KUB (kidneys, ureters and bladder) X-ray
- [ ] C   Refer under 2-week rule
- [ ] D   Start trimethoprim pending results of culture
- [ ] E   Treat with fluids and NSAIDs and refer for outpatient intravenous pyelogram

DATA INTERPRETATION QUESTION

15.34 A 78-year-old man comes to see you for his annual check-up. He has been treated for hypertension for some years and has always been well controlled. On checking his BP you find the systolic persistently raised above 170 mmHg. You arrange for some blood tests which show a reduced eGFR. An ECG is normal and urine dipstick testing is negative for protein. Reviewing his records there seems to have been something of a decrease in his eGFR over the last 2 years. He is otherwise well, apart from some nocturia, dribbling and poor flow, which he feels is normal at his age. A graph showing his recent eGFR results is shown on the following page.

Which one of the following is the most appropriate action at this point?

- A   Introduce a calcium antagonist to improve BP control
- B   Refer for renal ultrasound
- C   Refer to cardiology for advice on further antihypertensive treatment
- D   Start finasteride
- E   Start ramipril and repeat renal function test in 1 week

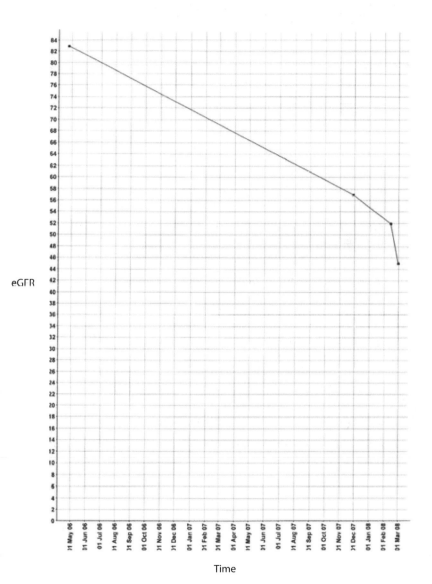

eGFR

Time

HOT TOPICS/EVIDENCE BASED PRACTICE

15.35 Regarding recent developments in nephrology, which one of the following statements is true?

☐   A   30% of patients in the UK currently have haemodialysis at home

☐   B   Impaired renal function is not a risk factor for cardiovascular disease

☐   C   Statins should be prescribed to all patients with chronic renal impairment

☐   D   Under the Quality and Outcomes Framework (QOF), patients with eGFR < 60 ml/minute only require treatment with an ACE inhibitor if they have proteinuria

☐   E   When investigating patients for labile hypertension or progressive renal impairment, a normal ultrasound excludes renal artery stenosis

ANSWERS

15.1 A: Childhood polycystic kidney disease is inherited as an autosomal recessive trait

Childhood polycystic kidney disease is inherited as an autosomal recessive trait, with an incidence of 1 in 40 000. Most children with the condition are diagnosed antenatally with ultrasound but, less commonly, they can present later in childhood with an abdominal mass. Prognosis is poor, with renal transplant the only realistic option for most patients. There are often associated hepatic cysts and subsequent portal hypertension and splenomegaly. Adult polycystic kidney disease is inherited as an autosomal dominant trait. It is less severe but 45% of patients will develop renal failure by the age of 60. It is always bilateral and can be associated with liver cysts; berry aneurysms are found in 40% of patients with the adult form of the condition.

15.2 E: Mild dehydration

This patient has a normal creatinine with a slightly raised urea level. This might be seen in the context of acute bleeding or heart failure, or in a catabolic state such as post-surgery or after starvation. It can also be seen sometimes in patients with a very high protein diet. Acute or chronic renal failure will cause uraemia but this would normally cause an elevated creatinine. She has no signs or symptoms of azotaemia so no further treatment would usually be necessary.

15.3 B: He should be referred for erythropoietin injections

NICE guidelines say that a target haemoglobin of between 10.5 g/dl and 12.5 g/dl is ideal, and patients should be referred to the renal anaemia team if their haemoglobin is less than 11 g/dl. If patients have low iron stores supplementary iron might be needed and this is usually in the form of parenteral supplements. Folate supplements are not necessary unless there is coexistent folate deficiency (eg due to poor diet or alcoholism).

15.4   A: All patients with chronic kidney disease (CKD) should have 5-yearly pneumococcal and *Haemophilus* immunisations

Patients with CKD should have 5-yearly *Haemophilus* and pneumococcal vaccinations. Patients who are likely to need renal dialysis or transplant (ie stages 4 or 5) should have hepatitis B vaccination.

15.5   D: Ureteric calculus

Renal tract calculi cause different symptoms depending on their anatomical location. Lower ureteric stones can impact at the vesico-ureteric junction and cause hydronephrosis. Other significant causes to consider in this case are tumour of the bladder or ureter. Prostatic hypertrophy (either benign or malignant) and urethral strictures can cause bilateral hydronephrosis. *Proteus* infections are associated with renal tract calculi. Schistosomiasis is a common cause of haematuria in North Africa but is not common in the UK.

15.6   D: Reduce BP to 135/75 mmHg or less using ACE inhibitors

Microalbuminuria occurs in both type 1 and type 2 diabetes mellitus. Damage to renal basement membranes, secondary to diabetes, allows excess protein to leak into affected nephrons. Patients with type 1 diabetes and microalbuminuria are at long-term risk of renal failure. The BP should be aggressively controlled to improve outcome and is more important than other factors, such as HbA_{1c} control. ACE inhibitors are particularly helpful as they control BP and can reverse microalbuminuria in affected patients.

15.7   B: A urine sample should be obtained for culture

This patient has symptoms consistent with acute prostatitis. Fever, arthralgia, low abdominal or perineal pain, and a urethral discharge are all common symptoms. Diagnosis is made by urine culture. Prostatic massage should be avoided as it can allow the infection to disseminate, and will be painful for the patient. Treatment with quinolone and aminoglycoside antibiotics is common.

15.8 D: Routine outpatient referral to the renal team

Patients who have an unexplained fall in eGFR might warrant routine referral to the renal team. An unexplained annual fall in eGFR of > 15% is considered significant by the Renal Association. NICE guidelines also suggest referral for patients with a fall in eGFR. Those with at least a 5-ml/minute unexplained fall in eGFR over 1 year (or less) should be referred. A renal ultrasound is also indicated in these patients.

15.9 B: Hyperphosphataemia

Phosphate is normally filtered and excreted by the kidney. Hyperphosphataemia is itself usually asymptomatic but is strongly associated with underlying renal disease. Retention of phosphate occurs when renal function is impaired. It is particularly problematic in stage 4 chronic renal disease if dietary intake is excessive. Patients with hyperphosphataemia and chronic renal disease have a high risk of osteoporosis and of vascular disease.

15.10 A: Fever

Lower urinary tract infections (cystitis) in women are common. Symptoms include pain on passing urine, urinary frequency and urgency, haematuria and suprapubic pain. Three days of antibiotic treatment is usually indicated in these patients. Upper urinary tract infections (pyelonephritis) cause fever, flank pain, nausea or vomiting. Urine should be sent for culture and antibiotic treatment is usually indicated for at least 7 days. Women who are systemically unwell might need admission to hospital.

15.11 A: A 15% or greater rise in serum creatinine following ACE inhibition is strongly suggestive of renal artery stenosis

Arteriosclerosis secondary to atheroma is the most common cause of renovascular disease in this country. Other causes include renal artery fibromuscular dysplasia and Takayasu's arteritis. Renovascular disease leads to hypertension in the majority of affected patients. Patients can present with severe, abrupt hypertension, which might be resistant to standard drug therapy. Patients with renovascular hypertension have underlying renal artery stenosis. Glomerular filtration is maintained despite reduced renal blood perfusion because efferent arteriole tone is increased by the renin–angiotensin system. If hypertensive patients with renovascular disease are given ACE inhibitors, blockade of angiotensin-II receptors reduces efferent renal arteriole tone, glomerular filtration falls and serum creatinine rises.

15.12   D: *Proteus* species

Renal calculi are common, affecting approximately 2% of the UK population, although most are asymptomatic. Symptomatic patients often present with severe, colicky abdominal pain that causes difficulty lying still. The pain often radiates to the testes or labia; haematuria is also a common feature. Most calculi are composed from calcium oxalate or calcium phosphate. Around 15–20% of renal calculi are known as 'mixed infective' or 'struvite' calculi. They are associated with chronic urinary tract infection. These calculi are composed of magnesium ammonium phosphate. Urease-producing bacteria break down urea to form this compound. *Proteus* and *Klebsiella* species produce urease enzyme and are common causes of struvite calculi.

THEME: LOIN PAIN

15.13   I: Retroperitoneal haemorrhage

Poorly controlled anticoagulant therapy results in bleeding into the renal and gastrointestinal tracts. Retroperitoneal bleeding is uncommon and can present as hip weakness due to femoral nerve paresis. A retroperitoneal haematoma might be palpable over the psoas.

15.14   E: Pyelonephritis

Ureteric reflux results in stasis of urine in the pelvicalyceal system and pyelonephritis is a consequence.

15.15   F: Renal adenocarcinoma

Renal-cell carcinoma is usually of insidious onset. Loin pain occurs when the renal capsule is stretched or invaded, and haematuria occurs when the tumour erodes into the pelvicalyceal system.

15.16   J: Ureteric calculus

Ureteric colic from calculus obstruction can present as an acute abdomen with normal serum inflammatory markers and amylase. There is usually microscopic haematuria.

15.17   B: Aortic aneurysm

A leaking abdominal aortic aneurysm can present as left loin pain radiating to the groin and can be mistaken for ureteric calculus obstruction. There might be guarding/rigidity and a pulsatile mass is sometimes present. An absent or diminished femoral pulse on that side with early signs of hypovolaemia should point to an impending catastrophe.

THEME: URINARY FREQUENCY

15.18   J: Vesicovaginal fistula

Vesicovaginal fistula results from ischaemic necrosis of the anterior vaginal vault and the adjoining bladder base and is a result of obstructed labour from cephalopelvic disproportion. Surgical repair of the fistula is required.

15.19   I: Urge incontinence

A common cause of urge incontinence is detrusor instability and this affects mainly elderly women. It is due to uncontrolled bladder contractions during filling overcoming efforts to inhibit micturition. Most cases are idiopathic.

15.20   F: Overflow incontinence

A neuropathic bladder in paraplagia causes overflow incontinence due to detrusor failure, resulting in incomplete emptying. This leads to raised intravesical pressures that eventually compromises renal function.

15.21   H: Stress incontinence

Stress incontinence is due to pelvic floor laxity caused by repeated birth trauma. It is also caused by neurological deficit and postmenopausal hormonal imbalance. Pelvic floor exercises, weight reduction and constipation resolution are sometimes effective but some patients will require surgical measures such as colposuspension and vaginal sling operations.

15.22   F: Overflow incontinence

Bladder outflow obstruction due to benign prostatic enlargement is the commonest cause of overflow incontinence. Acute urinary obstruction presents as an emergency with suprapubic pain and a distended, tender bladder.

THEME: PROSTATE CANCER THERAPY

15.23   D: Local radiotherapy

The patient was initially treated with gonadotropin-releasing hormone analogue for prostatic cancer. Metastatic spread to the bone suggests that either the disease was not hormone-sensitive (25% are non-responsive) or has stopped being sensitive. The treatment is palliative radiotherapy with pinning of the fracture.

15.24   G: Radical prostatectomy

Radical prostatectomy (removal of the prostate and seminal vesicles) aims to cure and is offered to the fit and relatively young patient with disease confined to the prostate gland. Metastatic disease must be excluded by CT and bone scans and by a PSA of < 20 ng/ml.

15.25   F: No specific therapy

Watchful waiting is permissible in the older patient with well-differentiated small tumours. They are kept under surveillance with PSA monitoring; a sustained rise would indicate the need for hormonal therapy.

15.26   B: Hormone therapy

Locally advanced (T3 and T4) and metastatic disease might respond to bilateral subcapsular orchidectomy or anti-androgen therapy (cyproterone acetate or flutamide) or inhibition of testosterone production (goserelin). Local radiotherapy and bisphosphonate is used to control bone disease.

15.27   D: Local radiotherapy

In this patient it is probable that a focus of prostatic carcinoma was missed during trasurethral resection (all chips are not subject to microscopy). Local radiotherapy would be the first line of treatment.

THEME: THE MANAGEMENT OF CHRONIC RENAL IMPAIRMENT IN PRIMARY CARE

15.28   J: eGFR > 60 ml/minute

15.29   I: eGFR 30–60 ml/minute

15.30   H: eGFR < 30 ml/minute

15.31   A: Aim for BP < 125/75 mmHg

15.32   B: Aim for BP < 130/80 mmHg

15.33   C: Refer under 2-week rule

This history is suspicious of a renal tract tumour. The lack of dysuria and frequency makes urinary tract infection unlikely and renal stones would normally cause colic. Clot retention from a bleeding lesion can cause colicky pain in patients with malignancies but the absence of colic makes a stone unlikely. Haematuria is very common in patients on warfarin and a drug history should be taken. The most likely site of a lesion in this instance is the bladder, and small lesions are not visible on plain X-ray or ultrasound.

15.34   B: Refer for renal ultrasound

Unexplained deterioration in eGFR or an unexpected change in the BP should prompt a search for causes of secondary hypertension. This patient had an enlarged prostate causing bladder outflow obstruction and progressive hydronephrosis. Management of the hydronephrosis followed by treatment of the prostatism restored renal function to normal.

15.35   D: Under the QOF, patients with eGFR < 60 ml/minute only require treatment with an ACE inhibitor if they have proteinuria

Currently, only 2.7% of dialysis patients receive haemodialysis at home in the UK. Many more should be able to do so and data suggest it is safe and effective, usually given as overnight dialysis. NICE guidelines recommend that all suitable patients should be offered dialysis at home. A recent article in the *BMJ* discussed assessment of patients in this category. A normal renal ultrasound does not exclude renal artery stenosis; magnetic resonance angiography is the investigation of choice. The QOF for 2008–2009 has been revised so that only patients with proteinuria and CKD (chronic kidney disease) need an ACE inhibitor to qualify for this payment criteria. Statins should be prescribed to patients with impaired renal function where there is an adverse cardiovascular risk profile, but there are insufficient data at present to support their use in all patients, although the SHARP (study of heart and renal protection) trial should provide this evidence when it is completed. Recent studies suggest that patients with a low eGFR have a relative risk of 2.5 for cardiovascular events.

CHAPTER 16 REPRODUCTIVE: MALE AND FEMALE
SINGLE BEST ANSWER QUESTIONS

16.1 A 30-year-old insulin-dependent diabetic has found out that she is 6 weeks pregnant. She is worried about the increased risk of congenital malformation associated with diabetic pregnancy. Which one of these is the most common malformation that her baby could have?

- ☐ A   Cardiovascular malformation
- ☐ B   Down syndrome
- ☐ C   Gastrointestinal malformation
- ☐ D   Genitourinary malformation
- ☐ E   Neural tube defects

16.2 A 26-year-old woman who recently had an ectopic pregnancy treated with laparoscopic salpingectomy visits her GP to discuss contraception. She is keen to try for a baby again but feels she should leave this for 6 months to get over the operation. Which one of the following is the most appropriate contraceptive method for her?

- ☐ A   Barrier method
- ☐ B   Combined oral contraceptive (COC) pills
- ☐ C   Copper intrauterine contraceptive device (IUCD)
- ☐ D   Depo-Provera
- ☐ E   Mirena coil

16.3 Which one of the following statements about the cause of subfertility is true?

- [ ] A A cause is found after standard investigations in only 30% of cases
- [ ] B Endometriosis is found in about 25% of cases
- [ ] C Ovulatory failure accounts for about 20% of cases
- [ ] D Sperm defects are found in about 5% of couples
- [ ] E Tubal damage is the most common cause in females

16.4 A 42-year-old woman who is hypertensive and has a BMI of 45 kg/m² presents with history of heavy periods lasting 7–9 days with occasional intermenstrual bleeding, her cervical smears are up to date and normal. An ultrasound scan shows a bulky uterus with a 4-cm fibroid. What should the initial management for this lady be? Select one option only.

- [ ] A Hysterectomy
- [ ] B Mefenamic acid + tranexamic acid + iron
- [ ] C Norethisterone
- [ ] D Referral for colposcopy
- [ ] E Referral for endometrial biopsy

16.5 A 56-year-old menopausal woman who presents with difficulty in passing urine has been treated with trimethoprim for two episodes of urinary tract infection (UTI) in the last year. Urine dipstick testing shows nitrites and leucocytes. On examination, you find a moderate cystocoele and atrophic vagina. How are you going to manage her? Select one option only.

- [ ] A Ring pessary and antibiotic
- [ ] B Ring pessary and local oestrogen cream
- [ ] C Start prophylactic nitrofurantoin
- [ ] D Treat with continuous low-dose trimethoprim
- [ ] E Urological evaluation and referral needed

16.6 A 25-year-old woman recently diagnosed with HIV after donating blood attends for her first smear. She is a non-smoker and is otherwise fit. With regard to cervical screening, which of the following is correct in this case? Select one option only.

☐ A Cervical smear 3-yearly

☐ B Cervical smears yearly

☐ C Colposcopy and smear every 3 years

☐ D HPV vaccination and 3-yearly cervical smears

☐ E Initial colposcopy and yearly cervical smears

16.7 When discussing the possibility of endometriosis with a 32-year-old woman with symptoms of dyspareunia, dysmenorrhoea and subfertility, which one of the following statements is most appropriate?

☐ A If the diagnosis is endometriosis, gonadotrophin–releasing hormone analogue is the best treatment for her symptoms

☐ B It can be an incidental finding on laparoscopy with no symptoms

☐ C It occurs mainly in the early twenties and gets better with age

☐ D It is a rare condition affecting about 1% of white people

☐ E The extent of disease correlates with symptoms

16.8 A 52-year-old postmenopausal woman presents with hot flushes. She does not wish to take hormone-based therapy. She would prefer to try some natural alternatives first. The use of which one of these products is evidence-based in the treatment of hot flushes? Select one option only.

☐ A Evening primrose oil

☐ B Ginseng

☐ C Liquorice

☐ D Red clover

☐ E St John's wort

16.9 A 15-year-old girl is attending with her 16-year-old boyfriend for contraceptive advice. She has been poorly compliant with the combined oral contraceptive in the past due to difficulty in taking it without her parents dicovering. She is Gillick competent, medically fit and has no significant family history. Which one of the following contraceptives is the least appropriate for this patient?

- [ ] A   Combined pills
- [ ] B   Contraceptive patches
- [ ] C   Depo-Provera
- [ ] D   Implanon
- [ ] E   IUCD

16.10 A 25-year-old woman with a history of dyspareunia, dysmenorrhoea, dyschesia and pelvic pain suffers from heavy periods. On examination you find a tender nodule in the pouch of Douglas. Which of the following tests is the diagnostic gold standard to confirm your diagnosis? Select one option only.

- [ ] A   Ca-125
- [ ] B   Diagnostic laparoscopy
- [ ] C   Histology
- [ ] D   Transvaginal scan
- [ ] E   Vaginal swab

16.11 Which one of the following statements about semen analysis is true?

- [ ] A   Analysis should be performed 10–12 days after the the last ejaculation
- [ ] B   Aspermia is invariably due to failure of sperm production
- [ ] C   Asthenospermia means abnormal morphology
- [ ] D   Motility is usually greater than 40%
- [ ] E   Normal volume is between 10 ml and 15 ml

16.12 A university student presents with a fever of 38 °C, lower abdominal pain and tenderness. She also complains of vaginal discharge for the past few days. She is using the combined oral contraceptive pill and her last menstrual period was 7 days ago. Which one of the following is the most appropriate initial management option?

- [ ] A Refer to hospital
- [ ] B Start amoxicillin + metronidazole
- [ ] C Start ofloxacin + metronidazole
- [ ] D Triple swabs + ofloxacin and metronidazole
- [ ] E Triple swabs + FBC and antibiotics accordingly

16.13 A 40-year-old woman has recently emigrated to the UK from Asia. At her new-patient check she reports that she has recently lost weight and feels tired. She is found to have leucocytes in her urine which persist despite antibiotic treatment. There is no significant bacterial growth on two consecutive urine cultures. What diagnosis do you suspect? Select one option only.

- [ ] A Bladder carcinoma
- [ ] B Bladder stones
- [ ] C Contamination from vaginal discharge
- [ ] D Interstitial cystitis
- [ ] E Tuberculosis

16.14 Non-gonococcal urethritis may result from infection with which one of the following organisms?

- [ ] A *Bifidobacterium*
- [ ] B *Chlamydia psittaci*
- [ ] C *Mycobacterium bovis*
- [ ] D *Mycoplasma hominis*
- [ ] E *Ureaplasma urealyticum*

16.15 A 23-year-old woman with chronic lower abdominal pain for 1 year complains of abdominal distension, pain relieved after defecation and occasional constipation. Her periods are regular and the pain is not cyclical. Based on current evidence, what is the best treatment plan that can be offered to this patient?

- ☐ A   Addressing psychological issues
- ☐ B   Adhesiolysis
- ☐ C   Antispasmodics
- ☐ D   Laparoscopy
- ☐ E   NSAIDs

16.16 A 45-year-old businessman complains of dysuria and discharge after returning from a business trip to Berlin. A swab confirms chlamydial infection but tests for other sexually transmitted diseases are negative. What is the single most appropriate treatment for this condition?

- ☐ A   Azithromycin
- ☐ B   Benzylpenicillin
- ☐ C   Ciprofloxacin
- ☐ D   Fluconazole
- ☐ E   Trimethoprim

EXTENDED MATCHING QUESTIONS

THEME: PREMENSTRUAL SYNDROME (PMS)

Options

A *Agnus castus*

B Evening primrose oil

C Hysterectomy

D Hysterectomy with bilateral salpingo-oophorectomy

E Progesterone on days 14-25

F Referral to a gynaecologist for a trial of gonadotrophin-releasing hormone analogue

G SSRI on days 14–25 of the menstrual cycle

H Symptom diary

I Vitamin B6

Select the most appropriate plan of management for the women with following presenting symptoms. Each option can be used once, more than once or not at all.

☐ **16.17** A 35-year-old woman presents for the first time with bloating, breast pain and premenstrual headache.

☐ **16.18** A 40-year-old woman who is currently on Cerazette for symptoms of premenstrual syndrome, and who feels out of control, with mood swings, tension and irritability affecting her life.

☐ **16.19** The above-mentioned lady, after trying two different treatments, demands to have a hysterectomy.

☐ **16.20** A 45-year-old woman with a symptom diary suggestive of premenstrual syndrome but who wants to try natural treatment.

☐ **16.21** A 40-year-old woman with premenstrual breast tenderness requests non-hormonal treatment.

THEME: EMERGENCY CONTRACEPTION

Options

A Barrier contraception

B Barrier contraception for 7 days + emergency contraception

C Continue combined oral contraceptive and barrier contraception for 7 days

D Depo-Provera

E Offer IUCD

F Pregnancy test followed by emergency contraception (levonorgestrel) and screen for sexually transmitted infections (STIs)

G Reassurance

H Screen for STIs, emergency contraception (levonorgestrel) and barrier contraception for next 7 days

I Sterilisation

Please choose the best management option for the each of the women described in the scenarios below regarding emergency contraception. Each option can be used once, more than once or not at all.

☐ **16.22** A 20-year-old student requests emergency contraception. She had unprotected sexual intercourse after a night out with friends 2 days ago. She does not remember when her last period was but thinks it was about 3 months ago. She assures you that she has had no other unprotected sexual intercourse since her last period.

☐ **16.23** A weight-conscious, married mother of three, whose last child was born only 3 months ago, does not wish to have any further children. She reports a burst condom 24 hours ago, and requests emergency contraception and long-term family planning advice.

CHAPTER 16 QUESTIONS

☐ **16.24** A 17-year-old girl had unplanned sex last night with a stranger. Her last period was 7 days ago. She is on the progesterone-only pill and she took her last pill 36 hours ago.

☐ **16.25** A 27-year-old married woman whose last period was 15 days ago is on a combined contraceptive pill. She forgot to take her last pill (which was due 12 hours ago) and had sex 3 hours ago.

☐ **16.26** A 30-year-old married woman on the COC pill has had an episode of diarrhoea and vomiting for the last 3 days. Her last period was 9 days ago. She has not had sex since being ill but wonders if it is safe to do so.

THEME: LONG-ACTING CONTRACEPTION

Options

A Depo-Provera

B Implanon

C Intrauterine contraceptive device (IUCD)

D Mirena intrauterine system

E Norplant

F Sterilisation

G Vasectomy

For each of the statements below, select the most appropriate option from the list above. Each option may be used once, more than once or not at all.

☐ **16.27** Should be changed every 3 years.

☐ **16.28** Frequently causes acne and irregular bleeding.

☐ **16.29** Indicated for women who have menorrhagia.

☐ **16.30** Effective for 5 years, it has a failure rate of approximately 2%.

☐ **16.31** Causes average weight gain of 2 kg over 12 months.

THEME: ANTENATAL TESTING

Options

A 20-week anomaly scan

B Amniocentesis

C Chorionic villus sampling (CVS)

D Fetal echocardiography

E Glucose tolerance test at 28 weeks

F Glucose tolerance test at 32 weeks

G Middle cerebral artery Doppler ultrasound

H Nuchal translucency

I Scan at 11–12 weeks

J Second-trimester triple test

Which of the above tests should be arranged for the pregnant women in the following situations? Each option can be used once, more than once or not at all.

☐ **16.32** A patient who is 8 weeks pregnant in her second pregnancy, with a history of previous termination because of anencephaly. The patient wants to confirm that this baby is not anencephalic.

☐ **16.33** A 40-year-old woman presents at 15 weeks and requests a diagnostic test for Down syndrome.

☐ **16.34** A 35-year-old woman presents at 9 weeks and wants to have first-trimester screening for Down syndrome.

☐ **16.35** A 30-year-old woman who previously delivered a 5-kg baby with great difficulty. Which specific test would be appropriate in avoiding a recurrence?

☐ **16.36** A diabetic woman is 16 weeks into her second pregnancy. Her first baby had a congenital cardiac malformation and required extensive surgery. She would like screening to minimise her risks of recurrence.

THEME: GYNAECOLOGICAL EMERGENCIES

Options

A Appendicitis

B Complete miscarriage

C Constipation

D Ectopic pregnancy

E Endometriosis

F Ovarian hyperstimulation

G Ovarian torsion

H Pelvic inflammatory disease

I Retroverted uterus

J Syncopal attack

K Threatened miscarriage

L Urinary tract infection

For each of the following scenarios, select the most appropriate diagnosis from the list of options above. Each option can be used once, more than once or not at all.

☐ **16.37** A woman who is 8 weeks into her first pregnancy and who had a small fresh vaginal bleed 2 days ago now presents with brownish loss. Her ultrasound scan performed in the early pregnancy assessment clinic 2 days ago showed an intrauterine gestational sac with a normal fetal heart.

☐ **16.38** A 20-year-old attends the out-of-hours treatment centre with abdominal pain and having fainted. Her last period was 5 weeks ago. Her urine pregnancy test is positive, her blood pressure is 70/40 mmHg and her pulse is 120 bpm.

☐ **16.39** An 18-year-old presents with right iliac fossa pain, diarrhoea and a temperature of 38 °C. Vaginal examination reveals slight tenderness on the right side with no palpable masses. She is tender in the right iliac fossa with guarding.

16.40 A 35-year-old being treated for infertility had embryo transfer 5 days ago. She now complains of feeling unwell and breathless. Abdominal examination shows distension and dullness to percussion in the flanks.

16.41 A 20-year-old primip presents with urinary retention. She also complains of tenderness in her loins. Urine dipstick testing is positive for protein. A booking scan 2 weeks ago showed a normal 12-week fetus.

ALGORITHM QUESTIONS

THEME: CHRONIC PELVIC PAIN

16.42–16.46

Options

A   Analgesics

B   Local anaesthetic injection

C   High-fibre diet

D   Laparotomy

E   Refer to infertility unit

F   Refer to specialist

G   Screen for STIs

H   Trial of combined oral contraceptive pill

I   Trial of progesterone

J   Ultrasound scan followed by diagnostic laparoscopy if needed

Please select the most appropriate option from the list above to complete the following algorithm for the management of chronic pelvic pain.

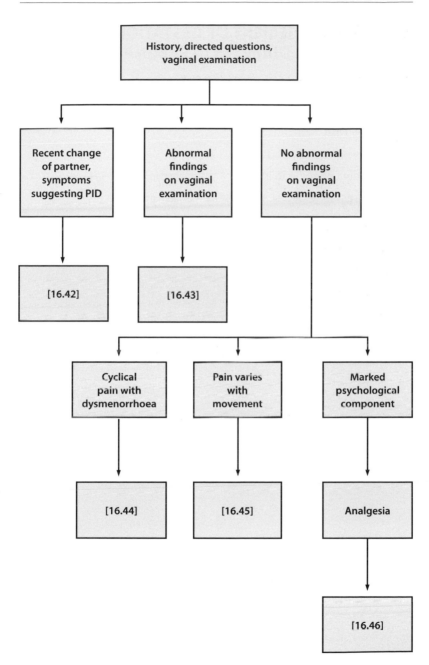

THEME: MANAGEMENT OF GESTATIONAL DIABETES AND DIABETES IN PREGNANCY

16.47–16.52

Options

A   Aim for $HbA_{1c} < 7\%$

B   Advice on exercise and diet

C   Consider changing to insulin

D   Glucose tolerance test at 28 weeks

E   Glucose tolerance test at 32 weeks

F   Increase dose of medication

G   Pre-pregnancy counselling

H   Terminate pregnancy

Complete the following algorithm for the management of diabetes and gestational diabetes in pregnancy and pre-pregnancy, using options from the list above.

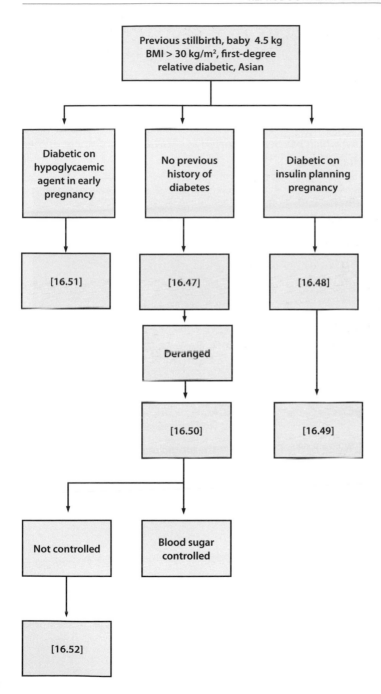

PICTURE QUESTION

16.53 A 30-year-old lady complains of several weeks of headaches. On further questioning she admits to secondary amenorrhoea of 12 months duration. She has had an X-ray performed (shown below) which has been reported as showing enlargement of the pituitary fossa.

Which one of the following is the single most likely diagnosis?

- ☐ A Cysticercosis
- ☐ B Glioma
- ☐ C Prolactinoma
- ☐ D Sarcoidosis
- ☐ E Tuberculosis

DATA INTERPRETATION QUESTIONS

16.54 A 35-year-old woman in her third pregnancy has a history of hypertension. Her previous babies were small for dates at birth and she is currently taking methyldopa. Dipstick testing of her urine shows protein. The growth chart for her current pregnancy is shown below.

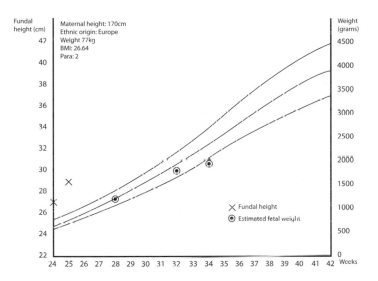

Which one of the following is the most appropriate interpretation of this chart?

- [ ] A The fetus is small but has normal growth
- [ ] B Growth is currently on the 50th centile
- [ ] C Growth is currently on the 90th centile
- [ ] D Growth is currently just below the 3rd centile
- [ ] E Growth is currently just below the 10th centile

16.55 A 28-year-old primip who is 32 weeks pregnant complains of epigastric pain, nausea and pedal oedema. Her BP is 140/90 mmHg and her urine is showing 2+ of proteins. She feels unwell. Blood tests are taken, the results of which are shown below:

Haemoglobin	10.0 g/dl
Haematocrit	0.35
WCC	$12 \times 10^9/l$
Platelets	$95 \times 10^9/l$
Bilirubin	20 μmol/l
ALP	250 U/l
ALT	76 U/l
Protein	6.6 g/l
LDH	550 U/l
Amylase	35 U/l
Creatinine	60 μmol/l
Urea	4.0 mmol/l
Uric acid	442 μmol/l
Na⁺	141 mmol/l
K⁺	3.5 mmol/l
Glucose	5 mmol/l

Which one of the following is the single most likely diagnosis?

☐ A Acute liver failure
☐ B Cholecystitis
☐ C Fatty liver
☐ D HELLP syndrome
☐ E Renal failure

HOT TOPICS/EVIDENCE BASED PRACTICE

16.56 A patient presents at 31 weeks of pregnancy with tightenings
every 3 minutes. On examination, her cervix is closed and
1 cm long. Which one of the following treatments to prevent
neonatal death does the evidence base support?

- ☐ A Antibiotics
- ☐ B Atosiban
- ☐ C Nifedipine
- ☐ D Two doses of corticosteroids, 12 hours apart
- ☐ E Two doses of corticosteroids, 24 hours apart

ANSWERS

16.1   A: Cardiovascular malformation

Diabetes and poor blood sugar control in early pregnancy are associated with increased risk of miscarriage and congenital malformation (higher levels of HbA_{1C} are associated with increased risk). The HbA_{1C} can be used as a guide of blood sugar control over the last few months (< 6.1% is ideal) – the higher the level, the higher the risk of malformation. Cardiovascular malformations are commonest, and therefore there is a need for fetal echocardiography at 22–24 weeks of pregnancy in these patients.

16.2   B: Combined oral contraceptive (COC) pills

IUCDs are not advisable for short-term contraception, and there is a theoretical increased risk of ectopic pregnancy. Depo-Provera is associated with secondary amenorrhoea and can cause delayed return to fertility. Barrier methods are less effective than the combined pill but can be useful if the contraceptive pill is contraindicated.

16.3   C: Ovulatory failure accounts for about 20% of cases

The main causes of infertility are shown below (remember that some couples can have more than one cause):

- Unexplained – 30%

- Sperm defects – 25%

- Ovulatory failure – 20%

- Tubal damage – 15%

- Others – 10%

- Endometriosis – 5%

- Mucus defects – 5%

- Other male problems – 2%

- Coital failure – 2%

16.4   E: Referral for endometrial biopsy

Hypertensive overweight women with intermenstrual bleeding should be investigated to rule out endometrial carcinoma. Patients with heavy bleeding who are under the age of 45 do not always need investigations before starting treatment with mefenamic acid and tranexamic acid but intermenstrual bleeding should always be further investigated. Colposcopic referral is appropriate when there is a history of postcoital bleeding and a suspicious-looking cervix.

16.5   B: Ring pessary and local oestrogen cream

Postmenopausal women often suffer recurrent urinary tract infections. Once obvious treatable causes eg diabetes have been excluded many of these ladies can be managed in primary care either with local HRT or prophylactic antibiotics. Failure to improve should prompt referral for specialist opinion, as in this case where repair of the prolapse may be appropriate.

16.6   E: Initial colposcopy and yearly cervical smears

HIV-positive patients are at increased risk of developing cervical intraepithelial neoplasia (CIN) and they can progress rapidly from CIN to cervical cancer. It is important to counsel these women adequately regarding the need for initial colposcopy and yearly cervical smears thereafter.

16.7   B: It can be an incidental finding on laparoscopy with no symptoms

Around 10% of white females have mild disease, the symptoms do not correlate with extent of disease and the incidence increases with increasing age (though mostly present in the reproductive age group, 20–35 years). Adenomyosis presents late in parous women. For this woman the best treatment is likely to be surgical, to relieve symptoms and increase her fertility chances.

16.8   D: Red clover

A few studies have suggested a benefit in hot flushes for red clover or black cohosh when compared to placebo. St John's wort is used for perimenopausal mild to moderate depression because of its antidepressant effect. Ginseng has not been proved to improve hot flushes, although parameters of wellbeing and depression improve.

16.9   E: IUCD

Depot injection is useful for short-term use in teenagers, particularly those who have been poorly compliant in the past with oral medication. It is not suitable for long-term use due to effects on bone density. An IUCD would be difficult to fit in nulliparous woman, although is sometimes inserted at the time of termination of pregnancy.

16.10   B: Diagnostic laparoscopy

The most likely diagnosis in this case is endometriosis. The diagnostic gold standard for endometriosis is diagnostic laparoscopy and the patient can be treated at the time of laparoscopy by resection of endometriosis.

16.11   D: Motility is usually greater than 40%

Asthenospermia is lack of motility. Retrograde ejaculation can cause apparent aspermia. A semen sample should be collected after a minimum of 3 days and a maximum of 5 days of abstinence. The sample should be brought to the laboratory within 1 hour of production and examined as soon as possible. Normal semen variables are:

Volume: > 2–6 ml

Density: > 20×10^6/ml

Motility: > 40% forward progression after 2 hours

Morphology: > 20% normal

White blood cells: <1×10^6/ml

16.12   D: Triple swabs + ofloxacin and metronidazole

Her presentation raises a suspicion of pelvic inflammatory disease (PID). It is best to start treatment based on this as delaying treatment increases the risk of long-term sequelae such as infertility. If she has confirmed PID, both she and her partner should be treated.

16.13   E: Tuberculosis

Persistent pyuria with negative cultures in a woman from a high-prevalence area should raise the suspicion of tuberculosis. Carcinoma and stones would present with haematuria and can increase the risk of UTI but cultures would be positive.

16.14   E: *Ureaplasma urealyticum*

Chlamydia trachomatis accounts for up to half of cases of non-specific urethritis. In the remainder, *Ureaplasma urealyticum* and *Mycoplasma genitalium* are pathogens, whereas *Mycoplasma hominis* is not. Bifidobacteria are commensal faecal organisms. *Mycobacteria bovis* causes infection in cattle and *Chlamydia psittaci* causes psittacosis.

16.15   C: Antispasmodics

Systemic reviews have concluded that antispasmodic such as mebeverine are beneficial in the treatment of irritable bowel syndrome where abdominal pain is the main symptom.

16.16   A: Azithromycin

Often patients are infected with more than one pathogen at a time and consideration should be given to treating accordingly. *Chlamydia* is sensitive to doxycycline and azithromycin. Any partners should be treated at the same time, as untreated *Chlamydia* can cause infertility in females by damaging the fallopian tubes. Aciclovir is a treatment for herpes; benzylpenicillin can be used to treat syphilis or gonorrhoea. A high index of suspicion for other sexually transmitted diseases should prompt screening for co-infection, including HIV. Ciprofloxacin is useful for the management of gonorrhoea but resistance is becoming a problem in some areas of the UK.

THEME: PREMENSTRUAL SYNDROME (PMS)

16.17　**H:**　Symptom diary

16.18　**G:**　SSRI on days 14–25 of the menstrual cycle

16.19　**F:**　Referral to a gynaecologist for a trial of gonadotrophin-releasing hormone analogue

16.20　**A:**　*Agnus castus*

16.21　**B:**　Evening primrose oil

For confirmation of a diagnosis of premenstrual syndrome it is essential to keep a symptom diary for 3 months before starting any medical or surgical treatment. SSRIs are effective for psychological symptoms related to PMS. A trial of gonadotrophin-releasing hormone analogue should be considered before hysterectomy. *Agnus castus* has been found to be effective for PMS symptoms in randomised controlled trials.

THEME: EMERGENCY CONTRACEPTION

16.22　**F:**　Pregnancy test followed by emergency contraception (levonorgestrel) and screen for STIs

16.23　**E:**　Offer IUCD

This is the most suitable long-term option in this case.

16.24　**H:**　Screen for STIs, emergency contraception (levonorgestrel) and barrier contraception for next 7 days

Patients missing one or more progesterone pills will need emergency contraception and 7 days of additional cover with barrier contraception, and should also be advised on future barrier contraception use along with pills.

16.25   G: Reassurance

Patients on the combined pill who forget their pill can take it up to 12 hours late without problems. If pills are more than 24 hours late or where antibiotics are being taken, the 7-day rule needs to be applied, with barrier precautions for 7 days.

16.26   C: Continue COC and use barrier contraception for 7 days

THEME: LONG-ACTING CONTRACEPTION

16.27   B: Implanon

Implanon is inserted above the elbow and releases etonogestrel, inhibiting ovulation. It can cause irregular bleeding but has a failure rate of only 0.1% over 3 years. Because it inhibits ovulation it is a safe choice in those who have had previous ectopic pregnancies.

16.28   A: Depo-Provera

Depo-Provera is useful in patients who are unable or unwilling to use oral contraception or a coil. It is often used in teenagers who are at risk of pregnancy but who cannot take the pill reliably. It can cause a delay in return to fertility (average 6 months) and must be given every 3 months.

16.29   D: Mirena intrauterine system

Mirena coils are licensed for contraception and for menorrhagia. Studies suggest that in some women they are a successful alternative to surgery where other treatments have failed. They are as effective as and contraception and provide 5 years of cover.

16.30   C: Intrauterine contraceptive device (IUCD)

Copper IUCDs prevent fertilisation and implantation. They have a failure rate of around 2%, can cause heavier periods and are associated with an increased risk of ectopic pregnancy.

16.31   A: Depo-Provera

Depo-Provera causes weight gain in most women, usually 2–3 kg over 12 months, and a reversible reduction in bone mineral density.

THEME: ANTENATAL TESTING

16.32   I: Scan at 11–12 weeks

Anencephaly can be easily diagnosed by non-invasive ultrasound at the booking scan.

16.33   B: Amniocentesis

Amniocentesis is a diagnostic test that can be offered at 15 weeks.

16.34   H: Nuchal translucency

Nuchal translucency can be offered in the first trimester, usually at the time of the dating scan, either on its own or as part of an integrated test with serum testing.

16.35   E: Glucose tolerance test at 28 weeks

A screening test for gestational diabetes should be offered at 28 weeks.

16.36   D: Fetal echocardiography

This can be offered at 22–24 weeks.

THEME: GYNAECOLOGICAL EMERGENCIES

16.37 K: Threatened miscarriage

16.38 D: Ectopic pregnancy

Any female with vaginal bleeding and a positive pregnancy test should be considered to have an ectopic pregnancy.

16.39 A: Appendicitis

16.40 F: Ovarian hyperstimulation

Ovarian hyperstimulation can present with pleural effusions and ascites.

16.41 I: Retroverted uterus

THEME: CHRONIC PELVIC PAIN

16.42 G Screen for STIs

16.43 J: Ultrasound scan followed by diagnostic laparoscopy if needed

16.44 H: Trial of combined oral contraceptive pill

Patients with cyclical pain should have a trial of suppression of ovarian function.

16.45 A: Analgesics

Non-gynaecological causes such as musculoskeletal pathology should be considered.

16.46 F: Refer to specialist

Where appropriate, referral to other specialities should be considered (eg psychiatry).

THEME: MANAGEMENT OF GESTATIONAL DIABETES AND DIABETES IN PREGNANCY

16.47   **D:**   Glucose tolerance test at 28 weeks

16.48   **G:**   Pre-pregnancy counselling

16.49   **A:**   Aim for $HbA_{1c} < 7\%$

16.50   **B:**   Advice on exercise and diet

16.51   **C:**   Consider changing to insulin

If a patient is on hypoglycemic agents other than metformin they should be switched over to insulin.

16.52   **C:**   Consider changing to insulin

Patients with poor control on diet and exercise should have insulin.

16.53   **C:**   Prolactinoma

Enlargement of the pituitary fossa suggests the diagnosis of prolactinoma. Other symptoms could include subfertility and galactorrhoea. A glioma would not normally cause amenorrhoea and would not show on a plain X-ray. Cysticercosis can cause central nervous system lesions but these are visible on computed tomography, not on plain X-ray.

16.54   **E:**   Growth is currently just below the 10th centile

This growth chart is showing tapering of growth between 32 and 34 weeks, falling to just below the 10th centile at 34 weeks. She should have Doppler studies and liquor volume assessment to confirm the wellbeing of this fetus.

16.55   D: HELLP syndrome

HELLP syndrome (**h**aemolysis, **e**levated **l**iver enzymes, **l**ow **p**latelets) is the diagnosis in this patient. The raised LDH and ALT, low platelets and raised bilirubin indicate the need for urgent action. Patients with pre-eclampsia can have this syndrome with even mild elevation of blood pressure. This patient should be delivered after starting on magnesium sulphate because if it is left untreated it is associated with high mortality rates.

16.56   E: Two doses of corticosteroids, 24 hours apart

Two doses of corticosteroids, given 24 hours apart reduce the risk of respiratory distress, neonatal death and intraventricular haemorrhage. Tocolytic agents delay the labour but have not been found to change the outcome.

CHAPTER 17
RESPIRATORY
SINGLE BEST ANSWER QUESTIONS

17.1 A 57-year-old man is newly diagnosed with cryptogenic fibrosing alveolitis. He comes to see you to discuss his condition and asks about his prognosis. Which one of the following statements is correct regarding this issue?

- [ ] A   He has a significantly increased risk of developing lung cancer
- [ ] B   Most patients do not experience any functional limitation
- [ ] C   The majority of patients respond to treatment
- [ ] D   The mean life expectancy from diagnosis is 6 months
- [ ] E   Treatment should be aimed at the underlying cause

17.2 A 22-year-old student has a 2-month history of weight loss and fatigue. He has had no cough or shortness of breath. He travelled to the UK from India to begin studying 4 months ago. He has a normal respiratory rate, but a dull percussion note and reduced breath sounds throughout the right lung field. What is the single most likely diagnosis?

- [ ] A   Melioidiosis
- [ ] B   Pneumoconiosis
- [ ] C   Psittacosis
- [ ] D   Sarcoidosis
- [ ] E   Tuberculosis

17.3 A 24-year-old woman complains of intermittent chest tightness and wheeze over the past 3 months. Her symptoms have been getting worse and are troublesome at night. She smokes cigarettes socially. She has a past history of hay fever. Her respiratory examination is normal. What is the next best action? Select one option only.

- ☐ A Ask her to keep a diary of her symptoms and review her in 2 weeks
- ☐ B Issue her a prescription for a salbutamol metered-dose inhaler and arrange a review in 2 weeks
- ☐ C Refer her to the hospital as an outpatient for a chest X-ray
- ☐ D Show her how to use a peak flow meter and request that she keeps a record of morning and evening readings for 1 week, then come for review
- ☐ E Show her how to use a peak flow meter and request that she keeps a record of morning and evening readings for 2 weeks, then come for review

17.4 A 10-year-old girl is reviewed by a foundation-year doctor at your practice. The girl has been using her terbutaline turbohaler four to five times a week over the past 6 months. She has reasonable inhaler technique. The doctor asks you for advice regarding her future management. Which of the following statements represents the best piece of advice? Select one option only.

- ☐ A Add a beclomethasone inhaler via a spacer to her treatment regime, at a dose of 100 micrograms bd; review in 6 months
- ☐ B Add a beclomethasone inhaler via a spacer to her treatment regime, at a dose of 400 micrograms bd; review in 3 months
- ☐ C Add a budesonide turbohaler to her treatment regime at a dose of 100 micrograms bd; review in 3 months
- ☐ D Continue with the current treatment regime and review her in 6 months
- ☐ E Continue with the current treatment regime and review her in 12 months

17.5 You are asked by the reception staff to issue a prescription for two salbutamol inhalers for a 16-year-old boy. You look at his medication record. He has been issued prescriptions for three salbutamol inhalers and two 100-microgram beclomethasone inhalers over the past month. What is the single best course of action you can take?

☐   A   Ask the receptionist to contact the patient and organise a review appointment in the asthma clinic by the end of the week

☐   B   Double the dose of his inhaled corticosteroid and leave a note explaining what you have done with the patient's prescription

☐   C   Increase the number of inhalers on the prescription, and issue the prescription

☐   D   Issue the prescription, but add a salmeterol inhaler to his prescription

☐   E   Issue the prescription, but ask the receptionist to book the patient in to your surgery in 1 months' time for review

17.6 A 40-year-old man has recently been diagnosed with mild obstructive sleep apnoea. He works as a handyman for a local school and part-time as a taxi driver. He attends for review. Which one of the following is the single most appropriate course of action?

☐   A   Advise that he need not inform his car insurance company of his diagnosis as his obstructive sleep apnoea is mild

☐   B   Ensure that he has been told verbally and in writing that he must inform the Driver and Vehicle Licensing Agency (DVLA) of the diagnosis

☐   C   Inform him that for now he should not work as a taxi driver. He might be able do so in the future provided he has no daytime sleepiness over the following month

☐   D   Inform him that he has a legal obligation to inform the school that he has obstructive sleep apnoea and will not be able to operate machinery until further notice

☐   E   Inform him that he is likely to require nasal CPAP treatment overnight

17.7 A 42-year-old ex-smoker complains of right shoulder pain and hoarseness for 4 weeks. Examination of his shoulder reveals a normal range of movement. His chest is clear, he is not breathless and he has no lymphadenopathy. His voice is hoarse. He does not have finger clubbing. The single most appropriate course of action is:

- ☐ A Organise a chest physician to review him urgently as an outpatient
- ☐ B Organise an urgent cervical spine X-ray
- ☐ C Organise an urgent chest X-ray
- ☐ D Organise a routine chest X-ray
- ☐ E Organise a routine X-ray of his shoulder and review with results

17.8 A 24-year-old secretary complains of a persistent dry cough. The cough has been present for the past 4 months. It is worse shortly after eating a big meal and she occasionally wakes at night coughing. She is a non-smoker. She is fit and well, with no other symptoms. A chest X-ray is organised and is normal. What is the most likely cause of her cough? Select one option only.

- ☐ A Bronchial carcinoma
- ☐ B Reflux cough
- ☐ C Psychogenic cough
- ☐ D Postviral cough
- ☐ E Pertussis

17.9 The practice nurse asks you to urgently assess a teenager who is in the waiting room. He has a history of asthma. On examination, his respiratory rate is 30/minute with prolonged expiration, he cannot complete sentences on talking to you, is tachycardic and has wheeze heard throughout his chest. What is the single most appropriate course of action, given the following options?

- [ ] A Give 5 mg salbutamol via oxygen-driven nebuliser and send home if he feels completely back to normal
- [ ] B Give oxygen via face mask at 10 l/minute and call an ambulance
- [ ] C Give salbutamol 6 puffs via a spacer and if the patient starts to improve send him home with a 5-day course of prednisolone
- [ ] D Give salbutamol nebuliser and prednisolone 40 mg orally; arrange hospital assessment
- [ ] E Give 10 puffs of salbutamol and 10 puffs ipratropium; arrange a review the next day with the asthma nurse

17.10 A 17-year-old girl has a 2-week history of malaise, myalgia and headache. She has recently developed a dry, hacking cough and chest pain on coughing. She has an urticarial rash on her limbs. Her chest is clear on auscultation. Which of the following organisms is the single most likely infective cause?

- [ ] A *Aspergillus fumigatus*
- [ ] B *Coxiella burnetii*
- [ ] C *Cryptosporidum* species
- [ ] D *Mycoplasma pneumoniae*
- [ ] E *Streptococcus pneumoniae*

17.11 A 45-year-old woman presents with increasing exertional breathlessness over the past 6 months. She has scleroderma. Spirometry shows:

	Measured	Predicted
FVC (litres)	1.98	3.51
FEV_1 (litres)	1.64	2.82
FEV_1/FVC	835	80%

FEV_1 = forced expiratory volume in 1 second; FVC = forced vital capacity.

Which of the following is the most likely diagnosis? Select one option only.

- [ ] A   Asthma
- [ ] B   Bronchiectasis
- [ ] C   Extrinsic allergic alveolitis
- [ ] D   Pulmonary fibrosis
- [ ] E   Tracheal stenosis

17.12 A 14-year-old boy is rushed into the surgery by his mother with sudden-onset abdominal pain and vomiting and an urticarial skin rash. On examination, you note he is very breathless with both stridor and wheeze. His lips and tongue are swollen. From the following options, what would the best initial drug management be:

- [ ] A   Administer nebulised 1 in 1000 adrenaline (epinephrine), 2 ml via oxygen-driven nebuliser
- [ ] B   Administer oxygen and give 1 in 1000 adrenaline, 0.1 ml intra-venously
- [ ] C   Administer oxygen and give 1 in 1000 adrenaline, 0.5 ml intra-muscularly
- [ ] D   Administer oxygen and give 10 puffs of salbutamol via a spacer
- [ ] E   Give nebulised salbutamol 5 mg via oxygen-driven nebuliser

17.13 A 54-year-old woman complains of episodes of productive cough and shortness of breath over the past 6 months. She is an ex-smoker. Her most recent spirometry shows that she obtains only 47% of her predicted forced expiratory volume in 1 second (FEV_1), and she finds that moderate exertion results in breathlessness. Her results are most consistent with the NICE classification of:

☐ A   Acute upper airways infection and asthma

☐ B   Mild chronic obstructive pulmonary disease (COPD)

☐ C   Moderate COPD

☐ D   Severe COPD

☐ E   Severe chronic obstructive and restrictive pulmonary disease

17.14 Your practice holds a clinic for the treatment of patients with known COPD. Some patients who are reviewed find they are still symptomatic despite taking single short-acting bronchodilators. According to NICE guidelines, what would the most appropriate next treatment option be? Select one option only.

☐ A   A 4-week trial of combination long-acting β agonist and inhaled corticosteroid

☐ B   Combined therapy of current short-acting beta agonist and theophylline

☐ C   Long-acting bronchodilator (β agonist or anticholinergic)

☐ D   Mucolytic therapy to reduce the incidence of dry cough

☐ E   Oxygen therapy via nasal cannulae at 2 l/minute for 15 hours each day

EXTENDED MATCHING QUESTIONS

THEME: MANAGEMENT OF ACUTE COUGH

Options

A   Amoxicillin 500 mg tds and erythromycin 500 mg qds for 1 week

B   Amoxicillin 500mg tds for 7 days and prednisolone 30 mg for 5 days

C   Amoxicillin 500 mg tds for 7 days and prednisolone 30 mg daily for 10 days

D   Amoxicillin 500 mg tds for 1 week

E   Contact the on-call team to arrange admission to hospital

F   Erythromycin 500 mg qds for 1 week

G   Erythromycin 500 mg qds for 1 week and arrange a chest X-ray

H   Levofloxacin 500 mg daily for 7 days

I   No prescription necessary

J   Salbutamol 6 puffs via a spacer and prednisolone 40 mg orally; call an ambulance

Choose the most appropriate management for each patient from the options listed above. Each option can be used once, more than once, or not at all.

☐ **17.15** A 66-year-old man is seen in his home. He has a productive cough and fever. On examination, his respiratory rate is 32/minute, he is lucid and alert, and his BP is 100/50 mmHg, SpO$_2$ 90% on air. He has coarse crackles on the right side of his chest on auscultation.

☐ **17.16** A 40-year-old non-smoker has been treated for mild community-acquired pneumonia with amoxicillin for the past 7 days. She still has a productive cough and fever and feels unwell. Her respiratory rate is 20/minute, her BP is 110/70 mmHg and she is lucid and alert. She has crackles on the left side of her chest.

☐ **17.17** A 45-year-old woman known to have COPD is seen at the surgery complaining of cough. Over the past 7 days she has felt increasingly breathless and her sputum has changed colour from white to green. Her respiratory rate is 20/minute and she has bilateral wheeze.

☐ **17.18** A 45-year-old woman who has no past medical history of chest problems is seen at the surgery. Over the past few days she has had a sore throat and dry cough and she complains of nasal congestion with purulent rhinitis. On examination, her chest is clear and her respiratory rate is 12/minute.

☐ **17.19** A 50-year-old businessman is seen at the surgery. He was previously fit and well. He has a productive cough and right-sided chest pain on coughing and he also complains of fever. On examination, he has coarse crackles on the right side, his respiratory rate is 18/minute, and his BP is 150/100 mmHg. He has recently returned from a business trip in France.

THEME: OCCUPATIONAL LUNG DISEASE

Options

A Asbestosis

B Chronic extrinsic allergic alveolitis

C Formaldehyde exposure

D Glutaraldehyde exposure

E Mesothelioma

F Occupational bronchial carcinoma

G Platinum exposure

H Psittacosis

I Siderosis

J Silicosis

Choose the most likely diagnosis for each patient described below from the options listed above. Each option can be used once, more than once, or not at all.

☐ **17.20** A 32-year-old nurse has a 4-year history of asthma. Her symptoms began in 2001, 6 months after she took up a new post in an endoscopy suite.

☐ **17.21** A 65-year-old woman presents with right-sided pleuritic chest pain and dyspnoea. Her symptoms have worsened over the past 3 months. Chest X-ray shows a right-sided pleural effusion. Her late husband worked in a naval shipyard.

☐ **17.22** A 40-year-old pet shop owner with a 2-week history of dry cough, dypnoea and malaise, has now developed a diffuse and severe headache and myalgia.

☐ **17.23** A 50-year-old man, originally from China, presents with gradual-onset shortness of breath and wheeze over the past year. He has lived in this country for the past 10 years but was employed China as a sandblaster for many years before that.

☐ **17.24** A 65-year-old retired builder presents with a chronic dry cough and progressive dyspnoea. On examination, you note he has finger clubbing and bilateral end-expiratory crackles. A chest X-ray shows bilateral pleural plaques and diffuse bilateral shadowing.

THEME: MOST APPROPRIATE INVESTIGATION

Options

A   Arterial blood gases

B   Refer for outpatient chest X-ray (AP view)

C   Refer for outpatient chest X-ray (PA view)

D   Methacholine challenge

E   None of these options

F   Serial peak flow readings once a day for 2 weeks

G   Serial peak flow readings twice a day for 2 weeks

H   Spirometry with reversibility

J   Throat swab

K   Venous blood gases

From the list of options above, choose the most appropriate investigation for each situation described below. Each option can be used once, more than once, or not at all.

☐ **17.25** An 18-year-old woman has had intermittent shortness of breath and wheezing over the past year. She is known to have eczema but has had no prior lung problems. Today, her respiratory examination is normal. At present, there is no significant change in her spirometry readings after β_2 agonists. She can return for review if necessary.

☐ **17.26** A 46-year-old man has had recurrent chest infections. He is a smoker. He had a normal chest X-ray 2 weeks ago. He attends again to report increased shortness of breath on exertion and a moist cough on waking. These symptoms have troubled him for the past 2 months. He is otherwise well and his weight is steady.

17.27 A tall 15-year-old boy is seen immediately as an emergency at a casualty department. On examination he is breathless, with a respiratory rate of 42/minute and has reduced air entry affecting his right lung field. His right-sided percussion note is hyper-resonant. His jugular venous system is distended. His symptoms began spontaneously 1 hour ago.

17.28 An elderly patient on the geriatric ward has become breathless and feverish over the past 36 hours. He had a chest X-ray 12 hours ago, which showed right lower lobe consolidation. The nursing staff are concerned because they feel that he has become confused over the past few hours.

17.29 A 19-year-old attends her GP surgery with a 3-day history of sore throat and cough. On examination, she has bilateral tonsillitis; her chest is clear. She is normally well.

CHAPTER 17 QUESTIONS

THEME: SHORTNESS OF BREATH

Options

A Bronchial carcinoma

B Bronchiolitis

C COPD

D Croup

E Metastatic lung disease

F Pneumonia

G Pneumothorax

H Pleural effusion

I Pleurisy

J Upper respiratory tract infection

Choose the most likely diagnosis for each patient described below from the list of options above. Each option can be used once, more than once, or not at all.

☐ **17.30** A 78-year-old man presents with cough, dyspnoea and weight loss over the past month. He has recent-onset haemoptysis and his nail beds appear spongy. He smokes regularly. On examination, his respiratory rate is 18/minute at rest and he has crackles affecting his right lung.

☐ **17.31** A 55-year-old man has had a productive cough for the past 3 days. He has right-sided chest pain and feels short of breath. He is a non-smoker. On examination, his respiratory rate is 20/minute at rest. Right low chest percussion is dull and he has inspiratory right lower zone crackles. His temperature is 38.5 °C.

17.32 A 60-year-old woman complains of a dry cough and sore throat for the past 3 days. She says that she feels breathless for a short while after coughing. She smokes 10 cigarettes a day. On examination, her oropharynx looks injected, her respiratory rate is 14/minute, her BP is 150/90 mmHg and her pulse is 70 bpm. Her chest is clear to auscultation and she is apyrexial. She has had no previous chest problems.

17.33 A man asks to see one of the nurses at your practice to get a 'cough bottle'. On further questioning, he tells the nurse that he has had a productive cough intermittently for the past 4 years. He is in his late forties. At present, he smokes cigars regularly and experiences shortness of breath when dressing or walking more than a 100 yards on the flat. His weight is steady. He sometimes wheezes on exertion.

17.34 A 6-month-old is seen at a general practice with a 3-day history of shortness of breath, reduced feeding and cough. On examination, the child has a respiratory rate of 30/minute and his chest examination reveals bilateral coarse inspiratory crepitations. He is afebrile.

ALGORITHM QUESTIONS

THEME: OXYGEN ADMINISTRATION

17.35–17.37

Options

A 100% oxygen

B 100% oxygen via non-rebreather

C No

D Target oxygen saturation 88–92%

E Target oxygen saturation 94–98%

F Yes

You are updating the practice resuscitation guidelines and wish to base the oxygen guidance on the current British Thoracic Society (BTS) recommendations. Complete the flow chart below regarding oxygen administration using the options above. Each option may be used once, more than once or not at all:

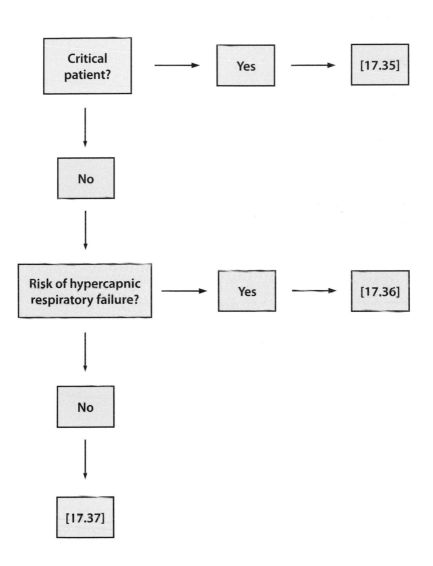

THEME: ASSESSMENT OF AIRFLOW OBSTRUCTION IN COPD

17.38–17.42

Options

A   Cough and sputum production common

B   Evening cough and sputum production problematic

C   50–80% predicted

D   50–70% predicted

E   33–49% predicted

F   30–49% predicted

G   < 33% predicted

H   < 30% predicted

I   Severe dyspnoea on minimal exertion

J   Severe dyspnoea prevents even minimal exertion

The following flow chart has been adapted from NICE guidance on classifying COPD.

For each stage of the flow chart, select the most appropriate option from the list above for measured FEV_1 and likely symptomatology. Each option can be used once, more than once or not at all.

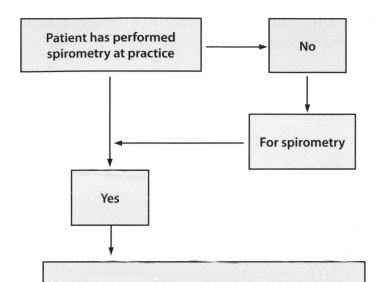

```
┌─────────────────────────┐         ┌──────────────┐
│  Patient has performed  │ ──────▶ │      No      │
│  spirometry at practice │         │              │
└─────────────────────────┘         └──────────────┘
              │                              │
              │                              ▼
              │                     ┌──────────────────┐
              │      ◀───────────── │  For spirometry  │
              ▼                     └──────────────────┘
      ┌───────────────┐
      │      Yes      │
      └───────────────┘
              │
              ▼
```

Mild airflow obstuction FEV$_1$ [17.38] predicted.
Moderate airflow obstuction FEV$_1$ [17.39] predicted.
Severe airflow obstuction FEV$_1$ [17.40] predicted.

Mild
- Little or no clinical signs usual at rest
- Morning cough

Moderate
- Dyspnoea on moderate exertion
- [17.41]

Severe
- [17.42]
- Productive cough and wheezing
- Life-threatening exacerbations

THEME: DIAGNOSIS OF CHRONIC COUGH IN NON-SMOKING ADULTS

17.43–17.45

Options

A Anti-tussive

B Bronchodilator

C Hiatus hernia

D Postnasal drip

E Rhinitis

F Silent reflux

The following flow chart has been developed to simplify the diagnosis of chronic cough in non-smoking adults. For each stage of the flow chart below, select the most appropriate option from the list above for condition or treatment.

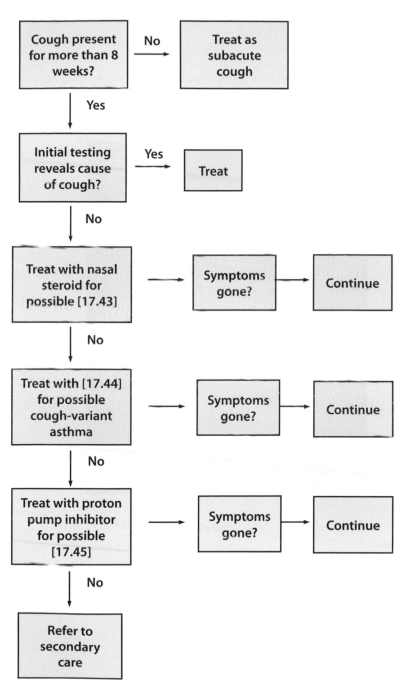

PICTURE QUESTIONS

17.46 This 64-year-old man has had a productive cough, shortness of breath and intermittent fever for the past week. He is a non-smoker. He has had a chest X-ray and this is the AP film:

What is the most likely diagnosis? Select one option only.

- [ ] A   Foreign body aspiration
- [ ] B   Pneumonia
- [ ] C   Pneumothorax
- [ ] D   Pulmonary oedema
- [ ] E   Upper respiratory tract infection

17.47 This 72-year-old woman has COPD. She has severe hypoxaemia ($Pao_2 < 7.3$ kPa) and receives treatment at home using the machine shown below.

To benefit from this treatment, she should use it for a prolonged period each day. What minimum treatment duration is required each day to significantly reduce mortality rates in COPD? Select one option only.

- [ ] A   8 hours
- [ ] B   12 hours
- [ ] C   15 hours
- [ ] D   18 hours
- [ ] E   22 hours

DATA INTERPRETATION QUESTION

17.48 A 20-year-old medical student complains of intermittent cough and breathlessness for the past 3 months. She was previously fit and well and takes no regular medication. She has been asked to keep a record of her peak flow measurements twice daily for 2 weeks; these are shown above. The peak flow rate readings show (choose the single most appropriate statement):

☐ A   Diurnal variation that is neither specific nor sensitive for a diagnosis of asthma

☐ B   Diurnal variation that is sensitive but not specific for a diagnosis of asthma

☐ C   Diurnal variation that is specific and sensitive for a diagnosis of asthma

☐ D   Diurnal variation that is specific but not sensitive for a diagnosis of asthma

☐ E   Normal results

HOT TOPICS/EVIDENCE BASED PRACTICE

17.49 Considering the recent TOwards a Revolution in COPD Health (TORCH) trial, which one of the following statements regarding mortality rate was demonstrated by the study?

- [ ] A   Mortality rate was not measured in this study
- [ ] B   Mortality was reduced in all patients receiving active inhalers compared with those receiving placebo
- [ ] C   Patients with COPD were more likely to die if they agreed to join this study
- [ ] D   There was a highly significant reduction in mortality for patients treated with combination therapy compared with other groups studied
- [ ] E   There was a trend towards reduced mortality in patients receiving combination therapy compared with other groups

ANSWERS

17.1 A: He has a significantly increased risk of developing lung cancer

Patients with cryptogenic fibrosing alveolitis have a 10-fold increased risk of developing lung cancer. Overall, the prognosis is poor, with only a small proportion responding to treatment and a 5-year survival rate of 40–50%. In most cases a cause cannot be identified, and where steroids and immunosuppression do not work lung transplant might be an option. For most patients, however, treatment is symptomatic, with oxygen when necessary.

17.2 E: Tuberculosis

TB often presents insidiously and patients can be asymptomatic despite having active TB. This gentleman has signs of pleural effusion, but he is not dyspnoeic. Dyspnoea is often a late feature in pulmonary TB and a high index of suspicion is therefore needed. NICE guidance advises chest X-ray as the initial investigation of choice in diagnosing suspected TB. This applies even when non-pulmonary disease is suspected, as there could be chest X-ray findings due to previous lung infection. NICE recommends screening for new arrivals coming from countries with a TB incidence of 40/100 000. The World Health Organisation (WHO) estimated that the incidence of TB in India was168/100 000 in 2004.

17.3 E: Show her how to use a peak-flow meter and request that she keeps a record of morning and evening readings for 2 weeks, then come for review

The history is suggestive of asthma and her past history of hay fever suggests atopy, supporting the diagnosis. A 20% or greater diurnal variation in peak flow on 3 days a week for 2 weeks is highly suggestive of asthma. She is unlikely to be able to use an inhaler effectively without training by a health-care professional. The British Thoracic Society (BTS) guidelines recommend objective tests to confirm the diagnosis of asthma before starting long-term therapy.

17.4   C: Add a budesonide turbohaler to her treatment regime at a dose of 100 micrograms bd; review in 3 months

Children using occasional-relief bronchodilators (Step 1, BTS guidelines) should be treated with regular inhaled corticosteroids (BTS 2) if:

- β_2 agonists are needed more than three times a week

- They have symptomatic asthma at least three times a week or are waking once a week at night

- They have had an exacerbation of their asthma requiring a nebulised bronchodilator or systemic corticosteroid in the last 2 years.

Spacer devices are recommended by NICE for the delivery of inhaled corticosteroid therapy to children aged 5–15 years. However, where the use of a spacer is unsuitable or inconvenient, a dry-powder inhaler can be used, providing the child can use it effectively.

Inhaled steroids should be started at 200–400 micrograms beclomethasone or equivalent a day. For most patients, a dose of 200 micrograms is sufficient. Treatment should be reviewed after 3 months and a stepwise reduction might be considered if control is adequate.

17.5   A: Ask the receptionist to contact the patient and organise a review appointment in the asthma clinic by the end of the week

This patient needs an early review. Using more than two canisters of a β_2 agonist per month is a sign of poorly controlled asthma. The nurse should check his inhaler technique and compliance with treatment and also eliminate any trigger factors if possible. Doubling the dose of his corticosteroid or adding salmeterol is futile if his inhaler technique is poor.

17.6   B: Ensure that he has been told verbally and in writing that he must inform the DVLA of the diagnosis

The Scottish Intercollegiate Guidelines Network (SIGN) have produced guidelines for the investigation and management of obstructive sleep apnoea (OSA). OSA can lead to an increased risk of the sufferer having an accident due to sleepiness. It is an offence to fall asleep at the wheel of a car and custodial sentences can be imposed. Patients with osbructive sleep apnoea can present reporting daytime sleepiness, but can also present with non-specific symptoms such as irritability and poor concentration. The Epworth questionnaire has been used in patients with suspected OSA to measure pretreatment sleepiness. Moderate to severe OSA is treated with nasal CPAP; weight loss should be encouraged in all patients. Patients should not drive if they report daytime sleepiness. Once diagnosed, patients should be told verbally and in writing that they must inform the DVLA. Those working with machinery or driving should be referred to a sleep centre for assessment.

17.7   C: Organise an urgent chest X-ray

The NICE guidelines for the diagnosis and management of suspected lung cancer suggest urgent referral for a chest X-ray in smokers and ex-smokers over the age of 40 with:

- Haemoptysis, or

- Persistent or unexplained (>3 weeks)

  - cough

  - chest/shoulder pain

  - weight loss

  - dyspnoea

  - chest signs

  - clubbing

  - hoarseness

  - cervical/supraclavicular lymphadenopathy

  - signs of metastatic disease.

17.8   B: Reflux cough

This lady has a chronic cough (duration > 8 weeks). All patients with chronic cough should have their chest X-rayed. Common causes of chronic cough seen in primary care include silent reflux, postnasal drip and cough-variant asthma. Adults can contract pertussis, as immunity from previous infection or vaccination wanes with time. Generally, the cough can last up to 3 months following pertussis infection. The disease is mild in these patients, but coughing adults and adolescents with pertussis pass the infection on to susceptible infants.

17.9   D: Give salbutamol nebuliser and prednisolone 40 mg orally; arrange hospital assessment

The patient has features of acute severe asthma and warrants referral. Features of acute severe asthma include:

*   Respiratory rate > 25/minute

*   Inability to complete a sentence in one breath

*   Pulse > 110 bpm

*   Peak flow 33–50% of best or predicted.

High-flow oxygen should be administered if available. Salbutamol or terbutaline can be administered by spacer or nebuliser as available, with oxygen-driven nebuliser the preferred method. D was the best option out of those given.

17.10   D: *Mycoplasma pneumoniae*

Pneumonia secondary to *Mycoplasma pneumoniae* occurs most commonly in children and young adults. It occurs in epidemics (approximately every 4 years in the UK). It has an insidious onset and often causes a persistent dry cough. Extrapulmonary manifestations include arthritis, haemolysis and myalgia. Dermatological manifestations include urticaria and erythema nodosum. In most cases the pneumonia resolves spontaneously over a few weeks. Treatment is with macrolide or tetracycline antibiotics.

17.11   D: Pulmonary fibrosis

Lung involvement in scleroderma is common and ultimately up to 80% of patients with the condition will develop abnormal pulmonary function tests. The spirometry measurements show a restrictive pattern (FVC and FEV_1 spirometry measurements are reduced and the FEV_1 to FVC ratio is normal).

17.12   C: Administer oxygen and give 1 in 1000 adrenaline, 0.5 ml intramuscularly

Gastrointestinal manifestations of anaphylaxis include abdominal pain and vomiting and are more common in cases of food allergy. This child has signs of respiratory compromise and should be given intramuscular adrenaline (epinephrine) and oxygen while an ambulance is called. An inhaled β_2 agonist might help if the bronchospasm does not respond to your initial treatment.

17.13   C: Moderate COPD

Airflow obstruction is classified as mild, moderate or severe on the basis of the measured FEV_1. Patients with COPD should have their disease state diagnosed by assessing their clinical history, physical examination and spirometry findings. This patient has both moderately impaired airflow obstruction and appropriate symptoms for moderate COPD.

17.14   C: Long-acting bronchodilator (β agonist or anticholinergic)

NICE guidelines suggest that patients who are not controlled with a single short-acting bronchodilator can be started on a combination of two short-acting bronchodilators or a single long-acting bronchodilator. Mucolytic therapy is used in patients with chronic cough productive of sputum. Oxygen therapy, inhaled steroids and theophylline are all considered, but as later more invasive treatments.

THEME: MANAGEMENT OF ACUTE COUGH

17.15   E: Contact the on-call team to arrange admission to hospital

This gentleman has community-acquired pneumonia with adverse prognostic factors. Several scoring systems have been developed to try and identify patients at greatest risk. The 'CRB-65' score has been endorsed by the British Thoracic Society and can be used with the information supplied in this scenario:

> **C** – New confusion?
>
> **R** – Respiratory rate > 30/minute?
>
> **B** – BP < 90 mmHg systolic or < 60 mmHg diastolic?
>
> **65** – Age > 65 years?

CRB-65 scores of 0 indicate a low risk of death and patients do not normally require hospitalisation.

CRB-65 scores of 1 or 2 indicate an increased risk of death and hospital referral and assessment should be considered, particularly with scores of 2.

CRB-65 scores of ≥ 3 indicate a high risk of death and patients require urgent hospital admission.

17.16   G: Erythromycin 500mg qds for 1 week and arrange a chest X-ray

The BTS guidelines for the management of community-acquired pneumonia recommend switching to a macrolide antibiotic if amoxicillin is not effective. The patient should be reassessed to ensure that they do not warrant admission, and a chest X-ray should be organised to rule out complications of pneumonia (lung abscess, empyema, etc).

17.17   C: Give amoxicillin 500 mg tds for 7 days and prednisolone 30 mg daily for 10 days

The patient has an exacerbation of her COPD – increased dyspnoea with purulent sputum. NICE guidelines recommend oral antibiotics and prednisolone 30 mg daily for 7–14 days in patients who have increased breathlessness. Past medical history, current clinical condition and social circumstances should all be taken into account in deciding where to manage the patient.

17.18   I: No prescription necessary

The patient has an upper respiratory tract infection. This is most likely to be viral and will not require antibiotics or steroids. Antibiotic treatments for both the common cold and for purulent rhinitis were reviewed in the Cochrane database and no benefit was noted in either case. The main issue here is appropriate patient education and over-the-counter medication.

17.19   D: Amoxicillin 500 mg tds for 1 week

Amoxicillin is the first-choice antibiotic for treatment of community-acquired pneumonia, provided there is no history of penicillin allergy. It should be given in adequate doses to cover intermediate resistance seen in some strains of *Streptococcus pneumoniae*. There are no features of atypical pneumonia here and the trip to France is of no significance. The patient should, however, attend the surgery in the near future for repeat BP measurement!

THEME: OCCUPATIONAL LUNG DISEASE

17.20   D: Glutaraldehyde exposure

Glutaraldehyde was, until recently, commonly used in endoscopy suites to sterilise endoscopes. The Health and Safety Executive has been implementing regulations to introduce substitutes. However, some of the substitute cleaning fluids have also been implicated as causes of occupational asthma.

17.21   E: Mesothelioma

Asbestos exposure is associated with mesothelioma. There is often a time lag of many years between exposure and disease. High-risk occupations include ship- and building construction, pipe fitting and insulation and demolition work. Family members have been exposed to asbestos through fibres embedded in the worker's clothing.

17.22   H: Psittacosis

This infection is caused by *Chlamydia psittaci*, contracted from infected birds. Budgerigars are a common source of infection, putting pet shop owners at particular risk! Severe, diffuse headache is a common complaint. Treatment is with tetracycline or erythromycin.

17.23   J: Silicosis

Silica dust is released during work with certain rocks and ores, sand and concrete. Sandblasting is a particularly high-risk occupation. Inhaling crystalline silica leads to pulmonary fibrosis and emphysema. With chronic exposure, symptoms begin after a long latent period, often 10–30 years after initial exposure. However, accelerated forms are recognised and carry a worse prognosis. The WHO reported that from 1991 to 1995, China recorded more than 500 000 cases of silicosis, with more than 24 000 deaths occurring each year.

17.24   A: Asbestosis

Asbestosis is the term used to describe pulmonary fibrosis secondary to asbestos inhalation. Finger clubbing affects a third of patients. Pleural plaques and thickening on X-ray provide strong evidence that fibrosis is due to asbestos exposure.

THEME: MOST APPROPRIATE INVESTIGATION

17.25   G: Serial peak fow readings twice a day for 2 weeks

Peak expiratory flow readings (PEFR) are measured twice daily to detect diurnal variation. A greater than 20% diurnal variation in PEFR for ≥ 3 days in a week for 2 weeks is highly suggestive of asthma. Patients with asthma can demonstrate diurnal variability below 20%. Serial PEFR is therefore a very specific but less sensitive test. Objective testing should confirm asthma prior to starting long-term treatment. Other tests include spirometry after prednisolone for 14 days.

17.26   H: Spirometry with reversibility

This man is a current smoker and has a 2-month history of shortness of breath on exertion. He is likely to have COPD. His recent normal chest X-ray and steady weight are both reassuring. Spirometry is likely to demonstrate reduction in both his FEV_1 and his FEV_1/FVC ratio. Medication will not change his spirometry readings back to the normal range.

17.27   E: None of the above

The patient has signs and symptoms consistent with a tension pneumo-thorax and staff in the casualty department will perform emergency needle thoracostomy. Performing a chest X-ray or other formal investigation first would delay treatment and increase his risk of death.

17.28   A: Arterial blood gases

An arterial blood gas is the most appropriate investigation available. This gentleman has had a recent chest X-ray which suggests pneumonia. Hypoxia, acidosis and hypercapnia could all contribute to his confusion and are demonstrated on arterial blood gas analysis.

17.29   E: None of the above

This patient has tonsillitis and a clear chest. Swabs could be taken but their usefulness is debated and they are not recommended routinely. Group A β-haemolytic streptococci might be cultured when taking throat swabs during tonsillitis. Unfortunately this could be due to coincidental patient carriage of the bacteria rather than to active infection with streptococci. The vast majority of patients will show a full recovery from tonsillitis without throat swab analysis or antibiotics.

THEME: SHORTNESS OF BREATH

17.30   A: Bronchial carcinoma

The patient has shortness of breath, haemoptysis and early finger clubbing. Non-small-cell carcinoma presents with finger clubbing more often than does small-cell carcinoma. He needs to be referred as an urgent outpatient.

17.31   F: Pneumonia

This 55-year-old has signs and symptoms consistent with right-sided pneumonia. His examination findings show that he should be managed in the community. He does not need further investigations such as a chest X-ray at present. A course of amoxicillin should be provided as long as he is not allergic to penicillins. The patient should be advised to rest and drink plenty of fluids.

17.32   J: Upper respiratory tract infection

The patient's chest is clear and her respiratory examination only shows injection of her oropharynx, which is often present during upper respiratory infections. Her upper respiratory tract infection only requires symptomatic relief but she should have her BP rechecked and should be encouraged to attend smoking cessation services.

17.33   C: COPD

This patient needs full investigation and management as he probably has COPD. If COPD is confirmed on further testing, he should stop smoking and is likely to need regular treatment to control his current symptoms.

17.34   B: Bronchiolitis

Bronchiolitis affects babies under 12 months of age. Infection with RSV is the commonest cause. It classically presents with coryzal symptoms, increased work of breathing, cough, and reduced feeding. Infants aged under 2 months can present with a history of apnoeic episodes. Treatment is supportive; referral is required if fluid intake is reduced to less than two-thirds of normal or if the child is showing signs of respiratory distress.

THEME: OXYGEN ADMINISTRATION

17.35   B: 100% oxygen via non-rebreather

17.36   D: Target oxygen saturation 88–92%

17.37   E: Target oxygen saturation 94–98%

THEME: ASSESSMENT OF AIRFLOW OBSTRUCTION IN COPD

17.38   C: 50–80% predicted

17.39   E: 33-49% predicted

17.40   G: < 33% predicted

17.41   A: Cough and sputum production common

17.42   I: Severe dyspnoea on minimal exertion

Patients with COPD should undergo spirometry testing as part of their diagnosis and also on at least an annual basis. Mild COPD usually causes minimal symptoms, but progression to moderate and severe COPD markedly affects symptomatology. Continuing to smoke is the major cause of disease progression; patients should stop smoking to limit disease progression as soon as possible.

THEME: DIAGNOSIS OF CHRONIC COUGH IN NON-SMOKING ADULTS

17.43   D: Postnasal drip

17.44   B: Bronchodilator

17.45   F: Silent reflux

Chronic cough is commonly seen in primary care. In some circumstances, coughing can be caused by serious disorders such as lung cancer or tuberculosis. However, in these scenarios, other signs and symptoms are present and a diagnostic cause is usually quickly discovered. In chronic cough which has persisted despite routine investigations being normal, the commonest causes seen in primary care are postnasal drip, cough-variant asthma and acid reflux. Appropriate treatment for these conditions aids chronic cough cessation.

17.46   B: Pneumonia

The X-ray shows consolidation within the right middle lobe and some patchy airspace consolidation adjacent to the horizontal fissure. The patient needs to be assessed using the CRB-65 scoring system and then treated at home or in hospital as appropriate.

17.47   C: 15 hours

This patient is receiving long-term oxygen therapy (LTOT) from an oxygen concentrator. NICE guidelines state that mortality is reduced in COPD patients with severe hypoxaemia ($Pao_2 < 7.3$ kPa) who receive LTOT (evidence level A). Patients with a Pao_2 between 7.3 kPa and 8.0 kPa and one other risk factor are also likely to benefit from LTOT (evidence level D). Treatment with LTOT needs to be given for at least 15 hours each day to significantly reduce mortality rate.

17.48   C: Diurnal variation that is specific and sensitive for a diagnosis of asthma

Asthma in primary care can be diagnosed through diurnal peak flow measurements or spirometry. Peak flow readings are measured diurnally for 2 weeks. Asthma is said to be highly likely where:

- There is diurnal variation in PEFR of $\geq 20\%$
- The variability occurs at least 3 days a week for both weeks
- The amplitude of change in PEFR is at least 60 l/minute.

Diurnal variability in PEFR is particularly common in asthma. A variability of 20% or more each day in diurnal readings is very uncommon in other lung disorders. This patient demonstrates variability of around 28% in PEFR each day for 9 days during the 2-week test.

17.49   E: There was a trend towards reduced mortality in patients receiving combination therapy compared with other groups

The TORCH trial looked at patients with COPD. All patients had a measured FEV_1 of less than 60%. The population was randomised into four groups: one group received placebo alone, one group received fluticasone, one group received salmeterol and the final group received both salmeterol and fluticasone. There was a trend towards reduced mortality in patients treated with combination therapy compared with other groups. Unfortunately this difference was not deemed statistically significant ($P = 0.052$). Authors in favour of combination therapy have suggested that this is because the study was underpowered.

CHAPTER 18 THERAPEUTIC INDICATIONS AND ADVERSE REACTIONS

SINGLE BEST ANSWER QUESTIONS

18.1 A 74-year-old woman currently in the local cottage hospital is taking morphine orally for bone pain from her myeloma. She has been constipated for 1 week despite enemas, Movicol and bisacodyl. She is in a great deal of discomfort. On examination she is constipated but there are no signs of bowel obstruction. Which one of the following would be appropriate in this situation?

- [ ] A Change morphine to oxycodone/naloxone
- [ ] B Fybogel
- [ ] C Lactulose
- [ ] D Methylnaltrexone
- [ ] E Sodium picosulfate

18.2 A 23-year-old woman attends your surgery to request help with smoking cessation. She tried to give up smoking 4 months ago but was unsuccessful. She wants advice because she is currently breast feeding. What does NICE recommend about smoking cessation in this situation? Select one option only.

☐ A That both bupropion and nicotine replacement therapy can be used by patients who are breastfeeding

☐ B That bupropion is not recommended in pregnancy but can be used by patients who are breastfeeding

☐ C That bupropion cannot be used because the risk of seizure is estimated at 1 in 100 in breastfeeding women

☐ D That if an attempt at smoking cessation is unsuccessful with treatment, then in general the NHS should not fund a further attempt with 12 months

☐ E That if nicotine replacement therapy (NRT) is prescribed, it should be discontinued if the patient starts to smoke again

18.3 An adult patient is started on a new drug and develops an itchy rash on their trunk. The drug is withdrawn and the rash subsides. The drug is new to the market and is marked with an inverted triangle next to the drug name in the *British National Formulary (BNF)*. What is the single most appropriate way to record this adverse event?

☐ A Inform the local pharmacy that the patient used it and discuss the adverse event at the next practice meeting

☐ B Make a record in the notes and contact the pharmaceutical company which makes the drug to inform them

☐ C Make a record in the notes and inform the local pharmacy that the patient used it

☐ D Make a record in the notes and inform the Medicines and Healthcare Products Regulatory Agency (MHRA) via the yellow card scheme

☐ E Record the adverse reaction in the patient's notes so that future prescribers will be aware

18.4 A 24-year-old woman has visited Vanuatu in the South Pacific recently. She returned 2 weeks ago. She has been taking doxycycline for antimalarial prophylaxis, but wishes to stop now she has returned to the UK. Choose the single most appropriate remaining antimalarial regime from the following options:

- [ ] A Stop taking all antimalarials now that she has been away from Vanuatu for 2 weeks
- [ ] B Take atovaquone 150 mg and proguinal 100 mg daily for a further 2 weeks
- [ ] C Take doxycycline 250 mg daily for 2 weeks
- [ ] D Take chloroquine 300 mg and proguanil 200 mg, both daily, for a further 2 weeks
- [ ] E Take mefloquine 250 mg daily for a further 2 weeks

18.5 An active 68-year-old patient with asthma and atrial fibrillation (AF) has been assessed by the cardiologists and diagnosed with permanent AF. They recommend rate control. Which one of the following statements about this situation is correct?

- [ ] A Digoxin can be used for first-line rate control in asthmatic patients with AF
- [ ] B Esmelol can be used for first-line rate control in asthmatic patients with AF
- [ ] C Nifedipine can be used for first-line rate control in asthmatic patients with AF
- [ ] D Rate control is not appropriate unless patient's ventricular rate regularly exceeds 130/minute
- [ ] E Verapamil can be used for first-line rate control in asthmatic patients with AF

18.6 **Regarding the prescribing of medications to children, which one of the following statements is true?**

- [ ] A Intramuscular injections are preferable to intravenous injections in small children because of the difficulty in achieving adequate cannulation

- [ ] B Quantities of medicine of < 5 ml should be given by syringe rather than by spoon

- [ ] C The small quantity of sugar in medicine is unlikely to cause tooth decay

- [ ] D The use of unlicensed medications in children is strictly forbidden

- [ ] E To ensure compliance with unpalatable medicines, these should be mixed in with food (eg mashed potato)

18.7 **Which one of the following statements about the use of medicines in paediatric palliative care is true?**

- [ ] A Children often require a higher dose of morphine related to their body weight than adults

- [ ] B Children tolerate strong opioids much better than adults

- [ ] C If children are unable to tolerate morphine, oxycodone is contraindicated

- [ ] D NSAIDs should not be used in children because of the risk of nephrotoxicity

- [ ] E Tricyclic antidepressants are contraindicated in children because of their effects on intraocular pressure

18.8 **Regarding drug treatments for osteoporosis, which one of the following statements is true?**

☐ A Bisphosphonates can only be given either daily or weekly

☐ B Calcitonin is taken orally

☐ C Patients with poor dental hygiene should see their dentist before starting bisphosphonate therapy

☐ D Strontium is taken as a once-weekly preparation

☐ E Teriparatide can be used to prevent osteoporosis in those at high risk

EXTENDED MATCHING QUESTIONS

THEME: ANALGESICS

Options

A Anticonvulsant

B Antidepressant

C Cannabinoid

D COX-2 inhibitor

E Non-opioid analgesic

F Non-steroidal anti-inflammatory drug (NSAID)

G Strong opioid

H Topical local anaesthetic

I Weak opioid

For each of the descriptions below, select the most appropriate option from the list above. Each option may be used once, more than once or not at all.

☐ **18.9** First-line treatment for children with pain and fever.

☐ **18.10** Has similar efficacy to codeine in chronic pain, but frequently causes psychomotor side-effects.

☐ **18.11** Associated with a 1% risk of gastrointestinal haemorrhage.

☐ **18.12** Topical treatment licensed for use in post-herpetic neuralgia.

THEME: SIDE-EFFECTS OF ANTIDEPRESSANTS

Options

A   Citalopram

B   Duloxetine

C   Fluoxetine

D   Mirtazapine

E   Paroxetine

F   Sertraline

G   Venlafaxine

H   All of the above

For each of the statements below, select the most appropriate option from the list above. Each option may be used once, more than once or not at all.

☐   **18.13**   Associated with the lowest incidence of sexual dysfunction.

☐   **18.14**   Can cause severe discontinuation reactions.

☐   **18.15**   Frequently causes sedation.

☐   **18.16**   Associated with reduced risk of suicide in the over-25 age group.

THEME: DRUG SAFETY

Options

A Anticonvulsants

B Carbimazole

C Monoamine oxidase inhibitors

D Prednisolone

E Roaccutane

F Selective serotonin reuptake inhibitors (SSRIs)

G Warfarin

For each of the statements below, select the most appropriate option from the list above. Each option may be used once, more than once or not at all.

☐ **18.17** Women taking this should be warned that they must ensure adequate contraception.

☐ **18.18** Patients taking this should be warned to report sore throats promptly.

☐ **18.19** Patients should be warned that abrupt discontinuation of this can cause severe withdrawal symptoms.

☐ **18.20** Patients should be warned not to eat food high in tyramine.

☐ **18.21** Patients should be warned that if they are taking these drugs for more than 3 weeks they should taper the subsequent reduction.

THEME: ADVERSE DRUG REACTIONS

Options

A	Amiloride	**F**	Diclofenac
B	Amiodarone	**G**	Indometacin
C	Azithromycin	**H**	Methotrexate
D	Bendroflumethiazide	**I**	Prednisolone
E	Colchicine	**J**	Sulfasalazine

For each of the scenarios decribed below, select the drug most likely to be responsible from the list above. Each option can be used once, more than once or not at all.

☐ **18.22** A man who is suffering from inflammatory arthritis starts a new medication but it has to be withdrawn promptly by the specialist when the patient develops a dry cough, fever and breathlessness.

☐ **18.23** A woman with rheumatoid arthritis starts taking a new daily medication but has to stop it after developing neutropenia.

☐ **18.24** A woman develops dizziness after starting a medication prescribed by her GP for an acutely swollen and painful metatarsophalangeal joint.

☐ **18.25** A patient develops severe diarrhoea after starting a medication prescribed for an acutely swollen and painful metatarsophalangeal joint.

☐ **18.26** A patient develops hypothyroidism 6 months after starting this new medication.

THEME: DERMATOLOGICAL ADVERSE REACTIONS

Options

A Chloasma

B Erythema multiforme minor

C Fixed drug reaction

D Jarisch–Herxheimer phenomenon

E Maculopapular drug rash

F Phototoxic skin reaction

G Photo-allergic skin reaction

H Stevens–Johnson syndrome

I Toxic epidermal necrolysis

J Type III immune complex reaction

For each of the scenarios described below, select the most likely dermatological reaction from the list above. Each option can be used once, more than once or not at all.

☐ **18.27** A patient has developed an erythematous, oval skin lesion on the dorsal surface of his left foot. He had a similar lesion 3 months ago after starting tetracycline antibiotics for acne which resolved on stopping the medication but has recurred on the dorsal aspect of his left foot 4 hours after restarting the treatment.

☐ **18.28** A 33-year-old patient sees you about a new rash she has noticed on her face for the past 3 months. She has developed brown macular lesions affecting both her cheeks and her forehead. The lesions are not uncomfortable but are becoming unsightly. She started taking the combined oral contraceptive pill 4 months ago.

18.29 A specialist has started a patient on carbamazepine for the treatment of trigeminal neuralgia 4 weeks ago. He is now unwell with a fever and sore throat and has developed a non-pruritic maculopapular rash, conjunctivitis and ulcerated genitalia. Overall, 9% of his skin is involved.

18.30 A 10-year-old boy has been given some amoxicillin suspension for a suspected lower respiratory tract infection by a colleague. He is bought back to the surgery after 5 days because he has developed an itchy erythematous rash affecting his trunk and arms. His chest is better and he is otherwise well.

18.31 A 55-year-old with heart failure has recently changed his regular furosemide to bumetanide. He subsequently developed a severe sunburn-like rash on his lower arms, face and neck while travelling outside on a sunny day. The rash was not itchy and did not involve areas of skin that were covered by clothing.

CHAPTER 18 QUESTIONS

ALGORITHM QUESTIONS

THEME: SUSPECTED ADVERSE REACTION

18.32–18.36

Options

A Black triangle drug

B Consider reporting

C No

D Paediatric drug

E Report under yellow card scheme

F Serious reaction

G Yes

The following flow chart illustrates the hierachy of actions that should be taken in the event of a suspected adverse drug reaction.

For each of the numbered spaces in the flow chart, select the most appropriate option from the list above. Each option can be used once, more than once or not at all.

PICTURE QUESTIONS

18.37 A 78-year-old lady with mild dementia is brought to see you by her carer after he noticed a rash on her back. He thinks she is on some medication for her dementia but is not sure what this is. The rash is shown below.

What is the most likely cause of her rash?

- ☐ A Contact dermatitis
- ☐ B Erythema multiforme
- ☐ C Erythema nodosum
- ☐ D Non-accidental injury
- ☐ E Shingles

THEME: INHALERS

Options

There are a number of different inhalers on the market for delivery of respiratory drugs. Some of these are shown above. For each of the statements below, select the most appropriate device from options A–E. Each option can be used once, more than once or not at all.

- [ ] **18.38** Can be used with a spacer.

- [ ] **18.39** Requires the user to insert a capsule before each use.

- [ ] **18.40** Has a dose counter, meaning that the user knows how many doses remain.

- [ ] **18.41** Primed by twisting the base.

- [ ] **18.42** Requires the user to coordinate activation and breathing.

DATA INTERPRETATION QUESTION

18.43 A 67-year-old woman who suffers from bipolar disorder has been taking lithium for 6 months. She attends for routine blood tests and the following results are obtained:

Lithium	1.6 mmol/l (normal range 0.4–1.0 mmol/l)
Creatinine	112 µmol/l (normal range 60–110 µmol/l)
eGFR	57 ml/minute/1.73m²
TSH	5.3 mU/l (normal range 0.5–4.5 mU/l)
FT4	13 pmol/l (normal range 10–24 pmol/l)

What action should be taken?

- [ ] A Check compliance
- [ ] B Increase dose of lithium
- [ ] C Reduce dose of lithium
- [ ] D Start an ACE inhibitor for chronic renal impairment
- [ ] E Start levothyroxine 50 micrograms per day and repeat thyroid function in 3 months

ANSWERS

18.1   D: Methylnaltrexone

For severe opioid-induced constipation not responding to oral or rectal treatment, an injection of methylnaltrexone is often helpful. This is a peripherally acting opioid antagonist that reverses constipation without causing withdrawal or loss of analgesic affect. It is given parenterally and works within 30 minutes. Once the acute constipation has been dealt with, changing to oxycodone/naloxone might be effective in preventing recurrence but this can take 1–2 weeks for the bowels to return to normal. Co-prescription of Fybogel, lactulose and Movicol is often helpful in patients who wish to stay on morphine.

18.2   E: That if NRT is prescribed, it should be discontinued if the patient starts to smoke again

Bupropion is contraindicated in pregnancy. Both NICE and the manufacturers of bupropion advise that it should be avoided in breastfeeding. Bupropion has been associated with a 0.1% risk of seizure and it should be avoided in people with a history of seizure disorder. NICE guidelines recommend that breastfeeding women wishing to use NRT should not do so but should be counselled by a health-care professional first. The levels of nicotine from NRT are likely to be lower than those in regular smokers, however. NICE recommends that if a smoking cessation attempt is unsuccessful, in general, a further attempt should not be funded for 6 months. If a patient starts to smoke again while using NRT, it should be discontinued.

18.3   D: Make a record in the notes and inform the MHRA via the yellow card scheme

New drugs are marked with an inverted black triangle next to the drug name in the *BNF*. This signifies that the drug is being intensively monitored for adverse effects by the MHRA (formally the Committee on Safety of Medicines). All suspected adverse events, including minor ones, should be reported using the yellow card scheme. The MHRA ask that serious adverse reactions to established medicines are also reported. All suspected adverse drug reactions in children should be reported, including minor reactions to established medicines, vaccines and herbal products.

18.4   C: Take doxycycline 250 mg daily for 2 weeks

Chloroquine and mefloquine are taken on a weekly basis. Other medications are taken each day. Atovaquone-containing treatment (Malarone) only needs to be taken for 1 week after leaving a malarious area. All other treatments should be taken for 4 weeks after leaving infectious areas.

18.5   E: Verapamil can be used for first-line rate control in asthmatic patients with AF

Patients with AF are at risk of stroke. AF is managed through either rhythm or rate control initially, depending on a patient's age, comorbidity and the length of time they have had AF. NICE guidelines recommend that many patients requiring rate-control treatment are given rate-limiting calcium antagonists or β blockers as first-line treatment. Only very sedentary patients should receive digoxin as first-line medication. It does not control heart rate on exertion.

18.6   B: Quantities of medicine of < 5 ml should be given by syringe rather than by spoon

The *BNF* for children has a wealth of advice on prescribing for children. Unpalatable medicines can be mixed with small quantities of food but not with a large amount because of the risk of not taking the full dose and the risk of developing an aversion to the food if there is an unpalatable taste. There is a risk of dental caries if frequent medication needs to be taken and sugar-free preparations should be used wherever possible. Many common medicines are unlicensed in children but their use is acceptable where there is a body of evidence that it is appropriate to do so and the prescriber accepts the professional responsibility and potential liability.

18.7   A: Children often require a higher dose of morphine related to their body weight than adults

NSAIDs are particularly good for bone pain, and should be used initially. Children are more susceptible to urinary retention and pruritus than adults. Nerve pain often responds to anticonvulsants or low-dose amitriptyline, and dexamethasone is often useful. Oxycodone is often tolerated where morphine is not and should be considered as a second-line strong opioid.

18.8   C: Patients with poor dental hygiene should see their dentist before starting bisphosphonate therapy

Strontium is taken as an oral suspension, 2 g a day. It is useful in those who who cannot tolerate bisphosphonates and promotes new bone growth as well as reducing resorption. Bisphosphonates are associated with osteonecrosis of the mandible and patients should have regular dental follow-up. Ibandronic acid is given monthly as an oral tablet or 3-monthly by intravenous infusion. Teriparatide is initiated by specialists and only in patients who are intolerant of bisphosphonates or where these have failed to prevent a fracture and who have either extremely low bone mineral density or have very low bone density and have had fractures and have risk factors such as low BMI. Calcitonin is taken as either an injection or a nasal spray.

THEME: ANALGESICS

18.9   E: Non-opioid analgesic

A non-opioid analgesic such as paracetamol should be used first-line in children. Where pain or fever persists despite adequate doses, an NSAID can be used.

18.10   C: Cannabinoid

Studies looking at a variety of cannabinoids suggest that they are moderately effective for pain relief but that side-effects are common.

18.11   F: Non-steroidal anti-inflammatory drug (NSAID)

Studies suggest that conventional NSAIDs are associated with a 1% risk of gastrointestinal bleeding, while COX-2 inhibitors are associated with a 0.5% risk. Co-prescription of a proton-pump inhibitor will reduce the risk to similar levels.

18.12   H: Topical local anaesthetic

Lidocaine 5% patches are licensed for use in post-herpetic neuralgia. They are applied to the site of the pain for 12 hours a day and can be useful where antidepressants or anticonvulsants are not tolerated.

THEME: SIDE-EFFECTS OF ANTIDEPRESSANTS

18.13   D: Mirtazapine

Mirtazapine is reported to cause sexual dysfunction in only 24% of patients, compared with 70–80% for selective serotonin reuptake inhibitors (SSRIs) and venlafaxine. Duloxetine is better than other SSRIs and serotonin and norepinephrine reuptake inhibitors (SNRIs) but still causes this side-effect in 42% of patients.

18.14   E: Paroxetine

Antidepressants with a short half-life cause the most marked discontinuation effects. Typically these are venlafaxine and paroxetine, but paroxetine seems to be more commonly associated with this side-effect, although it is possible with all of these medications.

18.15   D: Mirtazapine

Mirtazapine commonly causes sedation and weight gain, and can be helpful in patients with disturbed sleep.

18.16   H: All of the above

SSRIs and SNRIs increase the risk of suicide or attempted suicide in adolescents and young adults (relative risk, RR, 1.92) but reduce the risk in adults (RR 0.57).

THEME: DRUG SAFETY

18.17   E: Roaccutane

Roaccutane is often taken by young women at risk of pregnancy. It is essential they are taking adequate contraceptive measures and many units check pregnancy tests regularly

18.18   B: Carbimazole

Carbimazole can cause agranulocytosis and patients should be warned to seek medical attention if they develop a sore throat or other infections.

18.19   F: Selective serotonin reuptake inhibitors (SSRIs)

SSRIs such as paroxetine and serotonin and norepinephrine reuptake inhibitors (SNRIs) such as venlafaxine both have relatively short half-lives and can be associated with withdrawal symptoms on abrupt cessation.

18.20   C: Monoamine oxidase Inhibitors

Food high in tyramine (eg blue cheese, pickled herrings, red wine) can cause a hypertensive crisis in patients on MAOI drugs. They should also be warned about over-the-counter cold cures which might also interact with these foods, as well as prescription drugs.

18.21 D: Prednisolone

Doses of prednisolone of 40 mg od can be stopped abruptly after 3 weeks or less without causing adrenal side-effects as long as the patient is otherwise well and has not had recent steroid therapy.

THEME: ADVERSE DRUG REACTIONS

18.22 H: Methotrexate

Methotrexate can cause pneumonitis. This can be fatal and methotrexate needs to be withdrawn and corticosteroids administered under specialist supervision in hospital. Other side-effects of methotrexate include pulmonary fibrosis and blood dyscrasias.

18.23 J: Sulfasalazine

Sulfasalazine is known to cause blood dyscrasias, including neutropenia, particularly in patients with rheumatoid arthritis. Methotrexate is also used in rheumatoid arthritis and can cause neutropenia, but is given weekly rather than daily.

18.24 G: Indometacin

This patient has arthritis affecting her metatarsophalangeal joint, the classic joint affected by gout. NSAIDs are used in the treatment of gout. Indometacin can cause dizziness as a side-effect and the *BNF* recommends that patients are warned that this can affect the performance of skilled tasks (eg driving).

18.25 E: Colchicine

Colchicine is used in the treatment and prevention of gout. Nausea and vomiting and profuse diarrhoea are well-recognised side-effects.

18.26   B: Amiodarone

Both hypo- and hyperthyroidism are recognised adverse effects of amiodarone treatment. Thyroid function tests should be performed before commencing treatment and after 6 months.

THEME: DERMATOLOGICAL ADVERSE REACTIONS

18.27   C: Fixed drug reaction

Fixed drug reactions are well-defined lesions that occur in the same site. They occur within a few hours after taking a medication internally. Lesions are usually singular and can affect either the limb, genitalia or trunk. Avoiding the causative drug is important to prevent recurrence.

18.28   A: Chloasma

Chloasma is also called 'melasma' by dermatologists. A brown macular rash affects the face and sometimes the neck. Hormone-based contraception and pregnancy are two common causes and the skin rash affects women 20 times more commonly than males. Treatment with sunblock cream and bleaching agents can help to treat the condition but resolution is normally slow.

18.29   H: Stevens–Johnson syndrome

After starting carbamazepine this patient has unfortunately developed Stevens–Johnson syndrome and needs to be transferred to hospital. Erythema multiforme minor is a milder reaction and does not affect the genitalia. Toxic epidermal necrolysis involves similar damage to the skin and genitalia, but involvement is severe, with at least 30% of the skin involved and a much poorer prognosis.

CHAPTER 18 ANSWERS

18.30   E: Maculopapular drug rash

Maculopapular drug rashes are the most common adverse drug eruptions affecting the skin, and often occur after administration of β-lactam antibiotics. The skin reaction can be associated with moderate pruritus. Withdrawal of the causative medicine, application of topical corticosteroid cream and provision of oral antihistamines will usually lead to resolution of the condition over a period of several days.

18.31   F: Phototoxic skin reaction

Many drugs can produce phototoxic skin reactions when skin is exposed to UV light. Phototoxicity appears quickly after exposure to light and is confined to sun-exposed skin. The skin looks sunburnt; itching is not present in all cases. Photo-allergic skin is always itchy and classically occurs at least 24 hours after exposure to sunlight. Skin which has not been directly exposed to sunlight can also become involved.

THEME: SUSPECTED ADVERSE REACTION

18.32   F: Serious reaction

18.33   G: Yes

18.34   E: Report under yellow card scheme

18.35   D: Paediatric drug

18.36   C: No

18.37   A: Contact dermatitis

This lady is using rivastigmine patches and has had a reaction to the adhesive in the patch. This is a common side-effect of patches and can be reduced by rotation of sites but, as shown here, this does not always prove effective. Changing the patient to oral treatment results in resolution. Patients should be warned about this side-effect. With some drugs (eg transdermal buprenorphine) co-prescription of antihistamines is recommended initially.

THEME: INHALERS

18.38   E

This is the only one of these devices that can be used with a spacer.

18.39   C

This device has a button that punctures the capsule before inhalation.

18.40   D

The Accuhaler has an indicator that shows when it is almost empty, but no dose counter.

18.41   A

The turbohaler is primed by being twisted and untwisted. The Easibreathe inhaler is also primed but not by twisting.

18.42   E

Metered-dose inhalers are the most difficult to coordinate and often result in deposition of drug in the mouth.

18.43   C: Reduce dose of lithium

These blood tests show stage 3 chronic kidney disease and subclinical hypothyroidism with elevated lithium levels. Lithium is toxic to the thyroid and kidneys, and at higher dose causes increasing confusion, disorientation, hyper-reflexia and eventually convulsions and death. Regular monitoring of renal and thyroid function, together with lithium levels is necessary in all patients.

CHAPTER 19
QUESTIONS: CRITICAL APPRAISAL
SINGLE BEST ANSWER QUESTIONS

19.1 You attend a presentation by the local public health team at which the data are presented on the top three causes of paediatric deaths in your primary care organisation (PCO) over the last 30 years. The data are presented below, with the commonest cause of death first.

	1989	1999	2009
1st	Trauma	Trauma	Neoplasm
2nd	Infection	Neoplasm	Trauma
3rd	Neoplasm	Infection	Infection

Which one of the following statements is correct regarding these data?

A No conclusions can be drawn on changes in incidence

B The data confirm that child mortality is falling

C The data suggest that the incidence of childhood cancer is increasing

D The data suggest that the incidence of serious accidents is falling

E The decrease in mortality from infection reflects increased vaccination coverage

19.2   Consider the data shown below summarising the findings of a review of Symbicort SMART therapy compared with usual treatment.

Comparison of new inhaler vs inhaled steroid and long-acting beta agonist (LABA):

- Exacerbations of asthma requiring oral steroids: OR 0.83 (95%CI 0.66 to 1.03)

- Exacerbations requiring hospital admission: OR 0.59 (95%CI 0.24 to 1.45)

Comparison of new inhaler vs inhaled steroid alone:

- Exacerbation of asthma requiring oral steroids: OR 0.54 (95%CI 0.45 to 0.64)

- Exacerbations requiring hospital admission: OR 0.56 (95%CI 0.28 to 1.09)

(OR = odds ratio, CI = confidence interval.)

Which one of the following statements is true regarding interpretation of these data?

- ☐   A   None of the data presented are statistically significant
- ☐   B   SMART therapy is effective in reducing oral steroid use in comparison with alternative steroid/LABA therapy
- ☐   C   SMART therapy is more cost-effective than usual treatment
- ☐   D   SMART therapy is no more effective than alternative steroid/ LABA treatment
- ☐   E   SMART therapy is superior to inhaled corticosteroids alone in reducing exacerbations of asthma requiring oral steroids

19.3 Consider the graph below, which shows alcohol consumption and all-cause mortality.

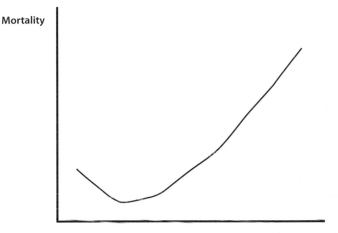

Mortality

Units of alcohol
per week

Which one of the following is a correct interpretation of this graph?

A Alcohol in moderate doses is beneficial to health

B Avoidance of alcohol is more dangerous than moderate consumption

C Heavy drinkers who reduce their alcohol consumption can reduce their risk of dying

D There is no question that high levels of alcohol consumption increase mortality

E These data demonstrate an association rather than a causal relationship

CHAPTER 19 QUESTIONS

19.4 The graph below shows the standardised (for age, sex and ethnic group) incidence ratios of three different cancers in patients followed up for 10 years after exposure to a potential carcinogen.

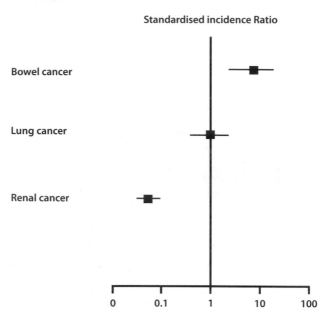

Standardised incidence Ratio

Which of the following statements is correct regarding interpretation of these data?

☐ A The confidence intervals for all three cancers are wide so there might not be a true increase in incidence

☐ B The incidence of all three cancers is increased

☐ C The incidence of bowel cancer is increased, while the incidence of renal cancer is reduced

☐ D The incidence of renal cancer is increased while the incidence of bowel cancer is reduced in this cohort of patients

☐ E These data confirm that the chemical causes cancer

19.5 Your local PCT has been piloting the use of a continence nurse service as an alternative to GP-led care for patients with incontinence problems. After the 6-month pilot the following results are obtained:

Which one of the following conclusions is correct?

- [ ] A   Continence nurse care is more cost-effective than GP care
- [ ] B   Continence nurse care produces a statistically significant improvement in symptom scores compared with GP care
- [ ] C   GP care is more cost-effective than continence nurse care
- [ ] D   More patients in the continence nurse group improved at 6 months compared with the patients in the GP care group
- [ ] E   More patients in the GP care group improved at 6 months compared with the patients in the continence nurse care group

19.6 After a 6-month pilot project to assess the impact of a nurse practitioner on the management of prostatic symptoms in primary care the following results for cost and impact on mean symptom score are presented:

	Cost per patient (£)			Symptom score		
	Nurse practitioner care	Standard care	Difference	Intervention	Standard care	Difference
Baseline	0	0	0	5	5	0
6 months	200	100	100	1	3	–2

Which of the following is correct regarding the cost-effectiveness of this service compared with standard care?

- [ ] A   The additional cost per unit change in symptom score is £200
- [ ] B   The additional cost per unit change in symptom score is £100
- [ ] C   The additional cost per unit change in symptom score is £50
- [ ] D   The data suggest the intervention is cost-effective
- [ ] E   There is a net reduction in costs

19.7 A study is carried out into drug use in the 3 months prior to an admission with acute upper gastrointestinal bleeding. The results of this are shown below.

	Drug A	Drug B	Ulcer-healing drugs
Incidence of gastrointestinal bleeding (odds ratio)	2.1	1.9	3.4

Based on these data, which of the following are valid conclusions?

- [ ] A Drug A is more likely to cause gastrointestinal bleeding than drug B
- [ ] B Drug B is more likely to cause gastrointestinal bleeding than drug A
- [ ] C These results are not statistically significant
- [ ] D The use of ulcer-healing drugs is likely to be a confounding variable
- [ ] E Ulcer-healing drugs are a proven cause of gastrointestinal bleeding

19.8 Consider the following data from the ACCORD study (BMJ 2009; 339: b4909) regarding the association between symptomatic severe hypoglycaemia and annualised mortality in type 2 diabetes:

	Mortality rate		Adjusted hazard ratio for no previous events vs at least one previous event (95%CI)
	No previous events	At least one previous event	
Intensive therapy	1.2% a year	2.8% a year	1.41 (1.03 to 1.93)
Standard therapy	1.0% a year	3.7% a year	2.30 (1.46 to 3.65)

Which one of the following conclusions is correct regarding these data?

☐ A   A history of previous symptomatic severe hypoglycaemia is associated with increased mortality in both treatment arms

☐ B   Intensive treatment is more hazardous than standard treatment

☐ C   Lack of previous symptomatic severe hypoglycaemia is associated with increased mortality in both treatment arms

☐ D   The data do not show a statistically significant difference between the two treatment arms

☐ E   These data suggest an increased mortality in patients on insulin therapy

19.9 Your practice is reviewing the prescribing of calcium and vitamin D in patients at risk of fracture. You decide to look into the data on fracture prevention with different preparations and come across the following data from the DIPART group (BMJ 2010; 340: b5463).

All trials   0.95 (0.90 to 1.01)

Calcium/D trials   0.92 (0.86 to 0.99)

Vitamin D trials   1.01 (0.92 to 1.12)

0.5   1.0   1.5

Risk of fracture (hazard ratio)

Which one of the following is a correct interpretation of these results?

- [ ] A Calcium alone will lead to a statistically significant reduction in fractures
- [ ] B Co-administration of calcium and vitamin D is necessary to prevent fractures
- [ ] C Meta-analysis of all trials of calcium and vitamin D confirm efficacy in preventing fractures
- [ ] D Vitamin D alone will prevent fractures
- [ ] E Vitamin D use is associated with a statistically significant increase in the risk of fracture

19.10 Consider the following data from a study of mortality and mean HbA$_{1c}$ levels:

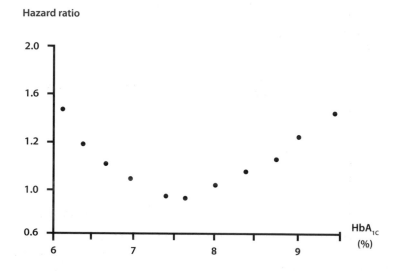

Hazard ratio

HbA$_{1c}$ (%)

Which of the following is a correct interpretation of these data?

- ☐ A   An HbA1C of 7.5% is associated with the highest mortality
- ☐ B   An HbA1C of 7.5% is associated with the lowest mortality
- ☐ C   Intensive glycaemic control is associated with lower mortality
- ☐ D   Intensive glycaemic control is associated with lower morbidity
- ☐ E   There is a direct relationship between glycaemic control and mortality

19.11 Consider the graph below from an 8-month follow-up of patients treated with either catheter ablation or antiarrhythmic drugs for paroxysmal atrial fibrillation.

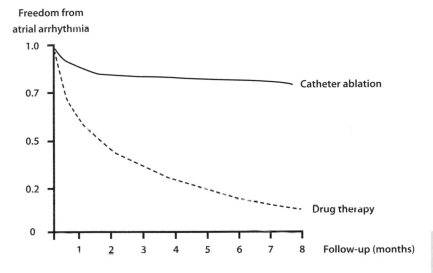

Which one of the following statements is a correct interpretation of these data?

☐ A   Catheter ablation is a safe procedure

☐ B   Catheter ablation is superior to drug therapy in preventing recurrence

☐ C   Drug therapy is associated with higher drop-out rates due to side-effects

☐ D   Drug therapy is superior to catheter ablation in preventing recurrence

☐ E   More than 50% of patients on drug therapy are free of recurrence at 4 months

19.12 A trial carried out to assess the impact of a very-low-energy diet on moderate and severe sleep apnoea in obese men (BMJ 2009; 339: b4609) gives the results below after a 9-week period.

	Intervention	Control	Mean difference	P value
Apnoea:hypopnoea index (AHI)	−25	−2	−23 (−30 to −15)	< 0.001
Weight (kg)	−18.7	1.1	−19.8 (−21.4 to −18.2)	< 0.001

Which one of the following statements about these data is correct?

A   The intervention improved daytime symptoms

B   The intervention improved night-time symptoms

C   The results suggest that weight loss is an effective treatment for snoring

D   Weight loss provides lasting relief of symptoms

E   Weight loss reduces long-term complications of sleep apnoea

19.13 A GP wants to audit dermatology care at her practice. She decides to look at viral wart treatment in children at the practice. At present, viral warts on hands or toes are initially treated in the practice using topical agents of various types. Patients are followed up at 3 months by some doctors; others advise patients to return only if their warts have not resolved after 3 months of treatment. When carrying out her audit, which of the following steps is most appropriate to follow?

☐   A   Define ideal practice and compare this with current performance at her surgery

☐   B   Ensure that all other clinicians are unaware that an audit is taking place

☐   C   Find out which is the cheapest topical treatment for viral warts and recommend that this is always used as first-line treatment

☐   D   Suggest that all doctors use different agents to ensure that patients receive the best care

☐   E   Write guidelines for topical treatment of warts based on current treatment at the practice

19.14 Which one of the following best describes absolute risk increase (ARI)?

☐   A   Control event rate (CER) – experimental event rate (EER)

☐   B   Control event rate (CER) + experimental event rate (EER)

☐   C   Experimental event rate (EER) – control event rate (CER)

☐   D   The likelihood of a positive result

☐   E   The proportion of positives accurately diagnosed with a disorder

19.15 Which of the following best describes the term 'external validity'?

☐ A The agreement between two raters using the same test at the same time

☐ B The consistency of a measure used on two separate occasions

☐ C The extent to which one can appropriately apply the results to other populations

☐ D The level of agreement between two or more raters using the same test on two or more separate occasions

☐ E The level of consistency between two separate halves of the same test

19.16 A novel oral hypoglycaemic agent has been developed to manage type 2 diabetes. You read a recently published paper that appears to show very favourable results for this drug. A brief extract is given below:

'Patients were recruited from outpatient clinics to receive drug B. A questionnaire developed by the trial coordinator was filled out by the clinician if he felt a patient might be suitable for the trial and these were collated by the trial coordinator. Baseline blood tests were taken at this time. Suitable patients were then selected by the coordinator and invited to join the trial. The group had the following characteristics: 32% female; 96% white, 2% black, 2% Asian. They were given drug B to take for a 6-month period. At the end of the trial questionnaires were given out to patients to evaluate side-effects and repeat blood tests were taken.'

Which one of the following statements is true regarding the trial described above?

☐ A The study design is free from bias

☐ B The study design is prone to inclusion bias

☐ C The study population is representative of the general diabetic population

☐ D The study was performed on an intention-to-treat basis

☐ E This study is a randomised controlled trial

19.17 You attend a lunchtime meeting sponsored by a drug company at which the drug company representative presents a novel treatment that has just been licensed for the treatment of osteoarthritis. He presents the following data comparing the new treatment (drug X) with standard treatment:

'One hundred patients with rheumatoid arthritis were randomised to receive either drug X 400 mg once daily or ibuprofen 800 mg three times a day for a 4-week period. They were instructed to stop their existing treatment 3 weeks prior to the trial to allow for an adequate washout period. To avoid bias, the patients were not told whether they were taking ibuprofen or the new drug. Each group was given a questionnaire to fill in weekly regarding side-effects and symptom control. In addition, the patients in the ibuprofen group were given a supplementary questionnaire on gastrointestinal side-effects. The questionnaires were administered by a trained nurse to standardise responses.'

Which one of the following statements is true regarding this trial?

- [ ] A The study design is not blinded, so the results are not valid
- [ ] B The study population was appropriate for the drug's indication
- [ ] C The trial was a randomised, double-blind, placebo-controlled trial
- [ ] D The use of a trained nurse to administer the questionnaires in this way excluded reporting bias
- [ ] E This study supports the use of drug X in the management of osteoarthritis

19.18 Which one of the following study designs most accurately describes a cohort study?

☐ A A study that aims to establish the normal height of 4-year-old children by measuring heights at school entry

☐ B A study that compares a group of children whose heights are below the 10th centile with a group of matched controls of normal height, aiming to identify possible causative factors

☐ C A study that compares two groups of 4-year-olds with similar characteristics: one group is given a drug and the other a placebo, and the growth of each group is measured following this intervention

☐ D A study that compares the height of a group of 4-year-olds living near a nuclear plant with the height of a group of 4-year-olds who live elsewhere

☐ E A study that looks at all children born at one hospital in 1 year and measures their height at intervals up to 4 years of age

19.19 Your local primary care trust (PCT) decides to audit its new, nurse-led, walk-in centre. It carries this out by doing semi-structured interviews with a nurse practitioner who works in the clinic. She selects 50 patients over a 4-week period and assesses their satisfaction with various aspects of their care. The results are shown below:

Number of patients completing the interview = 50

Number of patients expressing overall satisfaction = 49

Number of patients who found the visit satisfied their needs = 49

Number of patients who, when asked, felt that their visit was superior to normal GP care = 44

The PCT announce that on the basis of these results they will roll out the walk-in centres. Which one of the following statements is true regarding the validity of this study?

☐ A Extremely high satisfaction rates suggest inclusion bias

☐ B This methodology is a bias-free method of collecting data

☐ C The data confirm that nurse-led care is superior to GP care

☐ D The methodology is designed to ensure a representative range of participants

☐ E This study is a quantitative study

19.20 One of the doctors in your practice is an enthusiastic supporter of acupuncture for the treatment of chronic pain and wishes to introduce an acupuncture service into the practice. Unfortunately, however, the senior partner is of the opinion that this is mere quackery. Following a search of the available information on the Internet, a meta-analysis of acupuncture trials is identified to support the argument. The paper was published in the *Chinese Medical Journal* in 1997. It included all 256 trials that were published in peer-reviewed, Chinese-language journals between 1976 and 1996 and included trials of treatment for nausea, backache, migraine, abdominal pain and depression. Which one of the following statements is true regarding the interpretation of this paper?

☐ A Meta-analysis of this type can be considered as the gold standard of evidence-based medicine

☐ B The methodology of this paper is prone to bias

☐ C These results have been the subject of peer review and so can be assumed to be valid

☐ D This paper has followed the Cochrane Collaboration guidelines for meta-analysis

☐ E This paper includes a large number of trials and the findings therefore have high validity

19.21 A hierarchy of quality in evidence-based medicine exists, with study types ranked according to the strength of their data. The study types are listed below:

Case report (CR)

Randomised, double-blind, placebo-controlled trial (RCT)

Case–control study (CC)

Meta-analysis (MA)

Which one of the following correctly ranks the study types, with the most robust first and the least robust last?

☐ A   RCT, CR, CC, MA

☐ B   MA, RCT, CC, CR

☐ C   RCT, CR, MA, CC

☐ D   CR, CC, MA, RCT

☐ E   RCT, CC, MA, CR

EXTENDED MATCHING QUESTIONS

THEME: STUDY TYPES

Options

A Case–control study

B Case report

C Cohort study

D Double-blinded, randomised, placebo-controlled trial

E Meta-analysis

F Qualitative study

G Single-blinded, randomised, placebo-controlled trial

For each of the trials described below, select the option from the list above that most correctly describes the trial. Each option can be used once, more than once or not at all.

☐ **19.22** The Framingham Heart Study.

☐ **19.23** The Cochrane Collaboration.

☐ **19.24** The Scandinavian Simvastatin Survival Study.

☐ **19.25** A trial of sham acupuncture for period pains in which patients are allocated randomly to treatment or sham acupuncture.

☐ **19.26** A study of patients' experiences of bereavement.

DATA INTERPRETATION QUESTIONS

19.27 The results of a trial of treatment for arthritis with drug X compared with ibuprofen are shown below (CI = confidence interval; WOMAC = Western Ontario and McMaster Universities Index of Osteoarthritis):

Mean reduction in WOMAC score after 4 weeks:

Patients taking drug X = 2.4 (95% confidence interval [CI] 1.7–2.6, P value = 0.66)

Patients taking ibuprofen = 1.8 (95%CI 1.6–2.2, P value = 0.57)

Cumulative incidence of gastrointestinal side-effects after 4 weeks:

Patients taking drug X = 6% (95%CI 3.0%–8.4%, P value = 0.04)

Patients taking ibuprofen = 4% (95%CI 2.2%–5.4%, P value = 0.05)

Which one of the following statements about these data is true?

- [ ] A   Drug X has a significantly greater anti-inflammatory effect than ibuprofen
- [ ] B   Drug X has a superior long- and short-term safety profile
- [ ] C   Drug X improves quality of life to a much greater extent than ibuprofen
- [ ] D   Drug X is significantly safer than ibuprofen
- [ ] E   The reductions in WOMAC scores are not statistically significant

19.28 A new test to screen for cystic fibrosis carriers is being considered. Preliminary results for the test in 100 children, in comparison with the gold standard of chromosome analysis, are shown below.

	Gold standard	
	Positive chromosome analysis	Negative chromosome analysis
New test positive	4	8
New test negative	1	87

Based on this information, which one of the following claims about the new test are correct?

- A The accuracy of the test is 91%
- B The new test is better than the gold standard test
- C The positive predictive value is 80%
- D The sensitivity is 96%
- E The specificity is 87%

19.29 Consider the graph below, which summarises the relative risk of macrosomia for pregnant diabetic mothers according to the 20-week fasting glucose levels:

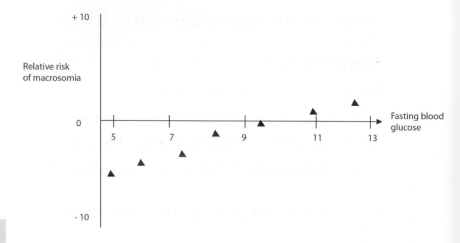

Which one of the following statements is true regarding the interpretation of these data?

- [ ] A   Caesarian section is significantly more likely in diabetic patients
- [ ] B   Gestational diabetes is becoming more common with time
- [ ] C   Glucose levels below 10 mmol/l are never associated with macrosomia
- [ ] D   Low blood sugar levels are associated with small babies, ie intrauterine growth retardation
- [ ] E   Tight control of blood sugar reduces the risk of macrosomia

19.30 A new statin has just been launched with the following advertisement:

'Lowers death rate from myocardial infarction by 33%'

Closer inspection of the original paper reveals the following data:

Number of patients in treatment arm = 200

Number of patients in control arm = 200

Number of patients experiencing MI in treatment arm = 6

Number of patient experiencing MI in the control arm = 7

Number of patients who die as a result of MI in the treatment arm = 4

Number of patients who die as a result of MI in the control arm = 6

Which one of the following statements about these data is true?

- A The absolute risk reduction for death by MI is 33%
- B The number needed to harm with the new drug is 100
- C The number needed to treat (NNT) with the new drug to prevent one death from MI is 3
- D The number needed to treat with the new drug to prevent one MI is 200
- E The relative risk reduction for MI is 33%

19.31 A trial is conducted to determine which symptoms and signs have the most impact on the diagnosis of pneumonia in patients with respiratory symptoms presenting in primary care. The results are presented below:

Symptom/sign	Likelihood ratio for diagnosis
Fever	0.94
Cough	1.00
Abnormal chest examination	1.25
Tachypnoea	1.34
Otalgia	0.07

Which of the following statements regarding these results is true? Select one option only.

- [ ] A An abnormal chest examination increases the probability that a patient has pneumonia by 25%
- [ ] B Tachypnoea has a negative association with the diagnosis of pneumonia
- [ ] C The presence of cough increases the likelihood that a patient has pneumonia by 100%
- [ ] D The presence of fever makes the diagnosis of pneumonia more likely in patients with respiratory disease
- [ ] E These results allow the diagnosis of pneumonia to be made without examining the patient

19.32 A trial is conducted of blood pressure treatment with homeopathic remedies. One group of patients is treated with homeopathic treatment while the other group has no treatment. Both groups are monitored by a nurse for BP and side-effects at monthly intervals. The data are shown below:

	Number of patients with raised BP in the homeopathy group	Number of patients with raised BP in the control group
Baseline	100	100
1 month	75	85
3 months	74	83
6 months	72	84
12 months	75	87

Which one of the following statements is a correct interpretation of these results?

- [ ] A Homeopathy has a statistically significant effect on BP
- [ ] B Homeopathy is well tolerated
- [ ] C The results in the control group are due to the Hawthorne effect
- [ ] D These data suggest that the effect of homeopathy on BP is purely a placebo effect
- [ ] E This trial is a randomised, double-blind, controlled trial and the results are therefore 'gold standard'

19.33 Consider the Kaplan–Meier survival plot below, taken from a paper comparing the use of a novel treatment for osteoarthritis with conventional treatment. The end point in the trial was the need for joint replacement.

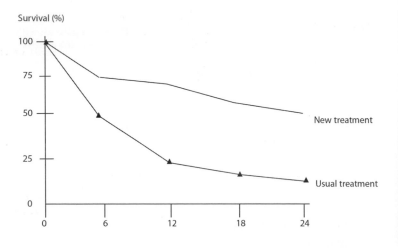

Which one of the following statements about these data is true?

A   At 12 months 75% of the usual treatment group have died

B   At 6 months 50% of the new treatment group have had joint surgery

C   At 12 months a patient receiving the usual treatment is three times as likely to have had surgery as a patient on the new treatment

D   The flattening off of the curves in later months shows that the effects of the treatments wear off with time

E   The new treatment is better tolerated than the usual treatment

19.34 The results of a meta-analysis comparing drug A with drug B are shown below:

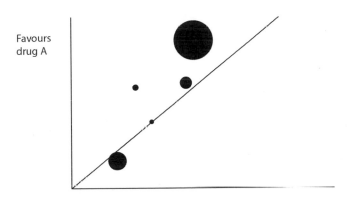

Favours
drug A

Favours
drug B

Which one of the following statements about these data is true?

- [ ] A   Because some of trial data cross the line of no effect, larger trials are needed to determine the true effect
- [ ] B   The majority of the trials suggest that drug B is favourable
- [ ] C   There is no difference between drug A and drug B
- [ ] D   The results unequivocally support drug A
- [ ] E   The size of the circles represents the size of individual trials

QUESTIONS: ADMINISTRATION

SINGLE BEST ANSWER QUESTIONS

19.35 A study compares the suicide risk in adolescents and adults who are taking two different classes of antidepressants. The standardised incidence of suicide is shown in the table below.

	Number of suicides in patients on drug A	Number of suicides in patients on drug B
Adolescents	150	100
Adults	50	100

Which one of the following statements regarding this data is correct?

- [ ] A The relative risk (RR) of suicide for drug A in adolescents compared with drug B is 1.5

- [ ] B The RR of suicide for drug A in adolescents compared with drug B is 3

- [ ] C The RR of suicide for drug A compared with drug B in adults is 2

- [ ] D The RR of suicide for drug A compared with drug B is higher for adults than adolescents

- [ ] E The results show a clear association with suicide for both drugs

19.36 A review of published papers for a new drug contains the figure shown below.

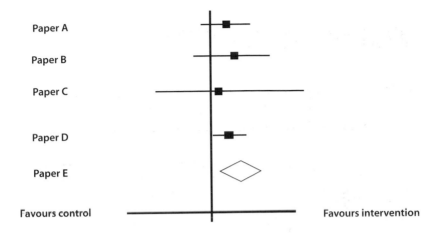

Which one of the following statements about this data is correct?

- [ ] A None of the papers shows a statistically significant effect
- [ ] B Paper E is randomised controlled trial
- [ ] C Pooling results from individual papers gives a statistically significant result
- [ ] D The individual studies are too small to give statistically significant results
- [ ] E The published papers all confirm that the drug is effective

19.37 A study looks at the association between certain symptoms and a disease to see if any of these are useful as a screening tool. The following results are obtained:

	Number with symptom	Number without symptom
Patients with disease (n)	60	40
Patients without disease (n)	40	60

What is the likelihood ratio that a patient with the symptom will have the disease?

- [ ] A 0.66
- [ ] B 1.5
- [ ] C 40%
- [ ] D 60%
- [ ] E 100%

19.38 Which one of the following statements is correct regarding Read codes in general practice?

- [ ] A Read codes are based on the ICD-10 database
- [ ] B Read codes are used for diagnoses only
- [ ] C Read codes are used to encrypt data
- [ ] D Read codes should be accompanied by free text
- [ ] E Use of Read codes is mandatory in the UK

19.39 Which one of the following statements about the Caldicott Principles is true?

☐ A Caldicott Principles apply only to clinicians

☐ B Caldicott Principles only apply where data is passed outside the NHS (eg insurance reports)

☐ C Every practice must have its own Caldicott Guardian

☐ D Every primary care organisation must have a Caldicott Guardian

☐ E The Caldicott Principles are part of the Data Protection Act

19.40 Which one of the following statements regarding the use of computer systems within general practice is correct?

☐ A Electronic transfer of prescriptions was implemented nationwide in 2007

☐ B Participation in 'Choose and Book' is mandatory

☐ C Practice computer systems are owned by the local PCT

☐ D The use of computer record systems is compulsory under the new General Medical Services (GMS) contract

☐ E Web-based primary care patient health records currently allow remote access for clinicians only (eg in hospitals)

19.41 Which one of the following statements about the Freedom of Information Act is correct?

☐ A General practices are covered by the Data Protection Act, so are specifically excluded from the Freedom of Information Act

☐ B Individuals can seek information on individual salaries of doctors working in the practice

☐ C Practices are able to question the motive for a request before deciding whether to comply with a request

☐ D Practices have 20 working days to respond to a request

☐ E The Freedom of Information Act allows patients to gain access to their medical records

19.42 Which of the following situations regarding the use of exception codes for the QOF would be appropriate? Select one option only.

- [ ] A A 23-year-old epileptic woman has frequent fits despite apparently taking her medication. She is removed from the practice register as 'unsuitable'

- [ ] B An 84-year-old woman with diabetes is housebound. She does not respond to three letters asking her to come into the surgery for a diabetic check. She is removed from the register as 'patient unsuitable'

- [ ] C A 24-year-old asthmatic woman has received three letters from the practice asking her to come in for an asthma check. She telephones the practice to say that she does not wish to be seen in the clinic. She is coded as 'informed dissent'

- [ ] D A 73-year-old man with stable ischaemic heart disease cannot take aspirin. He is coded as 'patient unsuitable' for the ischaemic heart disease register

- [ ] E A 79-year-old man with ischaemic heart disease is on warfarin for atrial fibrillation. In order to avoid adversely affecting the QOF performance for antiplatelet drugs, he is coded as 'H/O aspirin allergy'

19.43 A 15-year-old girl refuses to have a skin lesion removed. The lesion is thought to need treatment but does not require urgent removal at present. Her parents feel strongly that the lesion should be removed. You speak to the girl and find that she has done some research and is concerned about scarring. You feel that the girl is sensible and mature (in other words, you feel that she is 'Gillick competent'). Which one of the following is the single most appropriate statement in this situation?

- A Once the girl is said to have 'Gillick competence', this can be applied to any decision regarding her medical treatment
- B The girl is able to consent to and refuse medical treatment if she wishes
- C The girl is able to consent to but not refuse treatment
- D The parents' decision is final
- E You as the GP can decide if the girl is capable of making this decision

EXTENDED MATCHING QUESTIONS

THEME: LEGISLATION AFFECTING GENERAL PRACTICE

Options

A Data Protection Act

B Disability Discrimination Act

C Employment Equality (Age) Regulations 2006

D Equality Act

E Freedom of Information Act

F Human Rights Act

G Mental Capacity Act 2005

H Race Relations Act (RRA) 1976

I Sex Discrimination (Amendment of Legislation) Regulations 2008

J None of the above

For each of the statements below, select the most relevant piece of legislation from the list above. Each option can be used once, more than once or not at all.

☐ **19.44** Allows for positive discrimination.

☐ **19.45** Outlaws discrimination on the basis of sexual orientation.

☐ **19.46** Allows adults to make decisions on behalf of mentally handicapped children.

☐ **19.47** Prevents discrimination on the basis of pregnancy.

☐ **19.48** Allows access to medical reports.

THEME: CERTIFICATION

Options

A	Cannot issue statement	**E**	Med 5
B	Med 3	**F**	Med 6 and Med 5
C	Med 4	**G**	SC2
D	Med 4 and Med 5		

For each of the following patients select the most appropriate certificate from the options above. Each option can be used once, more than once or not at all.

☐ **19.49** A 36-year-old banker who is known to be HIV-positive has recently had a 2-week stay in hospital for treatment related to his HIV. He does not want his employer to know he is HIV-positive.

☐ **19.50** Mr Chester has been off work for 5 weeks following surgery, he is now fit to return to work, and his employer requests a certificate to confirm that he is fit to return.

☐ **19.51** Mr West has not been to work today (Monday). He has been unwell since Friday evening and you diagnose viral gastroenteritis and recommend that he does not return to work until 48 hours after he is better. In the past his boss has not been happy with absences for sickness so Mr West requests a certificate.

☐ **19.52** Mrs Shand is a flight attendant. She broke her leg skiing 3 weeks ago. Yesterday you saw a letter from the orthopaedic consultant, dictated 3 weeks ago, saying that her leg had been pinned and she was to be in plaster for the next 6 weeks. Mrs Shand phones to request a certificate to cover this 6-week period.

☐ **19.53** Mrs Ward is going through a relationship break-up and has financial problems. She is low and tearful and not coping at work. You decide that she would benefit from 2 weeks off work.

ANSWERS: CRITICAL APPRAISAL

19.1   A: No conclusions can be drawn on changes in incidence

The table shows relative incidence only, rather than absolute incidence. The decrease of trauma from first place in 1999 to second place in 2009 could be due to a fall in absolute incidence of trauma but could also represent an increase in the incidence of neoplasm.

19.2   E: SMART therapy is superior to inhaled corticosteroids alone in reducing exacerbations of asthma requiring oral steroids

The data show a statistically significant reduction in outcomes only for the exacerbations requiring oral steroids when compared with inhaled corticosteroids only. The results suggest a possible reduction in other outcomes in both arms but the confidence intervals are wide and exceed 1, suggesting there might not be a truly significant effect. No costs are given for treatment or admission so no conclusions can be drawn on economic grounds.

19.3   E: These data demonstrate an association rather than a causal relationship

These data appear to suggest that there is an association between mortality and alcohol consumption. It is not possible to say, however, that this is a causal relationship because of the need to remove confounding variables. Alcohol consumption could be a cause of increased mortality but it could equally be a surrogate marker for an unhealthy lifestyle. Drinkers are more likely to be obese, smokers, and take little exercise. There is also a possible confounding effect of class because alcohol consumption varies with social class. The graph is a population survey and does not give information on longitudinal outcomes, so conclusions cannot be made on the effects of changing consumption for individuals.

19.4   C: The incidence of bowel cancer is increased, while the incidence of renal cancer is reduced

Standardised incidence ratios (SIRs) compare the incidence of a condition between a patient under study with that of 'equivalent' patients. A standardised incidence ratio of 1.0 suggests that the incidence is the same as in an unexposed population. An SIR greater than 1.0 suggests an increased risk, while an SIR less than 1.0 suggests a reduced risk. The results of studies like this suggest association rather than confirm causation.

19.5   D: More patients in the continence nurse group improved at 6 months compared with the patients in the GP care group

The graph stratifies patients according to change in symptom scores at 6 months. An increase in a symptom score suggests symptoms have worsened, while a reduction suggests symptoms have improved. No data are given on statistical significance or costs of either treatment arm, so conclusions on significance and cost-effectiveness cannot be drawn. More patients have achieved reductions in symptom score in each of the groups in the continence nurse arm than in the GP care arm.

19.6   C: The additional cost per unit change in symptom score is £50

The intervention produces a reduction in average symptom score of 4 points, while standard care reduces the symptom score by 2 points, a difference of 2. The intervention cost, however, is £100 more per patient, making the cost per additional point reduction £50. These data cannot be used alone to judge the cost-effectiveness of an intervention because this requires agreement of an acceptable cost per improvement in symptom control that commissioners and patients would need to agree. There is a net increase in costs.

19.7   D: The use of ulcer-healing drugs is likely to be a confounding variable

Patients at high risk of upper gastrointestinal bleeding will often use ulcer-healing drugs because of previous bleeding or the development of new symptoms. The finding that the use of these drugs is three times more common in those admitted with an acute gastrointestinal bleed is therefore not unexpected, and use of ulcer-healing drugs is likely to be a confounding variable. There is unlikely to be a significant difference between drug A and drug B, although no comment can be made without information on confidence intervals and P values.

19.8   A: A history of previous symptomatic severe hypoglycaemia is associated with increased mortality in both treatment arms

These data suggest that increased mortality is seen in both intensive and standard treatment for patients with a history of severe, symptomatic hypoglycaemia. Furthermore they also suggest that the risk of death is lower in the intensive treatment arm in this subset of patients. There is no information on drug management, and although it could be surmised that hypoglycaemia is more common in patients on insulin this might also be seen with sulphonylureas. Lack of a previous hypoglycaemic attack is less harmful, but is still associated with a mortality rate of 1.0–1.2% a year. The confidence intervals suggest that this is a true effect, because neither group has confidence intervals which cross 1.0.

19.9   B: Co-administration of calcium and vitamin D is necessary to prevent fractures

The data suggest that trials of vitamin D alone show a non-significant increase in the risk of fracture, while calcium and vitamin D in combination will reduce fractures and this finding is statistically significant. There are no trials of calcium alone in the data so conclusions cannot be drawn about this. Meta-analysis of all trials shows a non-significant reduction in fracture rate.

19.10   B: An HbA1C of 7.5% is associated with the lowest mortality

These data show a U-shaped association between HbA1C levels and mortality, with the lowest mortality associated with an HbA1C around 7.5%, while higher mortality is associated with very low and very high HbA1C levels. Hazard ratios are higher in patients at higher risk of an outcome, in this case mortality, so the lowest mortality is associated with the lowest point on the graph. These data only apply to mortality, so conclusions on morbidity cannot be made. Again, conclusions on causation of this effect cannot be made because these data reflect all-cause mortality and this could include death from hypoglycaemic attack as well as from diabetic ketoacidosis.

19.11   B: Catheter ablation is superior to drug therapy in preventing recurrence

The figure is a Kaplan–Meier survival plot, where survival indicates the number of patients who have not suffered a recurrence. The rate of fall in survival is greater for drug therapy at each interval, suggesting that catheter ablation is more efficacious at preventing recurrence. There is no information on side-effects or on safety in this graph.

19.12   B: The intervention improved night-time symptoms

Obstructive sleep apnoea causes night-time symptoms of apnoea and wakening, which can be quantified with the apnoea:hypopnoea index (AHI), and daytime fatigue, which is assessed with the Epworth score. This study measured effect of a very-low-energy diet on the AHI rather than on the Epworth score. It is assumed that daytime symptoms correlate with night-time symptom severity and it therefore could be assumed that daytime symptoms are improved, but that has not been measured as an outcome in this trial. The data are only measured after 9 weeks and no long-term conclusions can be drawn. Snoring is a clinical entity that is distinct from sleep apnoea and it is not possible to draw conclusions on the effects of this intervention on snoring on the basis of these data. There are no outcome measures relating to complications in this study.

19.13 A: Define ideal practice and compare this with current performance at her surgery

To conduct an audit, the auditor needs to select a health-care topic. Standards are set which represent ideal practice in the topic area. Actual performance is then measured in the topic area. Any differences between measured and expected criteria measurements are reported. Differences between actual and ideal performance are tackled to try to reduce or eliminate poor practice. Performance is then re-audited at a later date to reassess health care in this area.

19.14 C: EER – CER

'Experimental event rate – control event rate' describes the absolute risk reduction (ARR) or the absolute benefit increase (ABI). Answer D is calculated by sensitivity ÷ (1 – specificity) and answer E describes specificity.

19.15 C: The extent to which one can appropriately apply the results to other populations

Answer B describes test–retest reliability, answer E is split-half reliability, answer A is inter-rater reliability and answer D describes intra-rater reliability.

19.16 B: The study design is prone to inclusion bias

The inclusion of patients on the whim of the clinician and coordinator will either consciously or subconsciously result in inclusion bias, with well-controlled, English-speaking whites more likely to be represented in the study. This is borne out by the demographic data, which are not representative of the diabetic population in the UK, with Asians and black patients under-represented. The study only followed patients who completed the trial, and those who dropped out due to side-effects are not included. The study was therefore not conducted on an intention-to-treat basis. There are no data showing whether or not the study was placebo-controlled.

19.17 A: The study design is not blinded, so the results are not valid

This study fails at a number of levels. Neither patients nor researchers are blinded as a result of both the different dosage regime and the supplementary questionnaire, which reveal the ibuprofen group. It is therefore prone to reporting bias by the nurse and the patients. It is randomised but not placebo-controlled. It is testing patients with rheumatoid arthritis, which is a different disease from osteoarthritis and the findings are therefore not relevant for the licensed indication. Furthermore, it uses a very high dose of ibuprofen, which would be expected to cause significant gastrointestinal side-effects, resulting in unfavourable comparisons with the new drug.

19.18 C: A study that compares two groups of 4-year-olds with similar characteristics: one group is given a drug and the other a placebo, and the growth of each group is measured following this intervention

Study A is a cross-sectional study. Study B is a case–control study. Study C is a cohort study. Study D is a controlled trial. Study E is a longitudinal study.

19.19 A: Extremely high satisfaction rates suggest inclusion bias

Qualitative studies are fraught with methodological difficulties and should be used only in appropriate studies, for example when canvassing opinions that cannot be quantified as hard data. Semi-structured interviews are frequently used but the study needs to be well designed to avoid reporting bias or leading questions. Patients should, however, still be selected on a structured basis to ensure subjects are representative of the wider population and are not selected on a whim, resulting in inclusion bias. A suitable model might be to enrol every third patient. Ideally, the people working in the clinic should not be aware that they are being audited in order to avoid 'playing up' to the study. The opinions of patients regarding their experience of care cannot be extrapolated to determine whether one form of care is superior to another because this was not studied.

19.20   B: The methodology of this paper is prone to bias

This paper is prone to bias on a number of levels. The first is publication bias: papers only published in Chinese journals are significantly more likely to be both submitted and published if they report positive results for acupuncture, a treatment deeply rooted in Chinese society. Papers with negative findings are therefore significantly less likely to be published than papers with positive findings. Secondly, the inclusion of all studies published in Chinese-language journals results in inclusion bias, because negative studies are far more likely to be undertaken and published in western journals. The inclusion of all studies published over a set time period also results in potential inclusion of poorly conducted trials, which could therefore influence the overall findings significantly. The validity of data is increased with bigger data sets, but only once poorly conducted and biased trials have been removed. The inclusion of non-peer-reviewed data in the trial also means that further publication of data in a peer-reviewed journal as part of a meta-analysis might give false credence to the data. The Cochrane Collaboration have extensive rules for the conduct of meta-analyses and these should be followed where possible.

19.21   B: MA, RCT, CC, CR

Randomised, double-blind, placebo-controlled trials are generally considered the most robust due to the near exclusion of bias. Case reports are considered to be the weakest because they do not test a hypothesis but describe observations which might happen by chance. Case–control studies attempt to match cases to similar controls but are prone to some degree of inclusion bias. Cohort studies collect longitudinal data which can be analysed at a later date.

THEME: STUDY TYPES

19.22   C: Cohort study

The Framingham Study was a cohort study that looked at a population living in the town of Framingham and provided much of our understanding of cardiovascular risk factors.

19.23   E: Meta-analysis

The Cochrane Collaboration is a network of researchers who use the strictest criteria for carrying out meta-analysis, excluding any trials that are prone to bias. It is therefore the purest form of meta-analysis.

19.24   D: Double-blinded, randomised, placebo-controlled trial

In the Scandinavian Simvastatin Survival Study the participants were randomised to either placebo or simvastatin. The trial was double-blinded.

19.25   G: Single-blinded, randomised, placebo-controlled trial

Sham acupuncture cannot be double blinded. The trials are therefore by definition single-blinded and prone to bias on the part of the clinician.

19.26   F: Qualitative study

This is a qualitative study. These studies are prone to different forms of bias and need to be interpreted accordingly.

19.27   E   The reductions in WOMAC scores are not statistically significant

The reductions in WOMAC scores (a quantitative assessment of symptoms and handicap) show a benefit for drug X but the 95% confidence interval is wide and the limits overlap those of ibuprofen, with P values greater than 0.05, meaning that the results do not achieve statistical significance. The results for gastrointestinal side-effects also overlap but the P value for drug X is 0.04 (ie the true result is likely to lie in the range of 3.0 to 8.4); again, these 95% confidence limits overlap those of ibuprofen and it cannot be said that there is a true difference between the two groups. A larger study would have greater power to detect these small differences. No long-term safety data are presented here, so no conclusions can be drawn in this area.

19.28   A: The accuracy of the test is 91%

	Gold standard	
	Positive	Negative
New test positive	a	b
New test negative	c	d

Accuracy is the proportion of tests which have given the correct result, ie

$(a + d) / (a + b + c + d)$, so $91/100 = 91\%$

Sensitivity is the true-positive rate, ie

$a / (a + c)$, so $4/5 = 80\%$

Specificity is the true-negative rate, ie

$d / (b + d)$, so $87/95 = 92\%$

Positive predictive value is the probability of having the condition, once the test is positive, ie

$a / (a + b)$, so $4/12 = 33\%$

Negative predictive value is the probability of not having the condition, once the test is negative, ie

$d / (c + d)$, so $87/88 = 99\%$

19.29   E: Tight control of blood sugar reduces the risk of macrosomia

These data support a link between the risk of large babies and fasting blood glucose levels. Large babies are associated with difficult labour and probably with increased caesarian section rates, but that observation cannot be confirmed from these data. Similarly, a low risk of macrosomia is not the same as a high risk of intrauterine growth retardation, because this would be based on an assumption that the same disease mechanisms apply to both clinical situations. These data do suggest an association between fasting glucose at 20 weeks and macrosomia, so it is reasonable to conclude that tight control of sugar will reduce macrosomia. These data do not provide any time frame, however, so no conclusions on incidence can be made.

19.30   D: The number needed to treat with the new drug to prevent one MI is 200

The absolute risk reduction (ARR) is the event rate in the control group minus the event rate in intervention group. The relative risk reduction (RRR) is (the event rate in the control group minus the event rate in treatment group) ÷ (the event rate in control group). The number needed to treat is 1/ARR. The number needed to harm cannot be calculated from this data as no adverse outcome data are presented. The results are therefore:

ARR for death by MI = 3%–2% = 1%

ARR for all MI = 3.5%–3% = 0.5%

NNT for prevention of death by MI = 1/0.01 = 100

NNT for all MI = 1/0.005 = 200

RRR for death by MI = 1/3 = 33%

19.31   A: An abnormal chest examination increases the probability that a patient has pneumonia by 25%

Likelihood ratios are used to determine the impact of a finding to the outcome. The results are expressed as a ratio: a score of 1 makes both outcomes (presence or absence of disease) equally likely, while a likelihood ratio of > 1 makes the diagnosis more likely and a likelihood ratio of < 1 makes the diagnosis less likely. In these results the presence of otalgia and fever have likelihood ratios of < 1, making them unhelpful in differentiating pneumonia from other chest infections, but the presence of tachypnoea and abnormal chest examination have likelihood ratios of > 1, making a diagnosis of pneumonia more likely. Cough alone has a likelihood ratio of 1.00, making a diagnosis neither more nor less likely, meaning that it is unhelpful in excluding or confirming a diagnosis.

19.32   C: The results in the control group are due to the Hawthorne effect

The control group have no treatment but are monitored. The phenomenon whereby observed outcomes improve merely as a result of being observed is called the 'Hawthorne effect' and is a form of placebo effect. The data presented do not provide any indication of statistical significance or tolerability. This trial is not blinded in any way.

19.33   C: At 12 months a patient receiving the usual treatment is three times as likely to have had surgery as a patient on the new treatment

The Kaplan–Meier curves demonstrate the proportion of patients who have not met the endpoint, meaning survival without treatment rather than true survival. The rate of decline in the new treatment group is slower than in the usual treatment group, implying that this treatment protects patients from reaching the end point of joint replacement. The flattening of the curves later on in the trial suggests that those patients who need surgery will have it early on. The study does not measure side-effects, so no comment can be made on tolerability. At 12 months, 25% of the new treatment group have had surgery, compared with 75% of the usual treatment group.

19.34   E: The size of the circles represents the size of individual trials

This is a L'Abbé plot. Each circle represents a trial and the size of each circle represents the size of the trial. The line bisecting the plot is the 'line of no effect'. Data to the right favour drug B; data to the left favour drug A. The further away from the line, the more significant the effect, so circles crossing the line do not show a net effect.

ANSWERS: ADMINISTRATION

19.35   A: The relative risk (RR) of suicide for drug A in adolescents compared with drug B is 1.5

The relative risk is the number of events in the treatment group divided by the number of events in the control group. In this example drug A has a higher RR of suicide in adolescents than drug B but in adults the RR is lower (1.5 in adolescents vs 0.5 in adults). No inference can be made as to causation because there is no true control group in this study, ie the rate in a control group might be higher than both groups if both drugs reduce suicide but by differing degrees.

19.36   C: Pooling results from individual papers gives a statistically significant result

This figure shows results from four individual studies and also a forest plot of pooled data, as would be found with a meta-analysis. This increases the statistical power of an analysis but also introduces potential bias because all the individual component studies might not be equivalent, either in terms of patient selection or follow-up measures. Papers A, B and C show a positive result but with wide confidence intervals which cross zero, while paper D shows a positive effect with confidence intervals which favour intervention, but only marginally.

19.37   B: 1.5

The likelihood ratio is the ratio of the probability that an individual with the target condition has a specified symptom (or test result) to the probability that an individual without the target condition has the same specified symptom. It is used to determine the validity of association between symptoms or tests and disease, eg headache and brain tumour. In this example the probability that the individual with the symptom has the condition is 60%, while the probability that a patient with the symptom does not have the condition is 40%. The likelihood ratio is therefore 60/40 or 1.5.

19.38   D: Read codes should be accompanied by free text

Read codes were developed to facilitate data collection. Read codes are a parallel system to ICD-10 but the Read code system includes all ICD-10 codes. There are Read codes for diagnoses, symptoms, procedures and occupations and they should be supported by free text to ensure an accurate clinical record. The use of these is not mandatory, although payment for the QOF is based on computer-generated audits of a standard battery of Read codes.

19.39   D: Every primary care organisation must have a Caldicott Guardian

The Caldicott Principles suggest the following: that all uses of patient data should be justified; that identifiable data should be used only when absolutely necessary, including when data is sent between different parts of the NHS; and that each practice should have a responsible individual who ensures compliance with good practice and the law, including the Data Protection Act.

19.40   C: Practice computer systems are owned by the local PCT

Computerised patient records are not mandatory but participation in the QOF would be very difficult with paper records. Since 2005 GP computer systems have been the property of PCOs, who maintain them and pay for software licences. Web-based records have been implemented for radiology services in most areas but not for patient records, although this is the intention. Electronic transfer of prescriptions was supposed to have been implemented in 2007 but has not yet been successfully introduced.

19.41   D: Practices have 20 working days to respond to a request

The Freedom of Information Act specifically includes general practices, which are expected to maintain a publication scheme containing policies and practice income. Individual salaries, however, are covered by the Data Protection Act. Practices cannot question motives, but a charge can be made. Failure to comply with a request will result in the practice being held in contempt of court.

19.42 **C:** **A 24-year-old asthmatic has received three letters from the practice asking her to come in for an asthma check. She telephones the practice to say that she does not wish to be seen in the clinic. She is coded as 'informed dissent'**

The use of exception codes is an area of misreporting in many areas and is one that PCTs are keen to investigate at annual QOF visits. Valid reasons for exception reporting include informed dissent or inappropriateness (eg people who are terminally ill), but being housebound or poorly controlled is not generally seen to be a valid reason. Caution should be taken when choosing the code to make sure that these are accurate. Individual indicator exception codes should be used wherever possible, rather than exclusion from the whole disease area.

19.43 **C:** **The girl is able to consent to but not refuse treatment**

The term 'Gillick competence' is used in relation to a child under the age of 16 years having the capacity to consent to medical treatment. Children aged under 16 years who are deemed to have a full understanding of the consequences are by law able to consent to medical treatment but not to refuse treatment. A child might be deemed to have the ability to give their consent in one situation but not in another. When the issue is a potentially serious one and when there are differences of opinion, expert advice should be sought.

THEME: LEGISLATION AFFECTING GENERAL PRACTICE

19.44 B: Disability Discrimination Act

The Disability Discrimination Act places a Disability Equality Duty on public service providers to take active steps to take account of disabilites even where this results in positive discrimination.

19.45   D: Equality Act

Since 2007 the Equality Act outlaws discrimination on the basis of sexual orientation.

19.46   G: Mental Capacity Act 2005

The Mental Capacity Act governs decision making on behalf of adults, where they lose mental capacity at some point in their lives or where the incapacitating condition has been present since birth.

19.47   I: Sex Discrimination (Amendment of Legislation) Regulations 2008

This amendment prevents direct or indirect discrimination on the basis of pregnancy now or in the last 26 weeks.

19.48   J: None of the above

The Access to Medical Reports Act allows access for patients to medical reports about them.

THEME: CERTIFICATION

19.49   F: Med 6 and Med 5

19.50   B: Med 3

19.51   G: SC2

19.52   E: Med 5

19.53   B: Med 3

An SC2 is used by employees to certify themselves as sick for the first 7 days of sickness for statutory sick pay purposes. For absences of more than 7 days: A Med 3 is used if the doctor signing saw the patient on the day or the day before issue; a Med 5 is used either to supply evidence of incapacity for a backdated period where you examined the patient on a previous occasion or to provide medical evidence without having seen the patient based on a report written in the previous 4 weeks by another doctor covering a forward period of not more than 4 weeks; a Med 6 can be used to provide an accurate diagnosis where a vague diagnosis is used on a Med 3, 4 or 5 if you do not want the patient/employer to know the true diagnosis.

INDEX

NOTES